CHIT > CONSCIOUSNESS > CHITTA > AWARENESS

Awareness to Consciousness

A Spiritual Journey

by

Sneh Lata Chakraburtty

First published in 2001 by
'Chitta-Chit' Publishers
129 Appleby Place,
Burlington
Ontario Canada L7L 2X2

ISBN: 0-9730057-1-8

Printed and bound by Thomson Press (India) Ltd

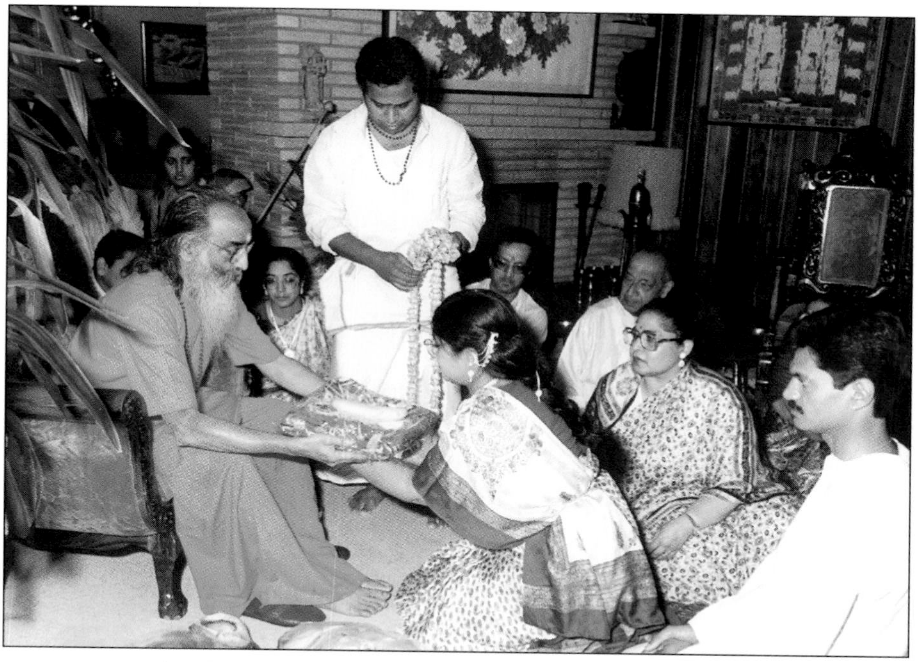

And This Wise Man brought with Him Gifts of Spirituality

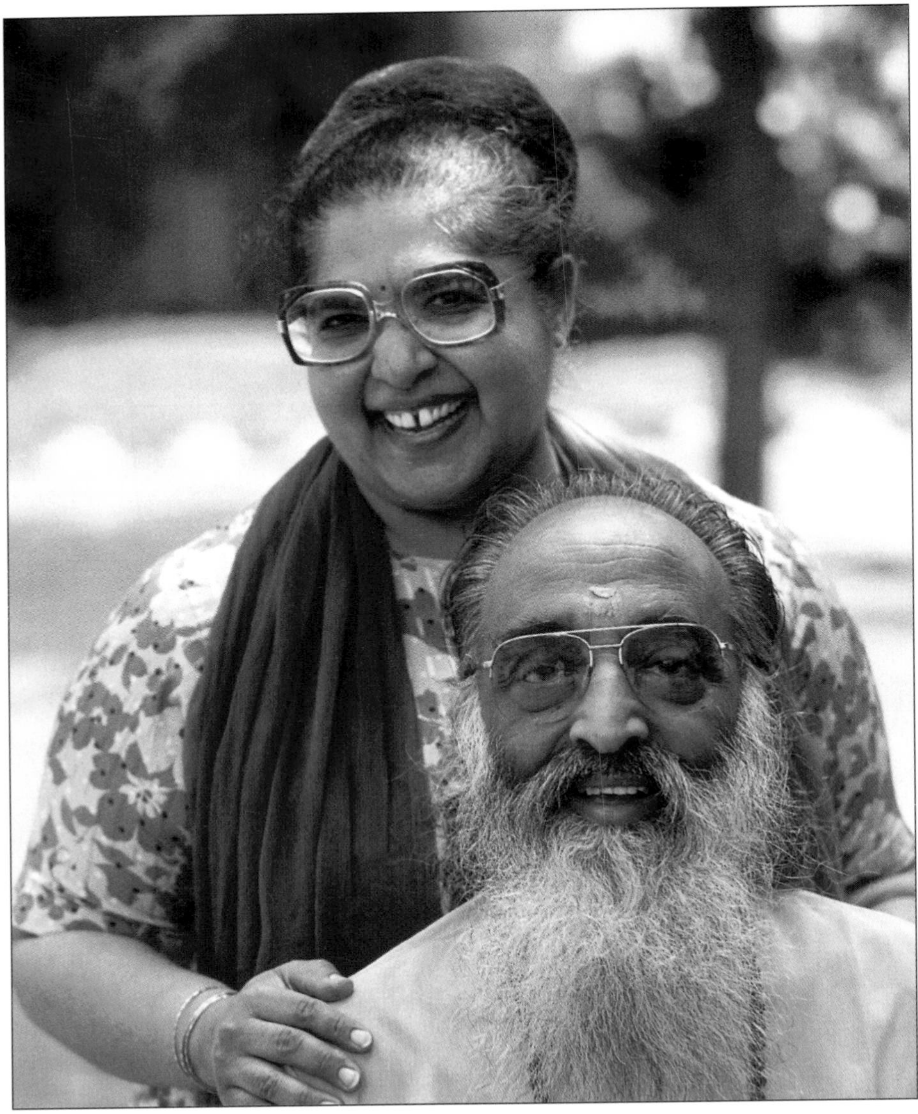

My best friend

A Note from the Author

Before opening this text to you, I offer this work at the feet of my bosom friend, guide, instructor, advisor, confidant, my ALL – Parampujya Swami Chinmayananda - who chiselled me from a rough rock to where I now am, still sadly imperfect, even after more than twenty-five years of study. Gurudev or Swamiji, as we lovingly called him, exposed me and my family to the world of seekers and the wise from every part of the world. They in turn, added special pearls to the wealth of our beingness as mere mortals.

Very early in my life with Swamiji, he admonished me in one of his infrequent but precious letters not to use the pronoun "I" in any writing, actions, or in speech: "You are never the doer", he said! Unfortunately, while seeking to honour my dearest friend and teacher, there is no other way to share my experiences with the reader other than to use this word.Perhaps by doing so, I am submitting to his criticism that I am still the same egoistic mortal that he tried so hard to mould. It is an ironic anomaly that his advice was the product of Eastern thought while the notes that are to follow are constituted in Western thought! These notes also trace my training while on a personal spiritual journey.

First of all, I want to honour my birth mother, Indravati Ahuja, who, as a young, naive seventeen-year-old wife of a thirty-year-old widower with two children aged seven and five from a previous marriage, moved from her home in India to Zanzibar, East Africa. She courageously adjusted to her new roles as wife and mother and also to a new cultural environment among Africans and Arabs. We grew together as we interacted intimately with different faiths and races. My mother possessed a profound grassroots wisdom and, in her mortal motherly all-loving and generous image, I was introduced to the existence of the Cosmic Mother. She has long gone, but I see her in every act of Mother Nature's frown, anger, and grace.

I also wish to honour my father and a daughter's best friend, Bansilal Ahuja who introduced me to meditation. I remember how I used to secretly watch him disappear each evening into the garden under the Zanzibar sky. One night, as a seven-year-old, I watched from the balcony, and saw him weep bitterly while he gazed at the full moon in the clear, tropical night. I can vividly recall a talk with him about why he was weeping. As he spoke, he attempted to explain death to me, weeping again as he described the loss of his sister, her husband, and their five children who had died in the massacre during the partition of India.

As he spoke, I recalled a black and white sketch of the face of a woman, lying on a horizontal crescent moon, which was in an autographed book of the poet and Nobel Laureate, Rabindranath Tagore. The caption under the picture read, "Death oh my death, come and whisper to me". And I imagined that all these relatives I had never met were now living up there in the moon where my father alone had the ability to see them. "They are lying on the lap of God while He massages their heads" my father said.

I was so moved by this experience that every evening I would go to my father in an attempt to console him. It is here that my interest in spirituality began. He started to teachme meditation for children, encouraging me to first listen to my own "inner sounds". This was the beginning of my journey into introspection. He next taught me to listen to my asserting mind and also my doubting mind. He identified the doubting as the sixth sense warning me against a particular action. This was my journey into the faculty of intuitiveness.

He showed me the face of the cosmic vision [deep infinity within the divine cave of the brain and spinal cord] in the dark sky between my eyebrows. When he found me dozing off during these sessions, he would encourage me to stretch my back. He then told me that the kneeling, stooping, and standing that the Arabs were practising during their prayers were to energise their awareness, and prevent them from falling asleep as they prayed: we lived above an Arab-owned Mosque and the activities of the faithful could be seen from our balcony.

Through him, I began to realise periods of silence and stillness. Every child and adult has the ability to connect with their own inner selves and to achieve a state of superconsciousness (an individualised beingness beyond wakeful, dream, and deep sleep states) through the practice of Yoga Meditation. These notes are a summation of all I have learned by drawing from all philosophies, both Eastern and Western. What follows describes my experience in this quest.

Our early education was influenced by the Roman Catholic teachings of nuns and priests at Convent Schools in Zanzibar, Dar-es-salaam, and Mombasa where my father started new trade schools: "Commercial Institute" is what they were called. Imagine my shock when at seventeen I arrived in Dublin and was assigned to live for the next few years in the YWCA in Mount Pleasant Square. Here, I made an incredible discovery: that there were many types of Christians!

My Goan schoolmate from Zanzibar, Grace Lobo, and I travelled together for the first time by air, stopping in Nairobi, Wadi Halfa, Malta, and London. Then we journeyed by overnight boat to Dublin. We were both very lonely, travelling so far and leaving the parental nest to pursue higher education.

Grace was the braver of the two of us. I dared not tell her that my firm feet had turn to crumbling sand. Given the chance, I would fly back home! I had spent a year urging my reluctant father to let me become a doctor. He took much persuading, feeling that medicine was a terrible life for his young girl; instead, he wanted me to become a lawyer, but none of my siblings took to that profession.

We took a taxi into Dublin's fair city. The taxi dropped Grace off at the Loretta Convent in St. Stephen's Green. My loneliness at seeing her leave moved me to tears, but I was a brave little teenager! I arrived at the YWCA in Mount Pleasant Square. It was breakfast time. The smell of eggs made me hungry as I lugged in my suitcase. A tall, stern lady met me at the door, and complained "You have arrived a day earlier than we expected you", and walked away in a huff.

My heart skipped a beat. Where, and how was I to find another place to stay? As I stood in the cold lobby, my mind raced in alarm. My thoughts were interrupted by the mutterings of another lady who had entered the lobby. I had not understood a word she had spoken. Finally, I heard the word 'breakfast' and realised she was asking me to come into the adjoining dining hall for breakfast.

She served me breakfast. She was very kind as she fussed over me. She spoke constantly but try as I did, I could not understand what she was saying. They speak Irish here, my mind cried in alarm! I became even more convinced: I must fly back to Zanzibar!!

Later, this lady led me up the stairs to my room which I was too share with a Nigerian student of Trinity College or University of Dublin. I was alone in the room, and I started to cry. My roommate suddenly walked in and inquired why I was crying. Through sobs I asked: "Must I learn Irish also"? We both laughed as she told me that my rescuer, the assistant to the English Director, was speaking English, but with a Cork accent!

My first Sunday Meeting at the YWCA was memorable. An Irish missionary had just returned from Kenya and she described the Masai tribe to the residents of the "Y"! She had to raise "Pennies for Black Babies" in Africa. Little white boxes with pictures of black babies on them were scattered all over the Hall. This was the first time I realised there were Protestants in addition to the Roman Catholics in the Christian world.

Young as I was, I also did not recognise much truth in what was being described by this missionary, having lived in Africa all my life! This was my first exposure to raising funds on the backs of sad stories of visible minorities in Third World countries. I bristled but was too young to do anything about it. My black Nigerian roommate let out a tirade when we got back to our room.

I often think of this incident. Later in my life, the Master would introduce me to back-breaking poverty and helplessness of illiterate women around the hermitages at the foothills of the Himalayas. Next, he would sendme to the draught-stricken wastelands of the Deccan plateau in Andhra Pradesh where families have lost their land, culture, and heritage to cruel changes in climates. Finally he would show me the devastation that accompanies industrialisation in semi-urban areas around the hermitage in Bangalore. Today, fund-raising in the West is an important part of my life. I have spent the last decade raising moneys in Canada for the Chinmaya Mission, working hand-in-hand with the Canadian

International Development Agency (CIDA). But I'm still of the opinion that using sad stories to make people guilty and raise funds is incorrect.

By the time I was nineteen, my younger sister, Saroj, and my childhood friend, Joti, had joined me in Dublin. By the time I was twenty, Joti and I were married. We both studied diligently, I medicine at the Royal College of Surgeons and Physicians on Stephen's Green, and Joti engineering at Trinity College. As undergraduates of medicine, we were not allowed to enter through the front door of the Royal College. However, Joti would storm through, announcing to Maxwell, the front gate security guard: "I am not governed by the laws of this York Street Technical College"! While waiting for me to finish classes, he and Maxwell would sit together to discuss the export of Irish education to the world.

Birth control was outlawed in Ireland. By the time Joti and I were both twenty-three, we had two Irish children. Meenakshi (Meena), the eldest, left me to return to live with my mother-in-law in Dar-es-salaam when she was thirteen months old (I had to do in-house training at Hospitals by then).

Finally, the course work and training were over. I stood with my classmates at the bottom of the stately stairs in the front lobby of the College to hear the final results-was I a doctor. As I heard that my five years of hard work had reached fruition, I fainted without warning. Binitha (Bina) had first made her presence known. She was my close inner-companion for the next nine months during Internship in the Limerick Regional Hospital and also the Jervis Street Hospital.

Bina was only three months old, and Joti was still studying Engineering, when I returned for Tanganyika [later to become Tanzania] to take my first daughter Meena back from my in-laws. Thirty-five years later, at a class-reunion in Dublin, my class mates asked me why I had fainted. They were belatedly told I was expecting my second child, Binitha.

For the next eight years of our professional lives we lived in Dodoma, Tanzania. The African illiterate elders whom I met as patients taught me humility. Grassroot men and women have the wisdom to detect ego. They would look upwards and were quick at reminding me that my education was a gift from *'Mungu'* (God).

As a family, we lived in India for one year in the late 1960s while my husband did his Masters in Water Resources Engineering, so important in arid Tanzania. At thirty, this was my first exposure to India. Until then, I had only heard of this ancient land through tales my parents had told me during my childhood.

It was an exciting time for me. My daughters were too young to be aware of this adventure. My husband had been in and out of India as a child and youth. For him, this was a time to discover India as an adult scientist checking irrigation projects and dams all over India. He was a proud tourist guide for his young wife and family. My recollection is one of a colourful people who were extremely resourceful and were experts at survival! The multitudes shocked me! I had never seen so many people in one place.

When I tired of these scenes, there was always an escape from the rigorous life at the University in Roorkee. New Delhi was not far away. My younger sister's husband was in the diplomatic service in India from Tanzania. 'Home' was always near by. It was so easy to escape and discuss the enigma: India!

Refreshed we would return to the University Residence where there were many graduate students with their families. They were from countries such as Sri Lanka, Malaysia, Africa, Mauritius, Indonesia, and of course the many States of India. All these young naive engineers were fired with the enthusiasm of 'saving' the world from drought and hunger!

While our husbands spent their days and evenings studying, we wives spent our time gossiping about our growing children, preparing for the many festivities of India, or introducing each other to the different traditions and cooking styles of their origin.

A Sri Lankan couple introduced me to *Sai Baba of Shirdhi* whose shrine burns with a mysterious eternal flame in *Aurangabad*, not very far from the caves of *Ajanta and Ellora in Madhya Pradesh.* Impressionable as I was, these discussions aroused a devotional connection in my own bosom. By this time my father had been dead for eighteen months, and *Sai Baba of Shirdi* became my silent companion and confidant.

We returned to Tanzania only to discover that our Irish-born children did not qualify to attend the International School for Expatriates because we, their parents, were local Tanzania-born citizens.

Wanting a good education for our children, we made the painful decision to leave Africa. As a Regional Water Resources Engineer for two regions (Dodoma and Singida) in Tanzania, Joti had for some years worked with Canadian Engineers from CUSO. My husband had already heard of the 'white ivory towers' of Canadian professional institutions! He knew we would face years of hardship. Our Irish qualifications would have to undergo the thrashing of an unforgiving economy and professional intolerance, and they did!

Thirty years later, it is interesting that Canada has not changed this intolerable narrow self-serving policy created by a few who head these ivory towers. Brilliant professionals from 'foreign' universities, in the thousands, are still unemployed because of professional arrogance. A few hundred individuals who lack a vision for Canada and her future spurn what is good for the Mother Country. Luckily, we were both very young, and we survived this temporary indignity! The vision and inclusiveness of Pierre Elliot Trudeau made it so much easier for us and perhaps many other visible minorities who had chosen Canada as their new home.

We lived in St. John's, New found land for the next ten years. We loved it there and still do. The local New found landers reminded us of the beautiful Irish people of our student years. Our doors were always open and neighbours came in and out of our homes, as they pleased.

Our first summer in Canada, I was working in our new home and getting acquainted with the unfamiliar plants in the garden, when I noticed my younger daughter dressed in her beach clothes spreading a mat on the grass of the back garden. The morning Newfoundland wind was cold and the sun behind the clouds was not very generous. I was sure she was copying the our neighbour to the left, who was a great "sunworshipper". Bina always had a mind of her own! We talked about the dangers of climatic exposures. She heard me out as she usually does, and then burst into tears. She had spent a terrible week worrying about living in Canada. A school-friend who had just returned from Disney World had lost her sun-tan. She did not want to suffer this disaster too! So life in Canada took some adjustment for all of us.

In the early seventies, I was enduring a private agony. New found land was fog-bound for days and I could not fly out of St John's. I had to ask Joti's childhood school friend and old neighbour from Dar-es-salaam, Nandi Jethi, to cremate my younger brother, Manmohan. He had sent the ashes to my father-in-law for disposal-rites into the Ganges in India.

It was at this time that I met *Swami Chinmayananda.* I was looking for a priest (whom some of us wrongly called a *swami)* to do the thirteenth day final funeral rite for my younger brother who had died days before in Vancouver. Until this time, I had only known bell-ringing priests who did birth, death, and marriage ceremonies in temples and homes.

Never before had I met a *swami* who was able to speak from the towering height of pure intellectualism and logic. His ten-day lecture series at Memorial University opened doors in my mind. I had arrived home. For years I had struggled with the books I had devoured from my father's library and with the experiences of my travels in India. I saw in *Swami Chinmayananda* a man of vast resources. However, I had the audacity to think that we were both on the same intellectual wavelength! He would teach me what was very wrong in my understanding and perceptions!

Madhuri Acharya who had spent her childhood in Bombay was now married to *Vipin Acharya* of St. John's. She had been a student of *Swami Chinmayananda* as a youth. Madhuri was familiar with *Swamiji's* ten-day lecture series *or yagnas* on the *Bhagavad Geeta. Madhuri* convinced her husband to urge Joti, my husband (the then chairperson of the Indo-Canadian Association of Newfoundland) to invite *Swamiji.*

The *Acharya* family hosted the Master for ten days. They were aware of our recent loss and our dilemma for a thirteenth day funeral rite. Imagine our surprise when *Swamiji* graciously conducted the funeral rite for my brother. It was a memorable celebration at our Reid Street home. He started the first *Bal Vihar*

[Sunday School for children] at our home. This was also the first *Bal Vihar* ever held in North America

It was at this celebration in the midst of a crowd of people, we officially connected with the Master. My two daughters, aged eleven and thirteen years, asked him to be their 'guru'. The eloquent *Swami* agreed, and the *Chakraburtty* family spent years nurturing the relationship between the girls and their chosen 'guru'! They knew little about what they had got themselves into. I had little time for this tall, regal, and handsome intellectual except during his visits to whatever City we lived in. He became a wonderful friend and urged me to run his cultural classes for children and youth. Weekly Study Classes with the parents of these children became fertile sessions of self-study and self-unfoldment.

As I grew in understanding, so did my ego! I now possessed a knowledge unlike anyone else! Now my friends and family had to deal with a new monster! I rejected the *Swami.* To me, he was a means to an end. I wanted to know what it was that made me tick!

It was at this time that he asked me if I would take him on as a *guru.* I rejected him outright. I informed him that I was emotionally connected to the *Sai Baba* of *Shirdhi. At* about this time I was troubled by a recurring dream of a banyan tree and a man in orange with an afro-style haircut whose face I could not identify. At a *satsang* (meeting with the wise) in Montreal, I mentioned this to *Swamiji.* He introduced me to a 'new' reincarnation of *Sai Baba* of *Puttaparthi.* Since this new *Sathya Sai Baba* had appeared to me in dreams many times, *Swami Chinmayananda* offered to take me to him in India.

I was convinced *Sai Baba* would recognise me! It was with great anticipation that I met *Sathya Sai Baba.* I had already been warned by *Swami Chinmayananda* that I would be disappointed with the meeting, but this young egoistic seeker had again taken no heed of his warning.

The meeting was a disaster! The 'miracles' performed by *Sathya Sai Baba* shocked and embarrassed me! I already had read about mystics performing miracles. And I also knew that this was one avenue that must be rejected by all serious seekers of Truth. I felt defiled and assaulted after this meeting. Confused, I asked *Swami Chinmayananda* to give me a chaperone to take me to the *Sai Baba* Institutions in *Whitefield* and *Puttaparthi.*

At *Puttaparthi*, I met with a retired pathologist who was staying in a room next to mine. We spent two days analysing my own violent reaction to the meeting with *Sai Baba* and came to the conclusion that my days of blind devotion to *Sai Baba*, had come to an end. I would have to ask *Swami Chinmayananda* to teach me *Vedanta.*

I returned to *Bombay. Swami Chinmayananda* heard me outwith genuine concern for my well-being! He knew I had rejected him as my spiritual teacher but he was generous enough to again offer his services for my own growth.

Looking back on this incident, I shiver to think at the picture of arrogance that sat before this mighty Teacher!

I challenged him to teach me. He gave me a schedule of the reading I was to complete. We would meet every year to discuss my questions. Over a period of ten years, we covered all the texts prescribed by him, except for the *Brahma Sutras.* Yet, when all was done, all I seemed to have accomplished was nurturing a gigantic ego! I was nowhere near what I wanted to become.

One day, during his visit to our home in Ontario, we were both seated at the window looking at the beautiful tall spruce trees swaying with the lake wind when I rudely interrupted his thoughts. "Now that you have made me go through this study, what do you want me to do with it"? He smiled knowingly. "Now, my child, read them all over again"! As he expected, I refused. After a long silence, he added "When you find your ultimate connection with the Cosmic Mother, you will have arrived".

I was angry. I avoided him for two years, convinced that he had set me up on a wild goose chase. My relationship with him was limited to ensuring that my two teenage daughters, who were flourishing beautifully under his care, would meet him each summer. These were dark days of a 'perpetual night on this spiritual journey'.

There were years of remorse and confusion. I loved him dearly. He had been a wonderful teacher. I had been an ungrateful seeker. He had been a gracious host every time I visited *India.* He refused to teach me any more, and I was too proud to ask him why! He knew his lecture series left me unmoved. He even told me to read the material he had covered and come to my own conclusions. In retrospect, I know now that everything he said left an indelible mark on my thinking.

Swami Chinmayananda had nurtured the girls as they moved from childhood to youth. He was now busy easing them into the independence of University years. I was busy studying and researching and he was alarmed when the girls were left to their own devices because I was of the opinion that they were now 'grown up'. He nurtured them through this too, acting as a mother to them.

As well, he played the role of a big brother, telling them tales of self-protection. Since they had no brothers, he taught them about the guile of young men! He knew that when their father was out of the country, they would need his fatherly advice and guidance. We can still think back and wonder: How did he ever know to be everything to everyone of us at one and the same time!

The girls adored him. I adored him for being so gentle, kind, and thoughtful. I could never get over the fact that in *Swami Chinmayananda* I had a wonderful friend. This giant of an intellectual, who had written and commented on over sixty books on Hindu Scriptures, had accepted and embraced this self-opinionated mother of two girls!

By now, it was eighteen years since we first met. At that time, I thought our meeting was an accident. Looking back, I now am convinced, that he had come for me and me alone! My inner *guru* had called for help and guidance and he appeared. I rejected him but he tolerated me!

My preoccupation with new positions and new knowledge was now waning. The girls had married and left the nest. I had mellowed. Dispassion had started to reign supreme in my life. My meditative efforts were becoming more intense.

It was at this time that *Swami Chinmayananda* summoned me to *Sidhbari*, at the foothills of the *Himalayas.* In his seventies, he had become frail. I decided to visit him for two weeks over the Christmas holidays and stayed with him for six weeks.

There in the quiet of the mountains, I reached an oasis. I spent days of regret. I just could not get over (and still cannot) that I had wasted two decades of my life rejecting this giant of a man! There were a lot of tears in the quiet of my room in the Monastery. Sometimes, I did not have the courage to face him in the morning.

Every time he missed me in the morning, he would gently prod me. A week before I left, he called me to his office. I sat at the foot of his desk. There was only silence between us. He was busy replying to letters that came to him in the hundreds from seekers from every part of the world where he had visited or lectured (270 centres around the globe).

"*Gurudev*, what took you so long to call me", I asked.

He dropped his pen. His kind eyes looked into my soul.

"*Gurudev*, did I hear you right"?

"Yes *Gurudev*", I replied. "What took you so long to call me to you"?

He stood up. I stood up too. Standing, I only reached his waist! He gathered me in his arms and said: "You were not ready for me, *Amma!* You were too busy acquiring name and fame".

As I wept in regret, this kind gentle soul apologised for not taking me any further. He told me his time was nearing its end. The rest of my spiritual journey would have to be without his physical presence.

I spoke with him for the last time in Canada only months before he left his physical body. In his usual soft tones he assured me that the path was clear. Intense study and meditation were all that was necessary. He also gently reminded me that without the initial years of work, it would be impossible to be where I was at!

Thirty years after meeting the Master, I have come to the conclusion that meditation is the ultimate path to finding spiritual fulfilment. Not only did, *Swami*

Chinmayananda teach my pragmatic intellect the logic of *Sankhyan* Philosophy but he also took me to other *yogis* and *yogin* is; some old and experienced, others youthful and wise.

Through him I met the great *yogini Swamini Sharadapriyananda* who opened my inner vision. She revealed to me the existence of the physical Universe on a substratum of the vibrating Holy Spirit Amen or Aum. In the bowels of Niagara Falls, she allowed me to meet Mother Nature in Her grandeur, although I had already seen the Falls with many a tourist! As a result of an intense spiritual experience she bestowed on me [to be discussed later in the text], from that time forward, I was able to balance my pragmatism with the higher faculty of intuition.

The Masters of *Yogoda Satsanga Ashram* of *Ranchi*, India and the Self Realisation Fellowship of California took me to the existence of the path of *Raja Yoga* which is the combined path of the four *yogas* in Eastern thought. Through my younger daughter, I read "Autobiography of a Yogi", by *Paramahansa Yogananda.* Later, a study of *Patanjali's Yoga Sutras* revealed and confirmed conclusively the experiences of my spiritual journey. It must have been divine intervention that I met *Swami Yogi Satyam* of *Allahabad, India.* He taught me the practical techniques of higher meditation.

In both the East and the West, meditation is practised with increasing interest. Its ultimate truth is that the experience of meditation has universal characteristics. The discovery of the ultimate truth in oneself requires a comprehensive understanding of one's own psychology, physiology (especially neurophysiology), and philosophy.

This understanding helps to explain the logic of acupuncture, ayurveda, and other ancient Oriental sciences of healing which relies heavily on the knowledge of the "flow of life-force" and kinetic-energy (ki-energy), along recognised fluid channels or *nadis. The* practice of meditation has an ultimate goal: the unification of the soul with the Spirit, in a state of superconsciousness. To achieve such a state, Yoga requires that the ego be completely dissolved.

Specific techniques, practised through *yoga,* are required to annul the ego. The practitioner needs to know how to deal with the various changes occurring in the beingness of the seeker. He or she also needs to know how to deal with the phenomena which accompany *samadhi (oneness* of "beingness" with "Beingness") in both the astral [subtle body of psychological-physiological energy] and causal dimensions [of thought]. This leads the practitioner gradually through to the "next stage" for meditation. The process of development involves moral training, physical training, and spiritual training.

The notes offer assistance in taming the wandering mind during the practice of meditation. The arrangement of the material is exactly as I learned it from the Master. First there is an *Introduction* to *Vedanta. Armed* with this material (which is both difficult at first and dry), it becomes increasingly easier to understand spiritual growth. At times the text reads as a teaching manual, and it is! I make no apologies. Only a serious seeker can read this book!

The text is divided into sections. Each section builds upon its predecessor and must be mastered before proceeding to the next stage. To facilitate this, each section contains questions which promote either individual introspection or group discussion. As each section is assimilated, it prepares you to move to the next. All of the five senses are analysed to their pure state. The purpose of this exercise is to fine-tune each faculty. The seeker now sees, hears, tastes, feels, and smells without the encumberance of past habits, likes-and-dislikes, and personal opinions.

Many techniques of meditation are offered. At the end of the day, the seeker devises what works best for him or her. But whichever path is chosen, it will be an exciting and rewarding journey.

The '*Introduction* to *Vedanta'* is my own personal note scribbled over many, many years. Without these notes to refer back to, it would have been impossible to keep disciplined and focused within the journey of self-unfoldment. What might have been significant in the earlier years, became part of my own natural understanding in later years. The notes are brief and succinct but adequate to understand what follows.

Every learning is based upon a foundation. On this foundation of universal values is what follows in the next chapter. Each chapter is a stepping stone to a specific measured growth.

One cannot embark on a journey unless the seeker understands what he or she 'meets' in the experiences of his meditation! Unless this is understood, the seeker complains of ending in a self-hypnotic void. That is not the intent of the text. Successful meditation is an intense experience and realisation that 'the boat of life has reached the shore of ultimate success'!

I have used Sanskrit in many places because there is no equivalent translation of the word in English; there is, however, a glossary at the end of the text.

While preparing the text, I realised that if my purpose was to share my spiritual journey with others who were unfamiliar with the subject of meditation, then I would have to tell my personal story. It became quite clear that I must speak of personal problems encountered in studying the Bible, the *Geeta,* the *Bhagvatam* and the *Upanishads*, and of my efforts, as an Indian born in East Africa, to understand the Indian culture. So, I also added stories of my own experience to the text, as well as excerpts from letters received by me from my Master, *Swami Chinmayananda*.

Originally, I began writing to share my spiritual journey of more than thirty years with my two daughters Meenakshi and Binitha, who in their own ways, also contributed to the journey. In time these writings matured into a study manual for students of meditation in the Niagara Peninsula. And as the manual gained a wider audience, itevolved even further to include how I came to these conclusions.

I am grateful to Carolyn Gray and Judith Tokar for consenting to edit this text. My special gratitude goes to Carolyn who edited the material over eight times and, along with my daughters, convinced me that the material needed to be "humanised". Carolyn thought it needed to be read by a fresh mind. A recent critique of this same material by Ann Edwards, convinced me that the writings would indeed have to "humanised."

I thought the manuscript was ready for publication, except for a feedback from Rachna Gilmore [a Canadian author of childrens' books who recently received the Governor General's Award for her book]. She has urged my intensely private persona to share my personal experiences and conclusions with this book. I thank her for this critique.

I would also like to thank my husband of over forty years, Joti Chandra Chakraburtty, who may not realise just how much he has contributed to my spiritual journey.

This text about spirituality entails a journey of exploration. My son-in-law recently said: "It is not sufficient just to have an address. A road map is necessary to reach one's destination." It is my hope that this book will aid you in your own journey.

In conclusion, I must admit that my life with my family and the many teachers the Master exposed me to has been an enchanting sojourn! My heartfelt gratitude to this Master.

Sneh Lata Chakraburtty

Table of Contents

SECTION SIX: AJNAA CHAKRA

Introducing the Master

Swami Chinmayananda has been my spiritual teacher for twenty five years. He too experienced a spiritual journey of his own. His thoughts give relevance to what follows in this text. I present the mind-state of a seeker embarking upon a spiritual journey in the Master's own words.

In the December 18, 1949 issue of the magazine "Champion" Swami Chinmayananda wrote about his own thoughts which led him on the path of spirituality. Here are some excerpts in his own words.

> "I was hiding from the British. I had become a fugitive in my own country. ... I was a law student from Lucknow University where I had led the students on an "Quit India" march against the British.
>
> "I found myself in Rishikesh on the banks of Ganga's Ananda Kutir: Swami Sivananda's Ashram. I was aghast at the institution and its various activities of guiding, instructing and encouraging his innumerable disciples from all over the world. We all watched silently. The more we watched the more we learnt. .....The cool confidence and sympathetic understanding with which he (Swami Sivananda) answered all our sceptical questions on God and a spiritual life gave us the courage to expose my curiosity.
>
> "Swamiji, may I ask a personal question?" I ventured bravely. "Certainly and why not?" smiled back Swami Sivananda. Knowing fully well that it was unpardonable for a *satsangi* (guest at the meeting with the wise) to ask any *sadhu* (monk) about his *purvashram* (premonastic life), I asked anyway: "Swamiji, why did you take *Sanyas* (renunciation from social ties)?"
>
> "There was visible tension on Swami Sivananda's calm face. He was on alert. His eyes wandered for a moment among the correspondence, files, typewriter and the many volumes that lay scattered around him. "What else do you expect any sensible man to do?" asked Swami Sivananda, "Would you have me," he shot back "marry, breed, fight and talk shop till wrecked with age and sorrow, until this body drops down dead?"
>
> "Menon (the future Chinmayananda-to-be) was already tired of living in his tomb (physical body), so he walked into the open to breathe, to bask in the sun, to work and to live. The unborn Swami was ablaze. None suspected that this frail body would contain such a consuming fire of earnestness. ... he sat out on the river-bank, looking into the glittering flow of the immortal river. It was a roar of "silence" that smothered the false values that lay heavy on his bosom (heart).

"The Chinmayananda-to-be returned to the meeting and dared to ask Swami Sivananda: 'But Swamiji, you have not answered my question. Why did you, an educated, young, efficient, smart, spirited physician kick away life and take to dressing as a monk?'.

"He thought about his own experience. From the University, Menon (Chinmayananda-to-be) walked away a proud peacock with his M.A. (English). His vanity had increased. His daring was supreme. He strode out to meet life, supremely confident that he could fix himself comfortably in one of life's 'luxury flats'. At the guarded 'entrance' to life's door, none were admitted unless of a healthy character, a good disposition, and a charming friendliness. He bustled his way onto the crowded veranda of life where men and women were busy doing nothing. ..... Without much difficulty he pushed himself into the stinking Hall of Life. Here, he met with unnatural values: impossible behaviour; stupid vanities; made to order laughter and sighs (as he studied smiles and tears); voiceless deep regrets; feigned friendships concealing stormy hatred, grudging sympathies; and, poisonous revelries. Each suffered and contributed lavishly to the 'Total suffering'. At the gates of life Menon realised that he was poor in real wealth'..

"However, Menon had to answer his own questions. 'Where to, you miserable stranger?' He took to meditation that had been taught to him as a youth at his paternal home. This decision was followed by intense study of the philosophy. ..." 'It now and then thrilled the intellect, but generally left the Spirit sorely disappointed'. The surging enthusiasm tore his insides and he thundered... demanding the freedom for self-expression.

"It was at this crucial moment in his life that he reached Swami Sivananda in Rishikesh ... 'more as a deserter of life than a discoverer of new shores'. He was led to Swami Tapovan near the origin of the Ganga (River Ganges). Breathing in the wholesome rejuvenating Vedantic (spiritually charged) air, Menon spent nine years in the Himalayas absorbing the Hindu Scriptures. He was given *sannyas* (monk-hood) as Swami Chinmayananda by Swami Sivananda on February 25, 1949."

A spiritual journey is not an easy destination. It is not easily reached. There are internal struggles. The mind and intellect thirsts for immortality in a field of change. The mind asks questions which cannot be answered. Only a fortunate few receive the gift of a Master to illumine the path as well as the journey. To my dearest friend and Master, I offer this adoration. I have used every note and paper saved during my tutelage under this incredible teacher.

tvameva mata cha pita tvameva tvameva bandhushcha sakha tvameva
tvameva vidya drivinam tvameva tvameva sarvam mama deva deva

You alone are the mother, father, kinsman and friend. You are the ultimate Knowledge and true Wealth. You are my all oh Lord and Master.

The BMI (body-mind-intellect) **Chart**

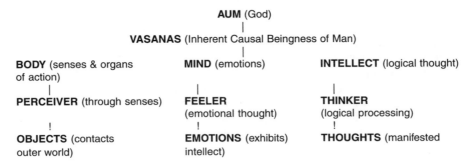

AUM (God)

|

VASANAS (Inherent Causal Beingness of Man)

|

BODY (senses & organs of action)	**MIND** (emotions)	**INTELLECT** (logical thought)
|	|	|
PERCEIVER (through senses)	**FEELER** (emotional thought)	**THINKER** (logical processing)
!	!	!
OBJECTS (contacts outer world)	**EMOTIONS** (exhibits) intellect)	**THOUGHTS** (manifested

The BMI Chart has been placed before 'Introduction to Vedanta' for easy future reference. The purpose of the Chart is to align Eastern and Western thinking so that we all understand the statements being made in this document.

All religions attempt to bring about self-transformation through self-mastery until the seeker's life is one of inner tranquillity despite outer circumstances. Ancient seers of the Truth identified the experiencer experiencing the world of objects, emotions, and thoughts [OET] through instruments of experience i.e. the body, the mind, and the intellect [BMI].

When identified with the body, a person becomes the *perceiver,* experiencing the world of objects. Identified with the mind, the person becomes the *feeler* of the world of emotions. Identified with the intellect, the person is the *thinker* who experiences the world of thoughts and ideas [PFT].

In truth, the experiencer is neither the BMI, nor the OET. Then who is the PFT? The principle behind the perceiver, feeler, and thinker [PFT] is the supreme Reality, God or *brahman.* It is the divine substratum, *aum,* which lends its light and energy to every being. This *aum* is the Holy Spirit or pure Consciousness, or pure Awareness.

The Divine Principle is one, yet appears as many when expressing through the various instruments of the body, mind, and intellect.

Vasanas [V] are innate urges, accumulated through past lives, influencing our minds and actions. They are our unmanifest unfulfilled desire-motivated tendencies. When they manifest, they become our unique personality which drives all our activities in the world.

> The Master explained the BMI Chart
>
> "..**BMI** (body-mind-intellect) are all caused by and function because of ***vasanas.*** This is called the Causal Body. This is the 'body' in which you exist in your 'deep-sleep state of Consciousness'.

B is gross body.. In waking state; **M+I** is the 'subtle body' in dream; and **V** is the causal body in deep sleep.

"..A tree is in the seed Causal Condition as ***Vasana*** **(Unmanifest)** in your deep sleep. When **manifested**, the seed condition bursts forth as a tree; when awake your unmanifest (V) bursts into your PFT (perceiver-feeler-thinker). Your PFT is in a 'seed condition' in sleep"....

"When M+I (mind-intellect) are transcended (when V is exhausted), PFT 'awake' gets 'enlightenment' of its Pure State, the *Aum-state*, the god-State of Consciousness. When you die, you leave B (Gross Body) and it is only a Subtle or Astral Body (M+I) and the Causal Body (V) that leaves. Even while you live, how can even your children and their father see your M+I?'......

Transformation through Meditation:

Aum the *Observer* or **Rishi** [cortex] with Total Knowledge. Silently **watches**

|

Vasanas the silent **Devata** [thalamus] **looks** and makes ***Observation*** of *transformation* in knowledge taking place through ***sadhana*** [spiritual effort]

|

Transformed **Neurohormones** [pituitary] & **Neurotransmitters** [hypothalamus]
from
Master Glands [Hypothalamus and Pituitary]

adjust all *perceiving-feeling-thinking*
to a specific transformed value with a specific or **Chhandas** quality

!

Perceptions of **PFT** [perceiver-feeler-thinker] through **BMI** [body-mind-intellect]

with **OET** [objects-emotions-thoughts] are

Actions of Service to *Prakriti or* **Mother Nature**

Making a study of *vedanta* at Study Groups and Sunday Schools is a seeker's attempt to understand all sacred texts. This can be taught at any school and university. Having studied it, the mind has been given esoteric facts. A sincere student may then embark on loving and feeling a devotion for this book knowledge. Neither of these have the ability to give us a realisation the Truth.

Truth lies beyond the instruments of the body and mind. To make Truth our own personal experience, meditation is necessary. The exercise of meditation requires the use of the mind, but the experience is both personal and beyond the mind! It is an inner realisation where self meets the Self!

Knowledge of the Scriptures cannot bless the seeker unless there is a gradual need and urgency to create new habits and concepts in the old mind. We need to see ourselves and identify with the pure self, not the body, mind, and intellect.

Repeated attempts have to be made to cut all identifications with the not-Self.

Over time and sincere meditation, a transformation is takes place at all levels of his personality. As the mind learns the new habit of focusing on one thought in meditation. This one thought signifies our own purity and limitless nature. Constant practice and contemplation makes the transformation permanent and the seeker sees a change in the way he uses his bodily equipments (BMI).

When the seeker becomes adept at contemplation and meditation, he or she becomes a witness and experiencer who watches without involvement. He is aware of the transformed experience and keeps looking and marvelling at the transformation. The inner experience of transformation makes the perceiver, feeler, and thinker (PFT) a transformed being. His interactions with the world of OET is a new type of experiencing.

In summary, the Pure Self or *rishi* watches all changes. The Causal self or *devata* looks at the incoming information, whether through reading, writing, contemplation, or meditation. Appropriate changes are recorded as information becomes ingrained in the psyche of the seeker. He now sees the world of objects, emotions, and thoughts from a different perspective and his worldly interactions have a transformed or *chhandas* quality. He begins to see the unity of the Self with the Cosmic Self.

Index to Vedanta:

Need for a Roadmap to the Destination

"I have been a student of the *Guruji* [teacher] for seven years, and I am still struggling with the concepts meditation is based upon" Ann said. " It has taken you less time to assimilate this".

"*Swamiji* feels his students will experience every possible knowledge within the folds of dedicated meditation. You need faith in what he is telling you" I said.

"When I started, I did not know whether Krishna and Arjuna were a city or a myth."

"The roadmap of *Vedanta* [philosophy of the Hindus] is necessary only to a point. Your *Guruji* is telling you that in the experience of *samadhi* [Oneness of self with Self] all knowledge must be shed" I replied.

"Having the roadmap in advance of a spiritual journey would have made my treading the path easier" she concluded.

Introduction to Vedanta

Vedanta is the philosophy of Hindu thought, which upholds the doctrine of either pure non-dualism (I am the Self) or conditional non-dualism (God and I are one).

This section attempts the almost impossible feat of summarising the philosophical thought in the four voluminous *Vedas. Vedas* are the highest, most ancient authoritative scriptures of the Hindus. They were not written by any one single person and are therefore free from the imperfections to which human productions are subject. If an experience is forgotten, they can be reproduced by *rishis* or seers of Truth, through intense meditation.

The section is purely informational. Diagrams have been added to assist the reader's understanding. Many of the examples provided illustrate the writer's own struggle as I ploughed my way into a spiritual journey, both fascinating and difficult. Included are excerpts from my Teacher in response to questions I had asked. These excerpts have been incorporated in the text to illuminate some of the problems encountered.

Included also comments made by a medical mind. These may be of no interest to some readers. These have been marked with asterisk [**] at the beginning and at the end of that section. These areas may be ignored by readers not interested in this field of science.

The Rational Quest for Philosophy

This text is based on the *Sankhyan* philosophy [one of the six schools of philosophy who accept the *Vedas*]. It is a fact of history that the Indian Culture is the oldest, most enduring, and most widely developed of all cultures. It was developed by disciplined sages and saints through a wide range of experiences and insights. Tireless inquiries led them to draw conclusions about Truth and Values of Life.

New ideas, generated through critical examination were not suppressed, but rather were answered, and the original views expanded and enlarged. The result is that *vedanta* grew and provided the widest cultural basis of Indian philosophy, religion, and ethic of Hinduism. It has, therefore, provided India with a perennial culture because it provides the basis for world civilisation. It recognises the common values of all religions.

The Sanskrit term for philosophy is *darshana* which means world-view. Its aim is a comprehensive understanding of the objective world, of the roles of rational consciousness, goodness, beauty, and their ultimate reality. There are sixteen major and minor systems of Indian Philosophy. Of the major systems, six are considered orthodox or *vedic systems* because of their professed allegiance to the *Vedas.*

Vedanta belongs to one of these six orthodox schools of Hindu philosophy. It is the most comprehensive and as such is the foundation and heart of Hinduism. *Sankhyan darshana* or world-view through reasoning or *Sankhyan* Philosophy uses reason, analysis, and reflection to make a comprehensive survey of Nature. Its founder is the sage *Chapel*, born in *Pushchair* in Nepal, over 4000 years ago.

The *sankhyans* discovered broad-based experiences through analysis and reflection. They discovered world interactions amongst physical conscious beings. These physical interactions seemed inter-related - joined together in a physical infinite common cause or primary *prakriti* or matter. This primary matter was seen to evolve into divergent things and processes. The divergence resulted in the world and the mind and intellect as awareness.

Evolution of the concept of matter or *prakriti* included intelligence (*mahat),* mind *(manas),* and intellect *(buddhi).* Logical reasoning by the intellect or *gyana* led the *sankhyans* to duty of right action or *dharma,* spiritual wealth or *aishvarya,* wisdom or *vigyana,* non-attachment or *vairagya,* and excellence in moral values. These were all evolutes of matter or *prakriti.*

They also discovered another independent reality, the spiritual self or *purusha.* Its characteristics were consciousness of the self, its individuality, and its will. Its individuality manifested as ego or *ahamkar* .

Sankhyans acknowledged awareness of inner feelings and mental thoughts. They reasoned that perception of outer objects was a function of the mind or *manas* which was the inner sense or *antar-indriya,* as opposed to external sense-organs.

Sankhyans insisted that *prakriti* is not substance but energy, which has all the potential for creative evolution. The Law of Qualities acknowledges three modes or qualities or *gunas* of energy. *Sattva* is the tendency for knowledge, goodness, brightness, and lightness. *Rajas* is dynamism, activity, surges of movement. If uncontrolled leads to sorrow. *Tamas* is a tendency towards inertia and dullness. These trends of energy determine the course of evolution in everything.

They also acknowledged the Law of Causality or cause and effect. Cause is the potential power and seed of effect seen in the future. Causation is therefore an evolution of cause!

Sankhyans insist that man is a product of his past. It is his past births which determines his present through the Law of Relativities or Duality. They determine the character fabric of the person in his present manifestation.

The *Sankhyan* philosophy of *advaita* or non-duality asserts God and I are One Infinite.

The reader is provided a roadmap to return to his Source, through intellectual understanding in tandem with meditation. It is this journey which gives meaning and answers to the eternal questions of Man: What are we here for? What is the purpose of my life? Why is there suffering in the world of a kind God? Why do we have disasters and phenomenon of mass destruction? Why must children suffer? Where is God? How do I find God?

These are questions that are perennial. We have all asked them. After years of thinking and asking, I have come to the following conclusion. All the answers are found in only three precepts. If a seeker remembers that the *Vedic* philosophy is based upon only three precepts, all questions about the mysteries of life and living are answered.

The seeker must first understand and assimilate these three precepts:

- Law of Qualities (*gunas*) as indolence *(tamas)*, passion *(rajas)*, and purity *(sattva).*
- Law of Cause and Effect or Causality (*karma).*
- Law of Relativity or likes-and-dislikes or Duality *(raaga-dveshaa)*

Logic of Meditation

Before attempting meditation, one must be clear about the macrocosmic universe, in whose "image" I, the microcosm, has been has been created. Is the Universe a closed-system with a boundary or an open-system reaching into infinity?

It is illogical to think of the Universe as a closed system that is finite. To assume that the Spirit is outside this system is an admission that Man's comprehension cannot fathom That which is beyond the tools (Body-Mind-Intellect) we use for analysis and assimilation.

Present-day scientists have decided that we live in a closed system where there is an equilibrium state of universal disorder or maximum entropy. We were once told by scientists that here, in this closed system, there exists a pressure-free end-state where no action is necessary or even possible. Recent thinkers have discovered the open system of millions of galaxies and there is a new understanding of the statement: 'Mother Nature is Infinite and beyond thought'.

The New Age scientists have also 'discovered' that atoms, molecules, and the Universe, are transcribed into solar systems and galaxies. They are seen to have a self-replicating system of organization, a self-renewing ability of universal order, all of which is within an open system of infinitude, beyond all boundaries. Here, they say action is necessary and possible.

The practice of meditation techniques is essential if one wishes to travel from the physical present to the infinite source. The inner journey is an experiential path enabling a progressive transformation. Terminology used by the ancient *rishis* or seers of Truth, must be learnt and proven concepts accepted in order for one to climb the spiral of dynamic energy and achieve an evolutionary progression.

At the beginning of my spiritual journey in the early 1970's, (after hearing him speak for the first time in Newfoundland), I wrote to Swami Chinmayananda. I told him that his lectures had lifted me as if I had graduated from University once more.

> Swami Chinmayananda responded to my letter,
>
> "Beloved one. . . . . When a sincere devotee calls out to her teacher and demands a way to guide, they come to her. If the talks we had. . . were revealing to you, I feel grateful for the Lord's Grace in He revealing Himself to you all".
>
> Thus, the tutoring began.

Man must know his real identity to maintain a proper and healthy relationship with the world at large. Every human being is constituted of physical, mental and intellectual equipment and the Conscious Principle which lends sentience to these equipments. Human development reaches its climax when man identifies with the Conscious Principle, the Spiritual Core in his own personality. (Please refer to the BMI Chart). Religion teaches us the art of focusing on the Spiritual Core.

Man is essentially divine, but his Divinity is veiled by an unbroken series of desires and thoughts. To remove the encrustations of desires and thoughts and unfold the Divinity inherent in man is the ultimate goal envisaged by the Scriptures.

The psychological being functions in three thought conditions under which the human mind functions. They are called in *Vedanta*, as the *sattva* or pure and noble, the *rajas* or passionate and agitated, and *tamas* or dull and inactive. Combinations of these *gunas* or qualities determine individual personalities.

Tamas is a mind state characterised by complete inertia, indolence and heedlessness where there is no consistency of purpose, softness of emotion, or nobility of action. *Rajas* is an agitated mind, which is agitated, stormy, passionate, ambitious, and constantly riddled with desires, emotions and activities. *Sattva* is the subtlest of the three: a state of mind with balanced joy and a serene creative poise; his human contemplation is available in its entire heritage.

These three types of thoughts form the material from which the human mind and intellect are composed. The difference in the mind and intellect is, only in their receptive functions. The mind is an instrument of feelings and emotions while the intellect discriminates and judges.

Godhood is experienced in the state of thought extinction. It is a state of being when the mind is totally transcended. Divinity is the very essence of man, but it lies covered under the encrustations of thoughts. Religion indicates different paths to this Reality. It prescribes different techniques for the extinction of thought.

A mind is merely thoughts just as river is merely water. It is the flow of water that makes the river. So too, it is the flow of thoughts which creates mind. It is the mind that veils the Divine Self within. It is the flow of thought which gives mind power and dynamism.

The human mind today is completely out of control and flowing in all directions. Our primary attempt in any spiritual effort is to prevent the flow spreading in all directions by controlling, harnessing, and regulating it. In the river of thoughts, it is the intellect that banks and determines the direction of flow. Therefore, the intellect has to be chastened and chiselled with the help of the Scriptures.

Thoughts can be changed by three methods: by reducing the quantity of thoughts; by improving the quality of thoughts; and by giving thoughts a different direction. By practising of one of the four *yogas,* or a combination of the four *(raja yoga),* the mind becomes purified and is rendered fit for meditative flights. The state of divinity acquired is not a mere personal achievement, but must culminate in a universal resurrection.

Fundamentals of Vedanta

Hinduism does not centre around any particular personality or books. Men of wisdom spent their days in the lap of Nature's beauty and grandeur. The valleys and forests of the Himalayas and the sacred Ganges were the teachers who kindled in their hearts a hunger to know the mysteries of the Power that gives life to the lifeless. The reflections and revelations of these perfect Masters formulated the scriptures which were later known as the *Vedas.*

The four *Vedas* are *Rig, Yajur, Sama,* and *Atharvana*. Each *Veda* is divided into three sections: *Mantra, Brahmana* and *Upanishad.* In the *Mantra* portion, we find ecstatic admiration of Nature's beauty expressed in lyrical poetry by these contemplative seers or *rishis.* The *Brahmana* portion deals with rituals and sacrifices. The last portion contains the philosophic wisdom known as *Vedanta.* Besides *Vedas* which are *srutis* or scriptural literature, there are other texts that deal with ethics, social sciences, laws of society, and so on.

The indifference to religion of the apparently educated man of today is not so much due to the futility or hollowness of the Science of Religion as such, but rather his own incapacity to understand the text-books of Religion in the world. True Religion never dies. Unfortunately we have come to identify Religion with stony edifices of temples, mosques, churches, synagogues, pagodas, and *gurudwaras* (sikh temples). We give endless personal interpretations to sacred books. Such misinterpretations lead to man-made inflexible doctrines. In the name of perfect Scriptures, we initiate painful quarrels resulting in violence and hatred.

It is reasonable to ask: "Why should a man hunt after knowledge of a greater Reality, of a greater Power behind the obvious?" The urge for spiritual freedom, the call from the depths within ourselves, is only experienced by man and even then it is not felt by all men!

No religion is possible in the world without a philosophy. In the East, philosophy is more than a view of life. The *rishis* or sages and the people demanded that the ideas and ideals be capable of being practised. It had to be a way of life as well. The topography and the route to be taken had to be offered in complete detail. What follows is this detail.

Sankhyan Philosophy

Sankhyan philosophy [also a *Vedic* philosophy] was propounded by the sage *Kapila* some 4000 years ago. He maintained that Consciousness and Awareness is our real nature and that evolution is completely fulfilled when we discover this state. *Vedanta* [philosophical portions at the end of the *Vedas*] asserts that this seeming world of sense objects is not real. It is only a finite appearance. It can be ended, just as a ghost is real to frightened man and the 'reality' of a mirage disappears with right knowledge. The Eternal alone is. The world and the egocentric ideas of our separative existence are superimposed upon the Truth.

Brahman or God before manifestation just IS as Existence-Knowledge-Bliss or *Sat-Chit-Anand.* He [God] is the Ultimate Source, the Infinite. Like the Sun or Spirit and the many Sun-rays or Matter, He or the Infinite decided to become many. The Unmanifest now becomes the Manifest.

Purusha or Spirit is conceived as male and stands in magnificent isolation, free of desire, emotion or activity. It is a perfect example of spiritual entropy - the Unmanifest Universal Psychic Principle which witnesses Nature, yet remains apart, uninvolved and immutable.

Prakriti or Matter or the Universal Physical Principle inherently possesses the power of ***maya*** or delusion which incorporates into it, the Law of Qualities or *gunas*, the Law of Cause and Effect *or karma,* and the Law of Relativities or dualities or likes-and-dislikes or *raaga-dvesha.* Being physical energy, Mother Nature is necessarily governed by the **Law of Qualities or *gunas*** *(rajas or activity, tamas or inertia, sattva or balance of activity and inertia). Prakriti* is conceived as female, dancing in all actions, thoughts and feelings. It is She who evolves into the world-of-multiplicity or the world of manifestation.

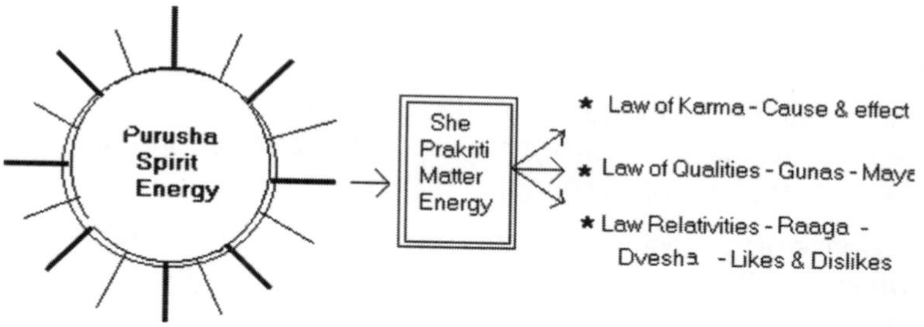

Figure 1. Purusha and Prakriti together are God or Brahman

She the Holy Spirit, is born of Him, the *Purusha.* She is *Prakriti* who as the vibrating *AUM* or Amen, is therefore the sole purpose of entertaining Him by virtue of the "powers" He vested in Her. In each *kalpa* or cycle-of-creation, She dances first away from Him, weaving Her magic of order, beauty, and love in the visible Creation.

She evolves to become the five astral [*prana* as energy], the elements of space, air, fire, water, earth as well as the universal mind and intellect. This astral clay [energy vibrating at different frequencies] is now converted into physical names and forms, All of these take their birth from causal seeds of previous births.

Prakriti which now is and always was the substratum of all names and forms, remains in connection with every atom and molecule through its feeling or mind and its thinking or intellect. Every wish and desire is possible because She records it in Her memory. At the end of the *kalpa* or cycle of creation, She dances back towards Him the *purusha*, until She collapses in Him in perfect unison or *pralaya* awaiting the next dance, but only after She has rested sufficiently.

This image is not of my creation. While visiting Andhra Pradesh in India we asked Swamini Saradapriyananda to tell us about the Dance of Creation.

This is what I understood:

With *pralaya* or dissolution of the visible universe, the cosmos merges into the unmanifest cosmic light energy. *Aum* or *Shakti* or *Prakriti. Prakriti* enters the Ultimate Substratum of Absolute Reality, who is *Purusha.* Together they become Infinity. .

After a period of rest, a new *yuga* or *Age* begins:

Shakti awakens to dance another 'dance of creation' on Her own substratum

Aum. Her magic holds Him (*purusha)* spellbound! She weaves her magic and dream while *Purusha* watches the splendour of Her creation in time and space. Her dance takes Her away from Him and She tires over time. The cosmos ages and She retraces Her dance steps towards Him until She enters *pralaya* and rests in His embrace until the next *Yuga.*

Prakriti or Nature is composed of the *essence* of the five gross elements (earth, water, fire, air and space). Their counterparts are the subtle senses (smell, taste, form, touch and sound).

The essence of the cosmic elements possesses the three qualities or *gunas* of *Mahamaya* of *Prakriti* that emanate from the Cosmic Intellect of *Ishvara, Mahat,* or *Ganesha*.

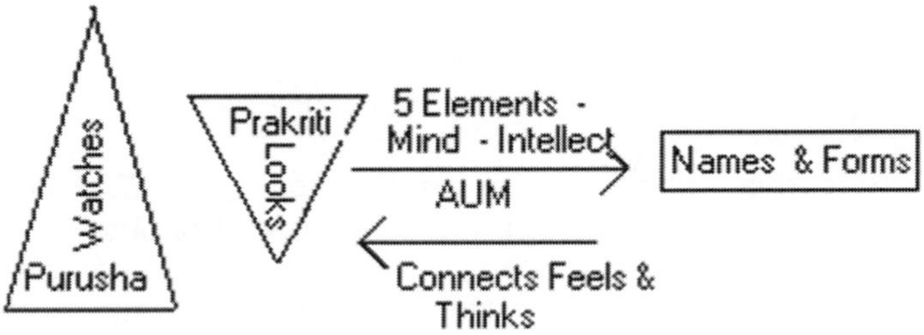

Figure 2. Purusha watches as witness and Prakriti looks to make the necessary changes

Together, the ego, the intellect, and the mind become the individualised awareness of a feeling or mood *(chitta)* that the individual intellect. The *chitta* or individualised ego-feeling is the microcosmic counterpart of the macrocosmic *Mahat* or Cosmic Intellect.

Mahat is the unevolved primary germ of Nature from which the material world is developed. Very like the microchip in the hard-drive of a computer, this seed has embedded in it. The records of every desire or *kama*, action or *karma*, likes-and-dislikes or *raaga-dvesha,* and tendency or *gunas*.

Also embedded in the primary germ of Nature are the twenty-five basic constructional elements or *tattvas* by which unmanifest desires are perpetuated in the manifested world. These are: *Prakriti;* the five gross elements; five subtle elements *(pranas);* ego; mind; intellect; five organs of perception; five organs of action; and *Purusha* as *chit.*

The blueprints or essence of: the five organs of perception (senses), five organs of action (ears, nose, eyes, skin, and tongue), five gross elements (space, air, fire, water, and earth), five subtle elements (*pranaya, apanaya, vyanaya, samanaya, udanaya)*, mind, intellect, ego, and *Purusha* as *chit* also exist here in Her Causal state.

Creation cannot take place without the Life Force coming into contact with the constructional units of creation or *tattvas.* All existence revolves around *Purusha* and *Prakriti.*

The mind acts as the bridge between the physical body and the soul. The sensory mind is imperceptible. As "Me", the soul fulfils its aspirations and pleasures through the mind that acts as a mirror. The body, in turn, serves as an instrument of enjoyment and attainment.

Sheaths Surrounding Self

According to *Vedanta*, there are three frames of body *(sharira)* enveloping the soul. They [the three bodies or *sharira*] consist of five interpenetrating and interdependent sheaths *(koshas).*

The three bodies or *shariras* are:

- Gross *(sthula sharira)* frame or the anatomical body;
- Subtle *(sukshma sharira)* frame or the physiological, psychological, intellectual body; and
- Causal *(karana sharira)* frame or the ideational body.

The **gross body** or *sthula sharira* is the anatomical sheath of physical atoms born of physical food or nourishment. It is called ***annamaya kosha*** or the gross food sheath.

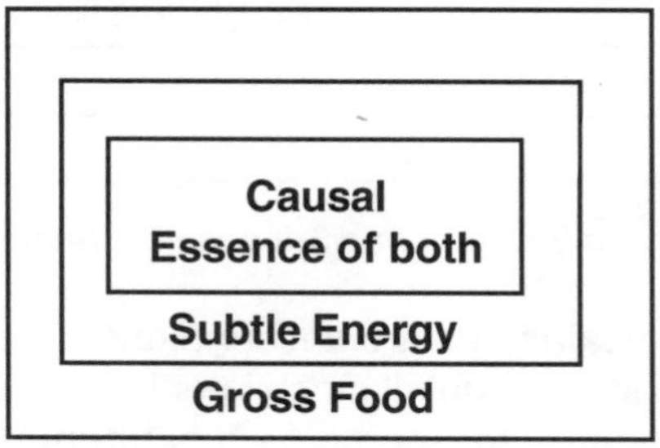

Figure 3. Three Bodies or *shariras*

The physiological *(pranamaya kosha)*, the psychological *(manomaya kosha),* and the intellectual *(gyanamaya kosha)* sheaths make up the **subtle body** or the ***sukshma sharira***.

These sheaths are composed of *prana* or subtle energy.

- ***Pranamaya kosha*** includes the respiratory, circulatory, digestive, nervous, endocrine, excretory, and reproductive systems.
- ***Manomaya kosha*** affects awareness with feelings and sense-desiring motivations; it does not depend upon any subjective experience.
- ***Gyanamaya kosha*** affects intellectual processes of reasoning and judgement; it depends and derives from subjective experience, both past and present.

The **causal body** or the ***karana sharira*** is the subtlest of the three bodies. It is an ideational sheath of joy (***anandamaya kosha***). It is composed of the essence of the gross and subtle bodies. It is made up of all the ideas of a mortal's past through his many lives. The experience of awakening after a refreshing sleep and the total absorption of the seeker in the subject of meditation is what is being alluded to when we speak of the joy of *anandamaya kosha.*

The skin encloses all these *koshas and shariras* (sheaths and bodies), which at different levels, are all intermingled with the Self.

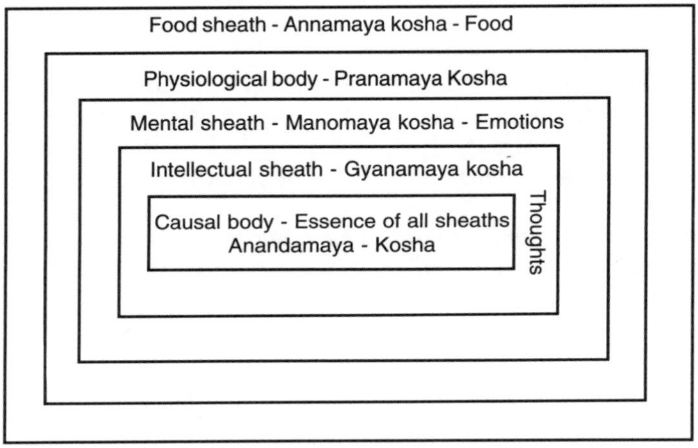

Figure 4. Three Bodies *(shariras) and* Five Sheaths *(koshas)*

There are two other sheaths that are encountered in the depths of meditation and will be referred to in more detail much later in the text:

- *chittamaya kosha* or the combined mind-intellect-ego complex of Awareness in *Prakriti;* and
- *chitmaya kosha* or the soul sheath of Consciousness in *Purusha.*

These seven sheaths were described by St. Theresa of Avila as the 'seven veils'. To reach the core of one's being, one needs to shed every one of these veils or sheaths.

Aims of Life

Man has **four aims in life**: ***dharma*** (duty), ***kama*** (pleasures), ***artha*** (wealth), and ***moksha*** (liberation).

- *Dharma* is duty; without ethical discipline, attainment is impossible.
- *Kama* or pleasurable desires are impossible without a healthy body. The Self cannot be experienced by a weakling.
- *Artha* is the acquisition of wealth for independence and higher pursuits in

life. It cannot give lasting joy.

- *Moksha* is liberation. The enlightened man realises that power, pleasure, wealth and knowledge pass away, and do not give freedom. He, therefore, rises above the *gunnas* or his physical tendencies .

Body, Mind and Intellect

All spiritual philosophies teach that the body is the abode of Brahman (or Infinite). Because it plays a vital role in attaining the four-fold aims of life, he must keep his body in good condition. Health is the delicate balance of body, mind and spirit. Only if this balance is achieved, can the body and mind come together in the performance of Yoga of Meditation.

It has taken me a long time to understand that I need to have a perfect physical body, free from the aches and pains of aging, so that I may be able to practice meditation. I know most of us do not have the expertise to care for the body and its exposures. The damages are done and one needs the tools to put things right. This also is possible. Energising exercises taught in *raja yoga* invoke the energy or *prana* of the astral body to transform every abused physical cell back to health.

Prana is the Vibrating Energy of *Prakriti.* It is the "mains" into which every name and form is connected. It is the substratum and life force that nurtures and holds every molecule in the visible Universe and beyond.

Sexual energy is the most basic expression of life force as *"ojas"* (perfected essence of healthy bodily tissues). It is immense and powerful and deserves respect and esteem. It finds expression in the warmth of our emotions, the passions of our intellect, and in our idealism. Just as our physical essence is the egg (sperm or ovum), our spiritual essence is the individualised soul that manifests as the essence of the mind *(prana)* and of the intellect *(tejas).*

Their relationship is basic and is based upon cooperation. It is a creative relationship of *Prakriti* with *Purusha.* Their synthesis which leads to freedom. Renunciation of indulgence-for-pleasure is a positive step of disengagement, not a sterile rejection. There is a moral aspect to sexual behaviour. It is the offensive and immoral use of this energy that is rejected in spiritual exercises.

"Me," the "self," the "intellectualised ego," is a devaluated state of pure perfect *Prakriti.* Mired in the delusion of *Maya* and triggered by the *gunas* or the physical properties of visible world, I begin to believe I am the physical being. The deluded ego does not even know that there is a life-force of Awareness or *chitta* and a Consciousness or *chit* that enlivens the inert physical body we worship so dearly.

Prakriti, to the traditional *vedic* mind, is the personification of the abstract spiritual truth as a *devi* or the Holy Spirit, the female consort of *Purusha* or God the Father. Together, *Purusha* and *Prakriti* are the Infinite *Brahman* or God. Spiritual ideas are given a concrete image in his ideal upon which the seeker experiences contact with higher spiritual truths. There is no contradiction in such an approach because it is based upon a deep comprehensive understanding and a personalised perception.

The *devi* is worshipped as *shakti* or female-power of life-force, born of a "still" and "silent" mind. *Prakriti* or *devi* is born of a void before space, like Life born out of a womb of power and energy: She enlivens everything within the mortal as well as in the universe. She is the power of wisdom and devotion, not outside oneself, and serves as a recognition of the power of one's own consciousness. *Devi* is the descent of divine **grace** which has the power of peace. She is energy, with the power and potency to create new life. She energises, beautifies, and delights in her creativity because she works behind all changes in the universe.

Depending upon the **inclinations of the seeker, *Shakti*** is worshipped through ***Tantra*** (physical worship), or ***Mantra*** (form of the *devi* as variations of the sound of Aum), or ***Yantra*** (geometrical designs of the *mantra)*. **Internalised worship** involves the use of speech, breath, and mind. Variations in the worship of the *devi* are manifest in various meditative methods utilised to understand the one inner reality.

Speech

According to *vedic* thought, Genesis began with the **Word**, and that Word was *Aum* (Amen, Amin, Hum). She is the Holy Spirit or *Shakti* or *Prakriti* who is Herself the beginning of every form of **Speech**.

Vedic thought recognises **four levels of speech:**

- **Audible Speech** spoken from the **throat** in the **waking state.** This is the coarse or literal speech which is a reaction to sensation.
- **Thinking Speech** spoken from the **heart.** It manifests as pure thought in the **dream state.** This happens while "thinking deeply" about something.
- **Illumined Speech** is spoken as a "gut feeling" from the level of the **navel** and manifests in its purity in the **deep sleep state** as perceptions of the "illumined Word" in the "light" of revelations made in deep meditation, through the act of the *devi's* (Holy Spirit's) "grace".
- **Transcendent Speech** cannot be put into words and is felt as a divine "word" of silence. It is a level of pure consciousness and realisation: *"Tat Tvam Asi"* (That You Are) and *"Aham Brahma Asmi"* (I am All That).

The **power of speech** must be understood from its root. The energy of awareness of speech must be allowed to achieve to its highest potential through meditation. It must be permitted to penetrate the depths of our being. The power of speech and the restless breath must be taken inwards through *mantra;* speech must be brought to the root centre of the subtle body. The navel, heart and throat *chakras* must all be conquered so that speech may enter the fourth level of illumined perception.

Meditation is a progressive learning process aimed at reaching the silent consciousness, the "I," the Self. The first stage involves harnessing both *tamas* and *rajas*, until complete equilibrium is reached in *sattva*. This physical-entropy is necessary to attain the goal of spiritual-entropy, in the discovery of "I," the Self. Meditation is *kriya* or action, which must be performed to reach such physical and spiritual stillness and silence.

Early in my *sandhana* (spiritual journey), I struggled to come to terms with the 'nature' of God. If God was a potent void before space, I asked *Swami Chinmayananda*, where was I to focus my meditation: on the void, on the bubble, or in the water?

> the Master *Swami Chinmayananda* wrote:
>
> ". . The example of the bubble and water: the bubble is only to show that water is the Reality; and when disturbed, a rippled dance of Joy. .. a bubble is formed. The bubble is nothing but water enclosing 'nothing' in space. When the bubble breaks, the water is water again and void is void again. . . .
>
> "Similarly, Consciousness alone Is: when it becomes 'conscious of' a thing (nothing but mental delusion) it becomes thought. Such 'thought flow' is mind. When we still the mind .... the objects disappear (nothing) and what remains is only Consciousness from which thoughts arose!!!
>
> 'Consciousness of things' is 'thought'. Objectless thought is Pure Consciousness. THINK ... REFLECT!!!"

What is Yoga?

No one knows the timeless Absolute One, or when the world came into existence. *Purusha* and *Prakriti* existed before Man. When man appeared, he developed and cultivated himself and began to realise his own potential. Through this, Civilisations were born. Words evolved. Concepts of God, Nature, Religion and Yoga developed.

The question kept coming back: How does one come to grips with the different faiths and yet see in them the unifying thread of Truth?

> and the Master wrote:
>
> ". . When I say Religion, I do not claim for it as an application only to Hinduism; it is as much true of Hinduism as of any other religion in the world today. Unfortunately we have come to define the term 'Religion', with stony edifices of temples and mosques, churches and synagogues, pagodas and *gurudwaras*, with different sacred books, endless and varying interpretations, confusing rituals and in their name painful mutual quarrels resulting in hatred and violence. This is often the result of the colossal ignorance of what is true religion.

> "Religion is to be understood essentially as a Science of Living, so that we may cull out of it a set of desirable values of life, upon which we can rebuild wisely our day-to-day existence. . . "

When man was caught in the web of pleasures, he found himself separated from both *Purusha* or Spirit and *Prakriti* or Mother Nature. He became victim to the polarities of pleasure and pain, good and evil, love and hate, the permanent and the transient. Amidst all of this, however, man intuitively felt the presence of a personal divinity which is free of all experiences.

This led man to seek the highest ideal embodied in the perfect *Purusha,* also called the *Ishvara* or Lord, the guru of all *gurus,* the Eternal Being. He began focusing his attention through concentration and meditation. In this very fundamental quest of life, man devised a code of conduct whereby he could live in peace and harmony with nature and his fellow beings. This is also *yoga*, the union of the individual self with the Universal Self. *Yoga* is the art that brings the incoherent and scattered mind to a reflective and coherent state. It is the communion of the human soul with Divinity.

According to *Patanjali* [a philosopher who lived over two thousand years ago], *Yoga* is the neutralisation of alternating waves in consciousness. More simply, it is the cessation of all thought and emotion, including the cessation of the *pranic* life force, the senses, mind, ego, and intuitive intelligence which he collectively called *chitta* or mood or feeling.

When the meditator abides in his own Self or soul, he attains oneness with the Spirit: this Oneness of soul-Spirit is *Yoga. Yoga*, as elucidated by the sage *Patanjali,* is the teaching process of union of the individual with the Universal Soul. To facilitate this, Man requires an unruffled mind under all conditions. Yoga is a goal of the awakening man. It must be preceded by a fervent devotion to strive for God or Spirit. It requires extreme dispassion towards the world of senses.

> To the early uninitiated seeker, the Master was asked to describe the steps towards the practice of meditation:
>
> "Yes, M+I+V (Mind-Intellect-Vasanas) must also merge: and that can happen in meditation. To meditate, mind must become quiet. To quieten the mind and make it alert and vigilant, do ***japa,*** prayers, pure living, clean habits, obedience to elders, service to the world etc., etc., Think . . . discuss with your husband in the presence of children".

What is the "Self"?

The Self is the soul or *chit* - the only abiding reality, my perpetual experience that "I am." It is a feeling that "I am" beyond all objects, emotions, or thoughts (OET) and that "I am" not my body, mind or intellect (BMI). Through the body I am the perceiver; through the mind I am the feeler; through the intellect I am the thinker (PFT). The PFT looking at the world of objects, emotions, and thought is a *bhoga* or a mere mortal enjoying the world.

But I also know that "I am" above being the ordinary perceiver, feeler, and thinker (PFT). Turned inwards, I am the *yogi* or spiritual aspirant who is a PFT on the inward path to understanding the self (unenlightened Awareness *chitta)* and the Self or soul (or *chit).*

Where is the Self?

One of my daughters wanted the physical location of the soul or Self:

> and the Master wrote:
>
> "After creating a world of names and forms, the Creator wondered where to hide the Self. A group of angels or *devas* suggested that It be hidden in the bowels of the earth; another group suggested It be retained in the Heavens. These suggestions were unacceptable.
>
> *Brihaspati,* the *guru* of the *devas* suggested the Self be hidden in Man himself, where he would least expect Its existence. The Creator agreed because He knew that Man would identify himself with the insentient Body, the emotions and senses of the Mind, the 'logical' thoughts of the Intellect, and the world-of-objects - the BMI and OET".

Awareness or Self exists in every atom and molecule of the person and in the Universe of Matter. It is found by withdrawing and ascending back towards the divine cave in the brain and spinal cord. This inward spiritual journey is called meditation. Only seekers who have the desire for immortality, abiding happiness, and infinite knowledge embark on this inward journey.

Why desire?

To achieve abiding satisfaction and happiness (my own eternal nature), yoga is the final end to all other extraneous desiring. Unfulfilled desires from previous manifestations are the hallmark of *vasanas. Vasanas* gives a manifestation its *personality.* They are why we are on this earth born again as mortals.

These desires express themselves through the unenlightened *chitta* or mind-intellect-ego complex by involving the body in all actions. The body expresses itself as an individual-specific mood or feeling or *chitta,* through the five senses and the five organs of action. It is the duty or *dharma* of every mortal to fulfil all his desires that caused his present manifestation. This is exhaustion of unfulfilled desires, needs, and wants.

Whenever wants-and-needs were discussed at *satsangs* or meetings with the wise, the Master would bid us good bye with a 'hurry home'.

> "Desires are *vasanas* and they are why you are here in this existence. When the

desires are exhausted and you have achieved what you came for, Hurry Home. . *Hari Aum*!"

The closest translation to the salutation *Hari Aum* is 'May the Lord be with you'. It is a greeting used at the beginning and end of a meeting. The Master used it to tell seekers to stop their constant indiscriminate desiring and 'Hurry Home to the Self'.

For a long time I was unclear about desires. Are desires to be fulfilled? How does one exhaust desires? Once exhausted, how does one continue living without an aim to achieve?

Swamiji encouraged each one of us to achieve the desires and aspirations we came with in this incarnation. Our *vasanas* or desires dictate our rebirth in the home and environment we have chosen. It is in these ideal circumstances that these desires will have fulfilment in the four aims of life.

Once these have been exhausted, man must return to his own inner roots to connect with his very source. Man is the only animal who can enter the altar of his divine cave of the brain and spinal cord through meditation.

Where is Self achieved?

Man is endowed with mind *(manas),* intellect *(buddhi)* and ego *(ahamkara),* collectively known as awareness or *chitta.* This is the source of all performing, feeling, and thinking (PFT). It manifests in our silence and also in our agitated beingness, as moods.

As the wheel of life turns, *chitta* as feelings and moods experiences the five miseries of ignorance *(avidya),* selfishness *(asmita),* attachment *(raga),* aversion *(dvesha),* and love of life *(abhinivesha*).

These leave the *chitta* in five states of "beingness": dull *(mudha),* wavering *(kshipta),* partially stable *(vikshipta)*, single-pointed *(ekaagra)* and controlled *(nirudha).*

Unenlightened *chitta* or feelings and moods, is like a fire that remains fuelled by desires *(vasanas).* In its pure state, *chitta* becomes the source of enlightenment.

The enlightenment of the *chitta* is, therefore, the quest for self-realisation. When this is secured, the full achievement and goal of life gains ultimate value because it defines the reason for living as a mortal.

When and How is Self-Realisation Achieved?

Self-realisation is achieved when one follows the path of *yoga* or union with the ideal goal of life, the Spirit, through the practice of *Yoga Sutras* or Yoga Philosophy.

The *sutras* are instructions to be followed. One needs to study the Scriptures to understand both the definition of God and His address.

> The Master had a simple instruction for practising the *Upanishadic* or philosophical teachings in our daily life. He repeatedly reminded us:
>
> ". . Be silent, alert, and vigilant"

This was his most frequently repeated sentence. The study of the scriptures required a silent and alert mind. Vigilance is necessary to prevent the seeker from falling back to old ways!

Why Yoga and how many types of Yogas are there?

Pain is the only reason why man seeks happiness. Although he is unaware of it at most times, he is actually looking for perfect happiness. In its ultimate form, he is looking for the Bliss of God. Pain, suffering, and other limitations are due to Man's identification with his body and mind. All of these, cause tumultuous agitation and excitation, taking the form of pleasure and pain. We are then rendered almost blind to the existence of our own inherent state of Bliss.

The most sensible way to free the Self is through *yoga,* which removes Man's identification with the body and mind. Until Man understands that he is born of the vibrations of *Aum*, the Invisible Life Force that upholds creation, he cannot enter "into the Kingdom of Heaven". The physical body of flesh is born of flesh; that which is born of Spirit is Spirit. Unless we transcend the flesh, we cannot realise the Spirit and eventually the Universal Spirit.

Swamini Sharadapriyananda and I met again at least twelve years after our previous meeting in the bowels of the thundering Niagara Falls. Seeking to confirm some conclusions made from my readings on 'Creation', I shared with her my vision and how my mind interpreted creation. I dared to ask! I already had a graphic concept which explained it in the following way:

> 'At first there was a void and there was only *Brahman* (God) and He was both, the Pure Witnessing Consciousness "watching" and Perfect Awareness "looking." Together and separated, they are *Aum the Pranava: Sat-Chit-Anand* or Truth-Knowledge-Bliss.
>
> 'Consciousness is *Purusha* and Awareness is the essence of *Prakriti,* the Mother or *Devi,* the *Mahamaya.* The 'first' audible 'Word' is the *'vibrating Aum'* which vibrates at different frequencies supporting matter from the subtlest to the most dense. It is this vibrating 'Word' that supports all of Creation, the Universe. She is in every atom and molecule and fills the void and the Universe?"
>
> "You've got it. Now become One with It," said *Swamini Sharadapriyananda*!

Although religions are many, they are characterised by practices that take the form of dogmas and doctrines. Often, followers of doctrines cannot understand why the in-faith does not give them spiritual satisfaction. They cannot comprehend the true import of these doctrines. They accept the outer meanings of such doctrines which over time, become conventions and rigid practices: this is the origin of sectarianism and religious intolerance.

In response to reports of violence and forced conversions in the news media, the Master commented on doctrines, and religious intolerance:

> "Every being is born in accordance with the Divine Plan of Creation. It is mortals themselves who want this changed. "

Swami Chinmayananda conducted seven-day *yagnas* or discourses three times a month in different cities and towns all over the world for forty-three years of his life. He invited persons of all faiths to hear discourses on the *Geeta* (the revered philosophical text of the Hindus) and *Upanishads* (knowledge portions of the *vedas* dealing with the ultimate Truth). He hoped that each individual attending would be a better person (whatever be their religion) after hearing him.

The deepest truths of all doctrines must be experienced and realised, not just understood by the intellect. The realisations and experiences are drawn from Man's own soul, the Self. At a *satsang*, a seeker asked the Master why there were so many interpretations of the Hindu Scriptures, each contradicting the other.

and the Master said:

> . . . . "To a trained scientist, the term 'boiling point' is a definition of unquestionable authority and experience; to a non-scientist, the term suggests a point in space where water boils spontaneously. . . ". . . . To an ". . To an untrained scientist, the term "boiling point," is a definition of unquestionable authority and experience; to a non-scientist, the term suggests a point in space where water boils spontaneously. .
>
> "Similarly, when untrained people take it upon themselves to comment on the Hindu Scriptures, there is bound to be a distorted opinion of Truth. The tragedy compounds itself further when uninitiated individuals begin to believe these commentaries written in English by non-Indian authors, who label his (Hindu) scriptures as books of undigested 'Truth Declarations', of a "Dead Philosophy'. ."

There are four practical ways to liberate the body-mind-intellect (BMI) from the world of objects, emotions, and thoughts (OET), depending upon the mental and intellectual tendencies *(vasanas)* of the practitioner.

He is the same perceiver-feeler-thinker (PFT) whether he looks outwards at the world of indulgences or inwards seeking the Self. Depending upon his innate tendencies, the seeker chooses a Spiritual Journey most suited to him. His inner call for a Master-teacher will also match his innate needs and wants. He will come across writings and happenings which are responses to his own specific inner calls. There are no accidents in Nature. Everything happens as it should!

The four paths or *yogas* are:

- ***Gyana Yoga*** where through the path of Knowledge, Man attains understanding of the self and objects of the world. In this gradual process of evolution of awareness, Man gradually frees Awareness from an awareness-of-body-mind to self-awareness, an evolutionary necessity. With the help of a *guru,* Man gradually distances himself from the world-of-things and beings to attain ultimate unity with the Thought-of-an-Ideal;

- ***Bhakti Yoga*** emphasises intense devotion to an Ideal which is a spirit of Love. In this way, Man is drawn into the Ideal of eternal Love;
- ***Hatta Yoga*** focuses on improving the body and mind with the goal of eliminating obstacles preventing the "self" from enjoying perfect union with the Ideal.
- ***Karma Yoga*** where there is reciprocity between action and reaction.

There are combinations of these four pure paths, for example:

- ***Raja Yoga or Kriya Yoga*** is a combination of the four paths already discussed above. Seekers of this path observe austerities of *yama* or restraints and *niyama* or adherence to pledges of restraints, study the scriptures, and learn to surrender the self through purificatory actions or *kriya.* This is the path chosen by the author of this text.
- ***Tantra Yoga*** bestows the seeker with *siddhis* or psychic-powers. Only a *tantric-guru* has the knowledge of this path. The *tantric-student* must already be endowed with faith, purity, devotion, dispassion, dedication to a *guru,* humility, courage, truthfulness, cosmic love, non-covetousness, and contentment. Absence of these qualities in the student leads him to the abuse of *Shaktism. Shakti* is the life-force energy in all manifestation.

Tantra Yoga is *Devi* worship of the Holy Spirit. It is an integral part of Hinduism. It [*shaktism*] is one of the most important systems of Eastern thought. *Tantra* is not witchcraft, mysterious formulae, and magic spells. They are scriptural practices based upon fundamental ideas and correct reasons.

In the West, *tantra yoga* is the newest toy used by ignorant seekers who understand it as a path of indulgences.

The Master always reminded us repeatedly that we, the seekers, suffered from *avarana or* intellectual veiling of the Truth. We operated with responses such as, 'I don't know,' or 'I can't understand,' or 'I have no experience' of the Self.

The Master admonished at a *satsang* or meeting with the wise. He was referring to the lack of true understanding that 'I am that divine being':

> "When the *tabla* beats, it beats constantly. . . . .
> *tat-tvam-eva, tvam-eva-tat:* That you are: you alone are That;
> *tat-tvam-eva, tvam-eva-tat:* That you are: you alone are That;
> *tat-tat-tat:* That - That - That;
> *tat-tvam-eva, tvam-eva-tat*: That you are: you alone are That. . . .
> **yet so few hear it. . . . . "**

Raja Yoga *of Patanjali* combines all the four paths or *yogas*. It involves a practical training in meditation as prescribed by sages of all times and climes. By sincerely learning and practising meditation, eventually the *sadhak* or seeker develops and experiences a calm, tranquil, and blissfully happy state of conscious sleep. He becomes free of all thoughts and bodily sensation and is overtaken by self-awareness.

Depending upon the *depth and frequency* of the practice of meditation, man can temporarily forget all thoughts, bodily sensations, and mental disturbances. It is as if he is in deep sleep. This is, however not the first nor is it the final state. In conscious sleep or meditation, we must learn to voluntarily control the senses and the organs of action that are automatically controlled in natural unconscious sleep.

In the early stages of meditative practice, disturbances of internal organs, such as lungs and heart seem beyond our control. The *sadhak* or seeker must gradually be able to shut off all bodily sensations and internal organs at will, as all of these sensations can trigger thoughts. To remain vulnerable to these disturbances is to remain uncontrolled at all times; each effort is a lost opportunity of self-awareness.

Controlling the inner organs and voluntarily controlling the mind-body requires training as devised by *Patanjali,* many thousands of years ago. Herein, the Self can be felt as a separate being from the body: an experience of death without final mortal death. Man's ultimate end is Bliss, felt intensely; its enjoyment is beyond the pleasures felt through the senses and the mind. The more man practices meditation, the more intense is his experience of Bliss and the longer is its duration.

The tranquillity of this supramental state permeates Man's ordinary day-to-day existence; the *sadhak* experiences his own truth and eventually the universal truth in each and every name and form. It is and always was there; he just had to discover it. Selfish interests recede to where they belong, and the *sadhak* discovers pure joy.

The Indian Civilisation and Some Sacred Texts

Before introducing *yoga philosophy and the yoga sutras* to the readers in the next section, it would be prudent to introduce Indian Civilisation and some texts held sacred by the Hindus. Many of these have become subject matters in plays, dance, and ordinary literature, for example the three-day play in New York: '*Mahabharata'!*

The following is being included for those not familiar with the historical and cultural evolution of Spiritual Thought in Indian Civilisation. This book will repeatedly refer to these subjects and the Master's words were thought to be the best means of clarifying such a subject:

and the Master writes:

"Civilisation of a society increases with culture and breaks down as cultural values deteriorate, as we have seen in the fall of Egyptian, Greek and Roman civilisations. *Vyasa* arrested the deterioration in Indian culture by compiling the *Vedas. Buddha* in his time, also revived the philosophy. Many years later the culture of the country had again deteriorated. When a culture deteriorates, there is increased barbarity and immorality, philosophy is misinterpreted and utter disaster follows. *Shankara* appeared at such a stage and brought about a great renaissance in Hinduism.

"Hinduism does not centre around any particular personality. . . In ancient India, men of wisdom spent their days in the lap of Nature's beauty and luxuriance. The valleys and forests of the great Himalayas and sacred *Ganges* were teachers who kindled in their hearts a hunger to know the mysteries of the Power that gives life to the lifeless. The reflections and revelations of these perfect Masters formulated the scriptures that later came to be known as the *Vedas.*

"The *Vedas* or books-of-knowledge are four in number, namely, *Rig, Yajus, Sama* and *Atharvana.* Each *Veda* is divided into three sections and these are called *Mantra, Brahmana and Upanishad* or *Aranyaka.* In the *Mantra* portion we find the ecstatic admiration of Nature's beauty expressed in lyrical poetry by these contemplative seers. The *Brahmana* portion deals with rituals and sacrifices; they are for mental integration and self-purification. The last portion contains the philosophic wisdom known as *Vedanta.*

"Besides the *Vedas* which are *Srutis,* the spiritual literature includes *Smrities, Itihasaa and Puranas* which contain philosophy, ethics, social sciences and laws of society and so on. . .

"The *Vedas* were not written by any one individual - they are inspired declarations of several *rishis* from the height of their intuitive experience. And when they were absorbed in the Transcendental Experience they had gone beyond the realm of 'I' and 'Mine'. This explains why they never appended their names to the holy texts."

The texts enumerated by Swami Chinmayananda here under, will be repeatedly referred to in this book. They need to be introduced to any uninitiated reader. Once more, the subject is best introduced to the readers through the Master's own writings:

and the Master writes:

"Upanishads are texts of philosophical principles discussing man, world and God. *Geeta* is a handbook of instructions as to how human being can come to live the subtle philosophical principles of *Vedanta* in actual work-a-day world.

"Srimad Bhagavad Geeta, the Divine Song of the Lord, occurs . . . in the *Mahabharata,* and comprises of eighteen chapters. This great handbook of practical living marked a positive revolution in Hinduism and inaugurated a Hindu renaissance for ages that followed the *Puranic* era.

"In The Song of the Lord *(Geeta),* the Poet-Seer *Vyasa*, has brought the *Vedic* truths from the sequestered Himalayan caves, into the active fields of political life and into the confusing tensions of an imminent war.

"Religion is philosophy in action. From time-to-time an ancient philosophy needs intelligent reinterpretation in the context of new times and men of wisdom, prophets and seers, guiding the common man on how to apply effectively, the ancient laws in his present life.

"*Upanishad* is a word indicating a literature that is studied by sitting or *shad,* near or *upa* a teacher, in a spirit of receptive meekness and surrender or *ni.* The contents of the scriptural textbooks are all over the world, always the same. They teach us that there is a changeless Reality behind the ever-changing phenomenal world of perceptions, feelings and understanding.

"The word *Yoga* comes from the word *yuj* - to join. Any conscious attempt on the part of the individual to lift his present available personality and attune to the higher, perfect ideal, is *Yoga,* and the science of *yoga* is called *Yoga Shastra.*

"The theme of philosophy and *Yoga* cannot be attractive to the ordinary men of the world because it is so scientific and it deals with imperceptible ideologies. But religion tries to serve all and the anxiety of all the prophets is to serve every one in all generations. "

Yoga Philosophy

Yoga Philosophy uses powerful psychological suggestion, free of superstition, to release mankind from his anxieties. It discerns things as they appear from things as they really are.

The *Yoga Sutras* written by Patanjali over 3000 years ago, consist of 196 sentences divided into 4 books, carrying a universal message, transcending both time and cultures. Their content is profound and enduring because it is humanistic.

Yoga Philosophy insists there is something ultimate and irreducible about the species, Man, and his intrinsic value.

'All *yoga* practised even today is based on the *Yoga Sutras.* These are a collection of aphorisms offered more than 2000 years ago by the Indian sage Patanjali. The *Sutras* were and still are the earliest and most profound study of the human psyche. In them, Patanjali describes the enigma of human existence. He shows how we can transform ourselves through the practice of *yoga.* He shows how one gains mastery over mind and emotions and overcomes obstacles to spiritual evolution. To attain *kaivalya* or liberation, one needs to free oneself from the bondage of desires and actions. '

from 'Light on the Yoga Sutras' by B. K. S. Iyengar

Patanjali's Yoga Sutras are considered the most authoritative texts of *Yoga* Philosophy. *Patanjali's Yoga*, often described as *Raja Yoga,* is based on *kriyas* or practices, which are gradually introduced and must be followed: it utilises all the four prescribed *Yogas* described previously.

The process of *Yoga* training consists of:

1. Moral or ethical training;
2. Physical training; and
3. Spiritual training.

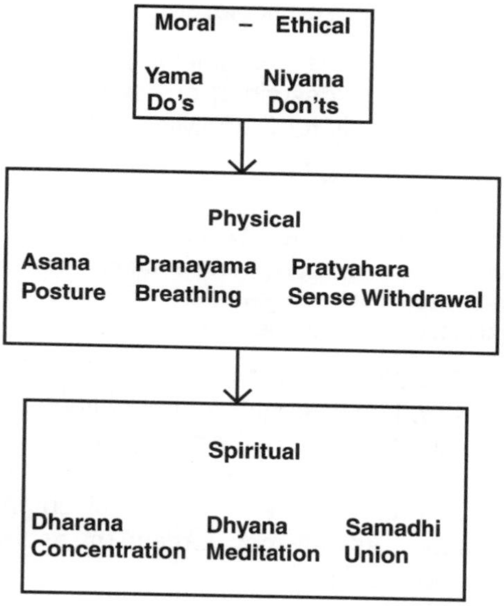

Figure 5. Patanjali's Yoga Sutras describe Eight Steps of Raja Yoga

Within these types of training, there are eight steps leading to spiritual growth. The meditator cannot hope to attain a higher stage without successfully completing the previous step. The last stage of training, composed of concentration, and meditation, takes the meditator to superconsciousness or *samadhi,* which is even beyond the causal state of being.

Eight Steps:

- The first two steps are for Moral or *yama* and Ethical Preparation or *niyama*; through them, one becomes morally fit to receive the instructions (through *Karma, Bhakti,* and *Gyana).*
- The next three steps are for control of body posture or *asana*, breathing or *pranayama*, and sense control or *pratyahara (Hatta Yoga*). Practitioners are taught that the Individualized Cosmic Energy lies in the base of the spine, in a latent state, and must be lifted.
- The last three steps presuppose that there is now control of the body. The mind is committed to controlling his attention and erasing all past memories or *dharana*. It is straight-thinking or *dhyana* and the seeker is desirous of

a Collective Good in *samadhi.* These steps are now the practitioner's chief preoccupation.

Raja Yoga is the most difficult but also the most direct path for reintegrating the pseudo-self or ego, as the ultimate reality. This is done by eliminating all irrelevant distractions. It is not an easy task and, unless there is total devotion to the steps to be followed, it cannot be achieved.

The Path through Spirituality is not simple to describe. The Goal is that of the Infinite which cannot be described or defined in words. Masters can only <u>indicate</u> That which is beyond Body-Mind-Intellect and yet permeates all of it.

> and the Master wrote:
>
> ". . Infinity is not a thing to be defined by finite words. Words can express at best a fraction of what we experience. How can such frail words express the Infinite? The Path of the seeker must be cleared by the seeker himself. When bogged down by the Intellect, nobody can help him. . . "

Psychic evolution takes place as a result of this effort. It involves desiring to become better. There are, however, natural frustrations on the path. Slipping back to the old ways is certainly one of them. Inability to practice the exercises despite a desire to do so, is another stumbling block. For those on the path who gain satisfaction may be troubled by desires for quick emancipation. These are often a seeker's frustrations. Anxiety may pervade the aspirant. These were my own stumbling blocks and still are.

But the self-ego is extremely aware of the body's weaknesses and how they cause 'self' miseries. The wise seeker toils truthfully and makes his gains over a long period of time. There is a gradual progression whereby the body and Self or soul, align their purpose. The pseudo-soul or ego continues to suffer until it finds freedom. The involvement of the pseudo-soul with the world of objects and desires is deep and complex. It has no power of its own to gain insight into this unhappy entanglement with the miseries of the world.

The soul is dependant upon the *chitta* or mind-intelligence-ego for the effort required to free the mind of senses from the pseudo-soul. But the *chitta* is matter *(Prakriti)*, and it has only two agendas:

- To eradicate itself; and
- To rid the soul of all desires, which is in fact the all-consuming desire of the aspirant.

To free the soul from all association with the body, the *chitta* must seek surrender to its own 'consciousness', that is, self-awareness must cease:

- The *chitta* or mind-intellect-ego must become latent for the soul to regain its isolation.
- Once it regains freedom from disturbing associations with body, mind and

desires, It or the enlightened soul becomes "Consciousness" instead of "Conscious of"!

The Achieving Man

Life today has become so complex that one becomes a pawn in the power plays underlying human relationships. To regain self-esteem and self-protection from the world, we often don the mantle of personality-traits.

It is both interesting and intriguing that James Redfield of the best-seller *The Celestine Prophesy* simplified humanity into four personality traits. These traits, he says, are often directed at controlling persons and things by:

- intimidation; or
- aggressive interrogation; or
- assuming an aloof stance to ward off the aggressor; or
- becoming the poor-me to get out of controlling situations.

According to Redfield, complex individuals may adopt two or more of these traits. Children reared amongst such adults and employees of such employers become victims of their behaviour. None of the players in these relationships even understand what they are doing to each other.

According to Indian thought, all power-plays are covert attempts to steal power and energy from each other, and, to energise themselves at the cost of others. The true source of power and energy (Aum, Hum, Amen, Amin or in Christian terms, the Holy Spirit) is not available to the modern extrovert man of science and technology who is unaware of the existence of such a subtle energy.

It is interesting that I have come to this conclusion. Entering the medical field was a dream to serve humanity. The reality of life and supporting a family tainted this idealism. Ego demanded that I remain abreast of all happenings in this field of science.

Over time, much of what I had read and concluded became redundant. The treatments had their own limitations. I soon realised that most times diseases take their origin from indulgences and neglect of the body. Temporary problems become permanent disabilities and man becomes a victim of his own creation.

How does he reverse this process? Meditation has the ability to transform every cell in the body. The neurone or brain cell is the most evolved cell in the body. Intense meditation has the ability to self-heal. The seeker must be able to enter the altar of God in the divine cave of the brain and spinal cord. The seeker requires a Master to show him the way. The gains are subtle and very personal. There are no tangible signs to show off these gains.

In the materialistic world touted by the Western Civilisation where success is gauged by position and possessions, life situations offer no lasting assistance to Man. The logic of the intellect alone cannot fathom this. The intellect or *buddhi* needs to be subjected to introspection, and the power of insight. Divine intelligence is sure to lead the intellect's knowledge or *gyana* to the threshold of wisdom or *vigyana,* to understand the Energy behind all actions and thought.

> and the Master wrote:
>
> ". . The secret of success behind all men of achievements lies in the faculty of applying their intellect (*buddhi to gyana)* in all their activities without being misled by any surging emotions or feelings (personal). The secret of success in life lies in keeping the head above the storms of the heart. . "

The deluded being:

- obtains power by manipulating science to create order in his own confused life; and
- obtains energy by aggression, intimidation, and interrogation.

The physical Universe itself is pure vibrating Energy (Aum) which creates both forms and substances, which we call multiplicity. To become aware-of and to know-how-to tap this force of Universal Cosmic Energy is the foundation for integrating Man's soul with Spirit, through the Yoga of Meditation. It also is the way to return to our inner core of "beingness".

Prana or Cosmic Life Force or Energy

The vibrating creative Light-Energy is the Unmanifest *Shakta-Shakti* (unmanifest and manifest Light-Energy or *Purusha-Prakriti*) or *Aum* or God. It is *Purusha* manifesting as the unmanifest witnessing Light of Consciousness. It is also *Prakriti* manifesting as unmanifest Energy or *Prana* who lovingly watches over the Universe as Mother Nature. She who is *Aum* the Holy Spirit, supports birth, sustenance, and the dissolution of creation, both in the microcosm and the macrocosm.

It is as difficult to explain *prana* or life-force, as it is to explain God! *Prana* is the principle of life and awareness. It is equated with the real Self or *atma.* It is the energy permeating the universe at all levels. It is physical, mental, sexual, spiritual and cosmic energy. All vibrating energies are *prana.* It is *Aum.* It is the breath of life of all beings in the universe.

Aum or Amen or Amin or Hum is the inherent power and energy in each of us. It silently enlivens every atom and molecule in the universe. To gain control of this energy source, one needs a teacher to show the what and how of tapping this mysterious *Aum.*

Once Man is made aware of the existence of the life-force, this wealth allows him to turn into a new "beingness", in search of the *Shakti* or Energy who is empowered by the *Shakta* or Light.

Countless universes are but the dust of Her feet, of this Cosmic Creative

Energy. She, the *Shakti,* leads Man's soul from plane to plane and unifies man, who is *Aum,* with *Sada-Shiva* or Consciousness in the *Sahasrahara.*

Man's physical body is a microcosmic manifestation of the macrocosmic *Shakti* or Energy. One needs the mortal body to reach the pseudo-soul or ego or individualised "beingness".

The seventh *sahasrahara chakra* is the final destination of Man's "beingness"; here, man sheds his physical beingness [atomic senses and organs of action], his astral beingness [life-force in mind and intellect or 'lifetrons'], and his causal beingness [*vasanic* 'thoughtrons' or desire ideations].

Here in the causal state, the practitioner intuitively understands the unenlightened *chitta* (mind-intellect-ego complex). He enters the sixth sheath or *chittamaya kosha.* Here he experiences Awareness of Matter *(prakriti).* His next step is to enter the seventh sheath or *chitmaya kosha* of Consciousness of Spirit *(purusha).* There now has to be the merging of the two!

Man's efforts at meditation end in progressive *samadhi* or Oneness of the Soul and Spirit. The realisation is that the Self is the Self in All and All is the Self - a personal knowing of the Universal Consciousness.

The manifested Universe has been likened to the Cosmic Mother and has been adored for thousands of years. Poetry and lyrics describe Her or *Prakriti* in all Her qualities of delusion *(maya)*, power *(shakti),* functions, beauty, and splendour. These traditions have become so ingrained in the psyche of Hindu thought over the thousands of years, that everyone accepts each and everyone's concept of the Cosmic Mother.

Seasonal adoration (*navratri and dushera* are ten-day celebrations during the Fall months of every year) to give thanks to Her abundance. The celebrations permeate every Province and society in India. Each home adores a particular form (traditionally nine of them) of the Cosmic Mother as *Durga* or Queen of the Universe.

> Hindus are accused of having 'thousands of gods' and a Wise-one wrote:
>
> "*Yoginidra or Maya* (yogic sleep) is that *shakti* or energy that it can even delude *Vishnu,* the Sustainer of the Trinity. With Her Will She thrusts each one of us into Her Great Plan for the Universe. By 'encouraging' the trait of egoistic attachments, She moves Her Universe through evolution in time and space, even if it is through the Power of Delusion or *maya.* When satisfied with Man's service, She bestows upon Man the Ultimate Knowledge for Liberation.
>
> "As *Kali* She is the Eternal Physical Universe. Because **phenomena** are Her 'visible' form, She manifests in many ways even though She is Unborn and Eternal. Some of Her recognisable manifestations include:
>
> - Cause of all actions;
> - Dissolver of all Manifestations only to rest in Consciousness;

- Perceiver of Thoughts and Repository of all Desires;
- The Creative Capacity and Mother of Dissolution;
- Perceiving Capacity and Queen of Cause, Sustenance, and Sleep;
- Mother of all beings and also the cause of Dissolution of worlds;
- Energy in all Sacrifices, Aum in all Uttering, and Hymn in all prayers and Rituals, and Time for all prayers;
- Both Pleasing and Terrible; and
- Serene Benefactress.

Many experience the Cosmic Creative Energy as the Divine Mother who reveals Herself in all Her splendour. One is left awed, and humbled. There are no words to express Her, but one tries to describe the indescribable!

The ultimate qualities of *Prakriti* or Energy or the Holy Spirit are: Divine Will, Wisdom, Universal Intelligence, Pure Love, and Life-in-Service. Each seeker must become acquainted with Her and embrace Her within himself, through self-effort or *sadhana.*

Sadhana or Spiritual Effort - The first step to self-mastery:

The first step to self-mastery is character building:

- The groundwork involves self-improvement or character-building so that one can be prepared for the Creative Energy when it stirs within.
- The first stage of evolution is to become aware that we have complicated and deep-seated beliefs, born of delusion or *maya*, and habits accumulated from many births originating from our causal or *karanic* beingness (*vasanas* in the BMI chart).
- This awareness exposes Man to the vast potential of released energy, power, increased perception, and awareness. There is a psychic feeling (mind and emotions) of release from one's own physical encumbrance, of carrying these beliefs.
- Release is a manifestation that happens when one becomes adept at dealing with the reflexive, or automatic responses to daily life.
- Once Energy is roused, it becomes a powerful tool for improving life's natural gifts for evolution and self-mastery.

There are many issues raised by seekers at our Study Groups. Some feel lost that their progress is too slow. Others experience bewilderment and a sense of loneliness during *sadhana.* Others are troubled by the experiences of phenomenon during deep meditation. Some feel they have slipped backwards.

Experience has always led me to conclude that I have not abided by the *yama* and *niyamas* or the do's and don'ts of personal conduct. At other times, surges of inner awakening with hitherto unknown energy are signs of personal progress. Fears of falling in voids are combated by regulated slow breathing.

There is so much written about the logic and necessity of Spirituality and yet so few hear the call. This enigma was posed to the Master, who wrote:

> "The necessity for religion, the urge for spiritual freedom, the call from the depths within ourselves is experienced only by Man and even then it is not felt by all men.
>
> "Why a glorious minority alone comes to feel the urge to face the vital problem has been exhaustively dealt with in our old texts and has been vaguely hinted at by Darwin in his theory of evolution.
>
> "If this biologist prophet be true in his conclusions, we have to accept that the ape-man lost his tail and started shaving daily to become the man of today.
>
> "But here again there has obviously been a period of transition wherein we find beings of animalistic instinct in the form of men behaving and acting as though they were no better than mere animals. . . To them, religion cannot have direct or immediate appeal at all.
>
> "But to those who have long since passed this stage and have grown through the turmoil of life into beings better developed mentally and intellectually, challenging questions begin to pose themselves: "From where did all these things come? Where do they go and why? Is there a mission and purpose in life or is life a mere accident?".
>
> "To these developed beings, religion has a meaning and a purpose and shows the path and the goal. No religion is possible without a philosophy. . . . And here indeed is the fundamental difference between the concepts of philosophy entertained by the East and in the West.
>
> "Extrovert by nature, philosophy to the Westerner is to a great extent an objectified science. . It points a view of life. The ideal may and does often change with the result that we have a new ideal in the West almost every decade.
>
> "In the East, philosophy means something more than a 'view of life'. . They (the seers) are practical men and they demanded that the ideas and ideals preached by the philosopher should be capable of being practised. . . it is a 'view of life' but also a 'way of life'."

Understanding Will - The second step to self-mastery

The second step to self-mastery is to understand "Will," "self-will", and "divine will":

- Will is the power behind all action. It must be distinguished from a wish (thought-desire in the mind), desire (mind-wish to possess), intention (intellectual-desire to possess by action), and volition (willed-act to possess).
- Self-will is the desire for result in accordance with one's own wishes.
- Divine will is action for the sake of a collective or higher benefit for the society at large. Some do it for the Cosmic Mother.

Will must be divided further into blind will (will governed by sense gratification and emotions) and thinking will (will governed by intellectual discrimination and laws of living). In most cases, our actions are dictated by my will or self-will.

Unless Self-Will is aligned with Her Will that is heard in the Silence of Meditation, one remains outside the domain of the Total Will of Creation - the *Hiranyagarbhaya.* To bring this willed action into fruition then becomes our *dharma* or duty.

Once this desire to know "Who am I" is acted upon, we must call upon our eternal saviour, - our own will, to perform the necessary actions. The seeker requires single-pointed perseverance to obtain such answers.

As the Master wrote

> "Fanatic consistency in doing anything has in it the assurance of success. This in a noble cause is perseverance. . . positive and creative. "
>
> Yet he recognised that when directed towards a bad cause, such perseverance ". . becomes obstinacy. . negative and destructive!"
>
> It is then, critical to. .
>
> ". . Choose intelligently. . . "

Love and Wisdom - The third step to self-mastery:

Detached from all will, in very deep meditation, the *sadhak* (seeker) undergoes subtle evolution: for it is Her/His *(Shakta-Shakti)* Eternal promise to return us into the embrace of their Perfect Love! This is a realisation reached through intuitive wisdom. This takes the seeker to the third step to self-mastery.

For the emotionally charged seeker who is able to spend his or her emotional energy in the embrace of this bliss, there is a change in the quality of his thoughts. The thought-flow is of a single direction. The seeker realises that wisdom is synonymous with loving the Self!

Intellect, Intelligence, and Persistence - the fourth step:

Most seekers confuse intellect with intelligence. Through intuitive understanding, the seeker is taken to the fourth step in self-mastery. He makes certain conclusions and they lead him to himself.

He understands that the Intellect is logical thought based upon known facts, past habits and opinions, and *raaga-dvesha* or likes-and-dislikes. The intellect functions in the domain of ego by motivating thoughts for "Me".

Intelligence is pure balanced knowing without the encumbrances of the present, past, or future. Intelligence is of form, unadulterated "I".

To assure this kind of controlled thought, clarifications must be made in one's mind. This is mandatory. Only by following prescribed exercises and acquiring skills, can intellectual awareness be purified and gradually elevated. This requires persistence.

Through persistence, the gains made through *sadhana* or self-effort, will assist the seeker in handling any experiences and changes without undue anxiety. One needs to control the senses, emotions, and even the intellect. There is emphasis on refining all the five senses, but especially the mind, which operates and controls all the sense perceptions.

Shakti or Prakriti's psychic energy (of the Holy Spirit) can only function in the realm of self-development as a Creative Energy. Experiencing lights or any other phenomenon are not the goals of meditation; they are merely an encouraging sign that one is on the right track. The seeker must press on. However, if they do occur, just observe them without involvement.

Exercises are prescribed to control desires and sense indulgences. Until there is a feeling of inner security that an awakening is taking place, the seeker suffers anxieties of impending "long journeys." The seeker is warned to remain vigilant. The Law of Karma or Cause and Effect is about past habits acquired through thousands of previous births or incarnations which have a habit of dragging the seeker to where he started, if not worse.

Man has no way to study the Creative Cosmic Energy of *Prakriti;* he can only study its manifestations. Whatever this Energy is, It [She or *Prakriti*] can and will reveal Itself when She merges in the embrace of the Light of Consciousness, the *Purusha.*

> As the *Chhandi* [an ancient text written over 2000 years ago, whose author is unknown] explains:
>
> "Mother Nature uses Her Divine Energy to work Her Plan of Creation. It is a struggle for the emergence of the Mind and Intellect residing in Man. His sense of Individuality (I, Me and Mine) is a devolutionary process. When Collective Will and Devotion works for the Universe, Her 'physical manifestation', individual likes-and-dislikes are put aside for a collective benefit and the evolution of man."

Three Bodies and Five Sheaths - Revisited

The human being is composed of three bodies: the body, mind, and intellect (BMI) or *Prakriti,* which function as vehicles for the inner Self or *Purusha.* Because all three are 'matter', they are called bodies, some grosser and some subtler.

The grossest body or *sthula sharira* has *sixteen* components: five senses, five organs of action, five subtle elements, and the mind. All are made up of the five gross elements derived from food. Within the *sthula sharira,* biological forces or main energetic forces, operate as the three humours: water or *kapha;* fire or *pitta;* and air or *vata.*

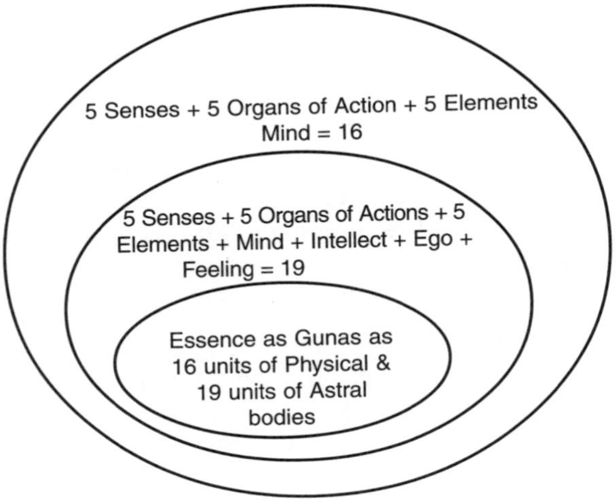

Figure 6. Building-blocks of Three Bodies *(shariras)* and Five Sheaths *(koshas)*

Within the gross body is the subtle or astral body or *sukshma sharira*. This is a pure form of energy composed again of the five senses, five organs of action, five subtle elements or *pranas [pranaya, apanaya, vyanaya, samanaya, udanaya]*, and the mind, intellect, ego, and feeling or *chitta.* It is made up of *nineteen* components of sensory impressions of the *tanmatras* or subtle elements.

Within this subtle body lie the seven *chakras* or astral energy centres that can be activated through meditation. The subtle body in the divine cave [the brain and spinal cord] has the whole astral universe represented in it. It is available for experience in meditation as pure energy. In this experience the seeker is freed from the inert inertia of his physical structure. He experiences himself without the *sthula sharira* or gross body . Its characteristic in meditation is that of luminosity with or without images, experienced in a dream.

Within the astral body is the subtlest or causal body, or *karana sharira*, characterised by the qualities of the three *gunas* of *Prakriti*. It is composed of *thirty-five* essences: nineteen units of the astral and sixteen units of the physical bodies. The *karana sharira* is the "source" of the other two bodies.

It stores within it impressions of all previous actions in millions of previous reincarnations. It is located in the centre of awareness located in the divine cave behind the spiritual eye of the brain. This is where the essence of food as *ojas*, the essence of life-force energy or *prana,* and the essence of the intellect or *tejas* concentrate to nourish the body-mind-intellect complex. Their powers are enhanced through meditation.

The *Purusha* or inner Self or pure Spirit, is encased in five sheaths: the food sheath *(annamaya kosha)*, breath sheath *(pranamaya kosha)*, emotional sheath *(manomaya kosha)*, intellectual sheath *(gyanamaya kosha)*, and the bliss sheath *(anandamaya kosha)*. The food sheath makes up the physical body; the breath, emotional and intellectual sheaths comprise the astral body; the bliss sheath is the causal body.

The breath sheath connects the physical to the astral body, and the intellectual sheath connects the astral to the causal body. The practice of meditation teaches one how to control breath and become breathless. The study of the Scriptures links a mortal to immortality.

Many seekers at Study Groups have asked questions such as: How does one live without breath? Why does the breathing become imperceptible or even stop? How can man live without oxygen? It is true that man must live by breath while functioning at a physical level. The more the meditator withdraws from his physical encumbrances, the more he withdraws from his automated respiration. Respiration is a response to physical activity. If the respiratory rate matches the physical needs of a body, then hibernating within the astral or the causal body, negates the physical factor. In this basal state, the mortal switches his mains to *prana* or life-force energy or the Holy Spirit or *AUM*. This is linking man's mortality to his own immortality.

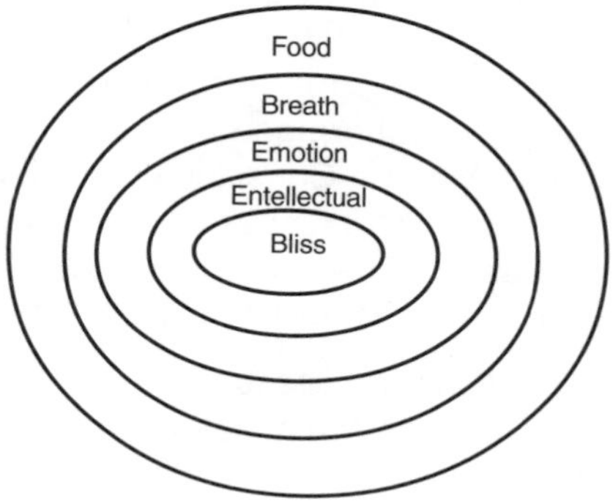

Linking the Three Bodies or *sharira*

Each of the five sheaths has its own density as matter or frequency of energy (Aum) vibration. Each sheath has its own specific processes of activity.

- The food sheath eats, digests, and excretes food that is composed of the five gross elements (earth, water, fire, air and ether).
- The breath sheath inhales and exhales breath and empowers physiological functions of the body through the five *pranas (prana, apana, samana, udana and vyana* - will be explained later*)*.
- The emotional sheath attracts and repels emotions by metabolising

impressions *(tanmatras)* to create sensory neuro-potentials of sight, smell, taste, sound, touch and ideation.

- The intellectual sheath attends to incoming and outgoing knowledge and processes this into thought, beliefs, opinions, and judgements of likes-dislikes.
- The bliss sheath processes incoming and outgoing bliss experiences and metabolises it to will, wisdom, intelligence, love, and joy of life-in-service, based upon the deepest experiences felt at this level.

Body's Supply of Energy

The body's battery and its energy supply reside in the medulla oblongata at the base of the physical brain. This battery requires constant recharging from a Cosmic Source of Life-Force Energy as the Holy Spirit *(Aum)* by the uncontrollable will-to-live.

The Source of Life Force is the Cosmic Intelligence of *Purusha* and the Cosmic Energy of *Prakriti - Aum* (both in fact are One). The body does not just live by food, oxygen, or the heat of the sun.

- Through the medulla, Cosmic Light-Energy breathes Life-Force up the brain and down the spinal cord within the divine cave. From here, the body is nourished by *pranic* energy: at first concentrated in the nerve plexuses, and then distributed to the body along nerve tracts and through neurotransmitters and neurohormones.
- In the waking state as Awaring-Conscious Mind, the physical body-mind-intellect (BMI) uses this Energy for its daily transactions. The transactions are processed at three levels: as an uninvolved *experiencer* or *rishi*, who silently watches every *experience* being processed.

  The incoming information is processed and recorded as an *experience,* in the brain by the *devata* [astral thalamus] who merely looks and makes the necessary changes of all actions as new and altered perceptions. The *experiencing* of the world of objects-emotions-thoughts (OET) depends upon the changes recorded in the *perceiver-feeler-thinker* (PFT) causal template, who is the pseudo-soul making contact with the world in the waking state. (Please refer to the BMI chart).
- In the dream state as Subconscious Mind, the life-force in the astral or psychological-physiological body of the brain and spinal cord becomes the perceiver-feeler-thinker (PFT). Here, the senses are withdrawn into the astral mind which is free to dream the astral dream of sensory-emotional-intellectual thoughts and experiences. Here also, the texture of the dreams depend upon the basic structure of the mind substance.
- In the deep sleep state as Unconscious Mind, the life-force rests in the causal state of beingness: it dwells in the *karanic* or causal brain as

memories of past experiences and impressions. It is experienced as a veil of darkness in the blissful deep sleep.

The discussion above allows the seeker to trace the life-force residing within the divine-cave of the brain and spinal cord or within the central nervous system: it is there *in all states of beingness.*

The Life-Force or *Prakriti* and the Light-of-Consciousness or *Purusha* is experienced in meditation within the centres of superconsciousness which is the substratum of all other levels of 'beingness'. While awake in meditation, it is the witness that *watches* all transformations. As awareness in meditation it *looks* and records all inputs of changes made in this meditative waking state; it looks at thoughts of the subconscious state as in dreams.

When all thoughts and images of past lives have been exhausted, awareness in meditation enjoys and *feels* the bliss. This was previously experienced as unconsciousness of the deep sleep state. Eventually, the Universal Energy of *Prakriti* or *Shakti,* which supports the physical, astral, and causal beings of the mortal, is experienced in meditation as a singular eternal vibrating *Aum.*

The **centres of superconsciousness** reside in the brain:

- *Kutastha Chaitanya* or Christ-Krishna Centre of Universal Intelligence or Universal Consciousness which is the repository of wisdom, intelligence, love and will of the enlightened *chitta.* This is located in the *ajnaa chakra* but reflects at the *bhrumadhya* between the eyebrows;
- *Ajnaa* in the medulla where Life-Force exists as awareness or *Aum* as it vitalises and awares or looks at all levels of beingness [physical, astral, and causal];
- *Sahasrahara* where Cosmic Consciousness is experienced as *sat-chit-anand* or Truth-Knowledge-Bliss in the crown of the divine cave and within the spiritual heart centre.

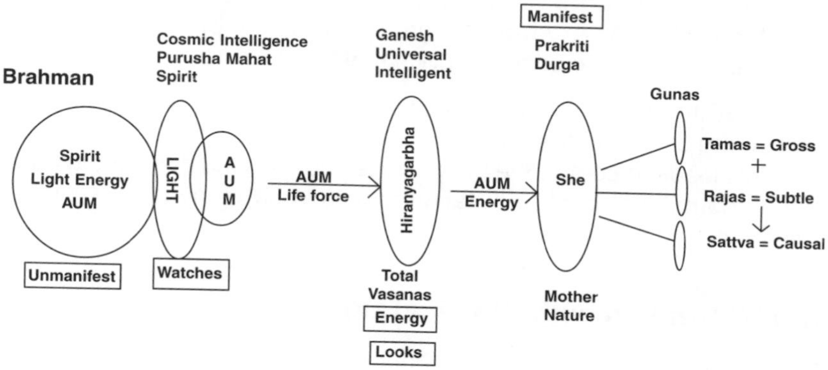

Figure 8. Unmanifest becomes Manifest on a Substratum of Aum

Brahman or God as pure Spirit works through *Purusha or Mahat* (Cosmic Intelligence - *Ganesh)*, acting on *Prakriti* (Nature or matter - *Durga)*, creating, beautifying and multiplying. Once we gain the knowledge of the Self or Spirit, we are able to transcend not only Nature (awareness), but also *Purusha* (Universal Consciousness or Intelligence) and merge with *Brahman* as pure Cosmic Consciousness.

Aum or the Cosmic Energy can be "willed" to energise all actions, whether motor, mental or intellectual, by directing the Life Force to where it is required. This is only possible through deeper and deeper meditation. Then, the intuitive knowing that "I and my Lord are One" can be held in the Infinite Cup of Consciousness in Meditation!

"Mind" as an Organ of the Body

Mind is *antakarana* or the inner organ, which as *chitta* is capable of three levels of function; from it, both motor and sensory organs eventually evolve:

- logic and reasoning as *buddhi* or intellect;
- emotion or sensory mind or *manas*; and
- ego or pseudo-soul or *ahankara.*

Mind or *manas* is atomic "matter" by nature, and therefore the atomic structure of creation. All of creation manifests through the mind. Because mind is matter, it can focus on only one thought at a time. This allows us to direct thought in a specific narrow direction at any given moment and can lead to attachments to points-of-view. Despite its atomic nature, mind can pervade, like an aura, the entire field of perception.

The mind is unstable, constantly changing in space as well as in time. It is really only a series of thoughts, which shift continually, both in the point of focus as well as in ideas. Because the mind is subtle, the seeker must devote intense attention to observe its movements, which both cause internal thoughts and express themselves as external thought stimuli. In the process, the mind can become caught up in and become a victim of thoughts.

This volatility makes the mind difficult to control; nonetheless, in yoga of meditation the control of the mind is of paramount importance. The inability to achieve this leads to control the mind causes sorrow and disease; in contrast. control of the mind through meditation results in harmony between the body and life-force.

"Mind" Connects with Physical Body

At the end of the first trimester of pregnancy, at week twelve, the 'mind' as *chitta* (mind-intellect-ego) or a seed of the causal body as soul enters the foetus in the womb; the foetus has already been energised by life-force *Aum,* through the fontanels of the skull and is alive. Prior to this time, the individual soul hovers around conceptions of the world, looking for a proper environment so its past *karmas* can be worked out in the coming life.

Pumsavana (or womb consecration of conception, or baby-showers, or *seemantam,* or *khoro-bharvun*) are ancient traditions dating from the pre-vedic period of *Prajapati* (ruler of all tribes) and the Laws of *Manu* (first laws of ethics ever written). The ceremony, called *Prajapatya,* was a celebration made with prayers for a healthy and wise child with excellent *samskaras* or prenatal tendencies carried forward from his previous existence.

During our lifetime, starting in the womb, the mind connects the body through the senses with the outer world. Our preoccupation with desires of the mind and pleasures of our indulgences makes us victims of all the changes in Nature. The external energy coming through the senses keeps the volatile mind constantly disturbed. At death, the astral-causal soul, along with the essence of impressions gathered in the present lifetime, leave the body.

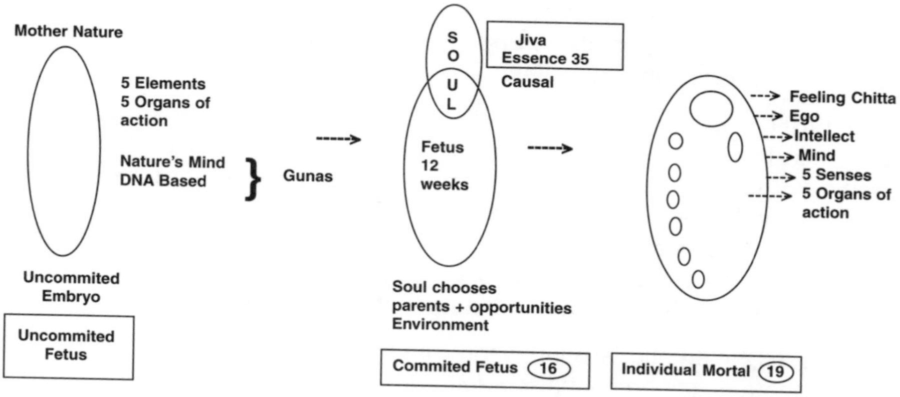

Figure 9. Mind as Chitta connects with Physical Fetus

Mind Functions at Four Levels

Patanjali recognises Mind's four levels of function:

- As the unconscious *chitta* or feeling of blind awareness of the mental field;
- As *manas* or the sensory and emotional mind;
- As *ahamkara* or self-conscious intellectual thought or "I am Me"; and
  As *buddhi* or intelligence or "I am I"

The **mental field** of the unenlightened *chitta* serves as a general backdrop of awareness, including within it the unconscious mind of the causal state with all its past memories and tendencies. *Chitta* exists in all of Nature, both animate and inanimate. It is responsible for the autonomic functions of the body as well as the organic structure of the functioning of the entire cosmos. In scientific terms, it is responsible for the physiological and psychological functions of the Total Mind, of which we are unaware.

Chitta functions as Collective-Unconsciousness, subtly imprinted by all the experiences in our body and in Nature. It functions even when we and Nature sleep. It acts as an organic memory recording the whole body of awareness in a latent seed state. In hypnosis, the mind is brought to the level of the *chitta* where we can recall everything that has happened to us. *Chitta* contains within it our deep-seated emotions, impressions, attachments, and habits. It is our own individual part of Nature or *Prakriti,* characterised by Her three *gunas* or physical qualities, functioning through the *tattvas* or element principle.

The **sensory and emotional mind** of our Personal-Subconscious-Awareness is called *manas* or mind. It is composed of two parts: the senses and the organs of action. The sensory mind is capable only of thoughts of desires, likes-and-dislikes, love-and-hate, emotions and imagination. It does not have any ability to stabilise, observe, and assimilate.

Mind is the efferent limb of the primitive animal reflex arc. It allows the outgoing mind to take into account the incoming information (afferent arc) and co-ordinating it with past habits and instincts [from past births]. Mind is not connected to awareness and thus is inarticulate. *Manas* has no principles or value systems. Through it, we become enmeshed in our emotions, victims of our outgoing senses which present as pleasures and aversions. This outgoing energy creates an inner darkness or *avidya* in our inner nature of awareness.

Manas, as the emotional mind, cannot be transcended except by stilling and silencing thought and emotions. In *sadhana,* a still and silent mind is an inward movement of divine energy, moving towards the altar in the Divine Cave. The extrovert mind uses the same energy to justify the existence of his ego as the "I am Me. "

The **self-conscious mind** or ego or *ahamkara* is also under the influence of the *tattvas* or matter. It functions as "I am Me" and is characterised by conceit, and pride of one's own self image. It is the "Me" behind all thoughts of intellectualism. It is the cause of the fragmentation of the lower and higher minds because it thrives on division, strife, jealousy and "Me and Mine. " It has a substratum based upon habits, opinions, likes-and-dislikes. It gives energy to the reactions of emotional-sensory mind.

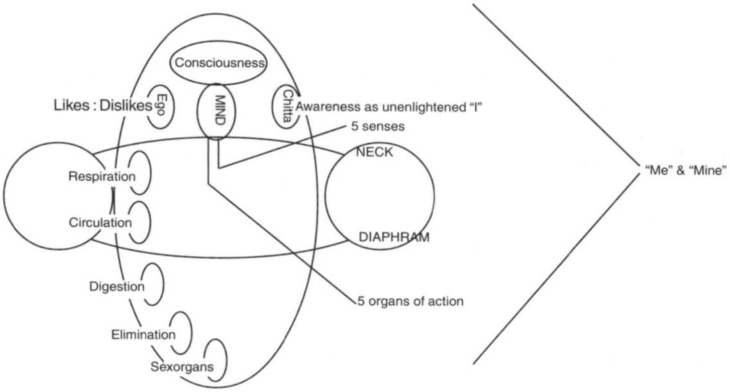

Figure 10. Mind as *chitta* in different roles from different levels of identification

Ego connects the inner world of *raaga-dvesha* or likes-and-dislikes with the outer world of the sensory mind. Its narrow focus to acquire and achieve becomes the most important thought process. Because of pride, the "Me" narrowly identifies with caste, creed, race, religion, country and opinions. "Me" looks down on everyone and everything and is the basis of all worldly conflicts and personal separation and unhappiness. Through the sensory mind, "Me" wants to feel connected and happy with indulgences. Thoughts are emotions directed by desires and only the owner of his thoughts knows the turmoil within.

The Master often picked my thoughts. He was a man of few words. When he spoke, his words were always pearls of wisdom. On one such occasion, I was mulling over what he had said about the *chitta* the little 'self'. I debated if I should question him about how he picked my thoughts. I also wondered what he would think of my silly question. He responded to both my queries!

> "It is I admit, a great wisdom to know others and their thoughts. . . but, it is pure Enlightenment to know your own Self: the Lord Shiva in you, by whose grace you live, work and think. . "

The ego can focus and be controlled by its ability to discern and differentiate. Because the energy of "Me" is more outward than inward, "Me" lacks harmony with the inner intelligence that would lead to harmony.

The rational mind is the **intellect;** that, is an individualised portion of the Universal Intelligence in *mahat* or Cosmic Intelligence. It has the ability to rationalise, discriminate and ascertain truth from falsehood, good from bad and the real from the unreal through detached observation.

By nature, the rational mind has the ability to evolve. When its energy is directed outwards, it gives actual reality to all ideas of sense pleasures and their purpose in life. Because it is characterised by Wisdom in its evolved state, it refuses to become enmeshed in ideas of status and possessions and rejects all justifications of emotions and beliefs. When this energy is directed inwards, it gets directed towards the Inner Spirit or Self.

The **individualised soul** or reincarnating "consciousness" as *"jiva"* is the individualised portion of the Cosmic Consciousness. Intelligence leads us back to a higher identity with the self, through the *gyana* of self-knowledge. The *gyana* state of the mind is the purest level of reflection of the Nature of Reality. It requires intense spiritual practice and meditation.

Diseases and the Mind

Ayurveda claims that all disease results from failure of wisdom and incorrect usage of the intellect. We believe we are here to enjoy the worldly pleasures. We use the body and senses to exploit Mother Nature or *Prakriti;* wilful and unintelligent self-indulgence leads to selfish pleasures. The false belief that "Me is" places the body under the sway of the ego. The energy is a downward-flow towards decay and disease.

Meditation is an optimistic desire for an upward-flow of the same energy, but requires hope, laughter, and concerted effort.

> and the Master said:
>
> ". . The healthy optimist laughs to forget while the diseased pessimist forgets to laugh. . "

The Lotus

The lotus *or padma,* is a symbol of meditation in Buddhism as well as in Hinduism. The spiritual centres of the divine cave in the brain and spinal cord are referred to as *chakras.* They bear a resemblance to the lotus. *Padma-asana* or lotus-pose is a meditative posture which will be referred to while describing techniques in meditation.

The lotus is a symbol of duality as well as transcendence, Each petal of the lotus represents a vital portion of our own spiritual understanding, while the stem symbolises that we are well anchored into the earth.

The lotus also symbolises growth in our understanding, that we come from humble beginnings in soil and water. It takes birth in "fertile muck" that not only makes it grow but allows an ascent, through its fertile but filthy beginnings, to achieve the blossom of beauty.

The healing-force comes from within the practitioner, from the body, the mundane "Me". While using the force for self-healing, the seeker is developing the spirit, the "real" me, the "I"; thus, the lotus represents the duality of both "I" and "Me".

One day, while travelling with the Master from Bangalore to Mysore in India by car, my eyes feasted on the beauty of the massive lotuses floating on the murky waters of the ditches along the road. While contemplating on a verse from *'Bhaja Govindam'* (a conversational poem by the sage *Shankaracharya* and his disciples), the Master intuitively picked my thoughts and added:

> ". . The foolish think I emanate from the filth. . . I am in the world but not of it. I remain untouched like a drop of water on the petals of the lotus. I am *Narayana (God)."*

He reminded me that I am indeed the pure Self encased but unaffected either by my body, mind, or intellect (BMI), or the world of objects (OET). I am indeed the pure perceiver, feeler, and thinker (PFT) when identified to super-consciousness.

The Duality of "I" and "Me"

From the first breath at birth, one lives with the duality of the spirit, which dwells in the physical shell of the body as the "I" the soul, and the "Me" the pseudo-soul. In many ways, these two parts are in conflict, yet each needs the other. After all, it is "I" as life-force that enlivens all matter equipment's, such as the body (B) and all its senses and organs of action, the mind (M) as emotions, and intellect (I) as thoughts!

"Me" (Self, filtering through BMI or body-mind-intellect) is the source of physical demands, constantly demanding attention. In contrast, "I" (pure Self as pure PFT or perceiver-feeler-thinker without the matter equipments) has no need for things and comforts. "Me", the ego or pseudo-soul, knows it is nothing without

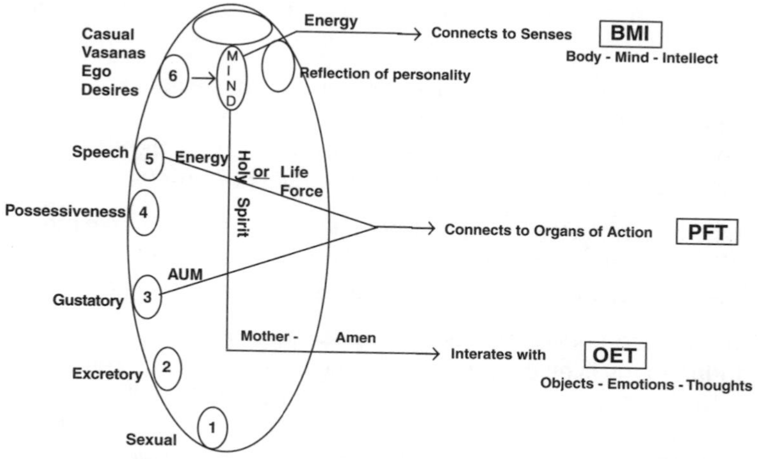

Figure 11. The 'Me' is perceiver-feeler-thinker (causal PFT) filtering through matter equipments (BMI) body-mind-intellect

the "I", (life-force) but "I" gives in to "Me" all the time, because of his causal beingness or *vasanas*. These *vasanas* are old habits, desires, concepts, demands and are the reason for taking a new birth in this present body. This expresses itself as a desire to exist and to be immortal!

The desire to be alive at all times is the innate urge to be immortal and be happy. "Me" the pseudo-soul, searches for immortality in name, fame, position, possessions, and comforts. It realises that in the school-of-life of knocks-and-bruises, there is neither immortality nor abiding happiness. In the silence of his being, the seeker knows there must be another way and he discovers meditation!

The purpose of meditation is to first separate "Me", the pseudo-soul, from "I", the soul. After developing each one separately, efforts are made at merging them in meditation.

Strengthening the introspective "Me" is done by developing the "Will" through self-control and abstinence from indulgences. This is realised through the appearance of dispassion or *vairagya* for things that the seeker once desired, born of the discovery of the Self in meditation.

To succeed in meditation, "Me", the ego, must be convinced to stop desiring mundane things from the world of objects, emotions, and thoughts (**OET**). "Me" the pseudo-soul or ego, must stop wanting to be the individualistic being as the egocentric perceiver-feeler-thinker (**PFT**).

In the silence of our inner selves in the causal-being or desire-ridden "Me", there resides "I" as *devata,* a deity who gives the worshipper or mortal whatever he seeks and is therefore worthy of worship. (Please refer to the chart 'Transformation through Meditation' on Page 5). The "Me" or ego must become transformed and, in the transformation, must become both still (body-mind) and silent (intellect).

As long as the "Me", the ego or pseudo-soul, is busy with its demands at its own "beingness, "I" as life-force or *devata,* is too busy assisting in the demands being made. In such a situation, "I", the Self or *devata* or *prakriti* or *aum* or life-force can never communicate with "Itself", the *rishi* or *purusha.*

In this type of a mundane human transaction, the *rishi* or seer in me remains the eternal witness and therefore 'watches' the goings on of the "Me", and the *devata* or deity "I" constantly 'looks' and caters to the demands of "Me".

"Me", the pseudo-soul or ego, is a 'tough customer': it has been looking out for itself during many lives as a desiring-being or *vasanas* and refuses to "die". "Me", the pseudo-soul or ego or causal being or *vasana*-impelled-being, has to convince "I", the *pure* perceiver-feeler-thinker (PFT) or "I" as *devata*, that "Me" is not a threat to "I". By submitting to "I", he actually elevates "Me," the ego.

The Master once used a parable by Jesus, to emphasise the need to become desireless of the pleasures of this world, if there was to be success in efforts at meditation.

> On purging the *vasanas* or 'Me', the Master said:
>
> ". . It is as difficult for a 'rich' man to enter the Gates of Heaven as it is for a camel to enter the eye of a needle. The riches of mortal existence are the bundles of desires as *vasanas* we carry with us from one existence to another. "

Why Meditation?

Ultimately, meditation is an attempt to 'plug into the mains' of the great Cosmic Consciousness as well as the Cosmic Energy.

The goal of meditation is to bring the two halves (the "I" and "Me") of the self in contact with each other and merge into one (1 + 1 = 1). It also reaches upwards and outwards to obtain guidance and answers for problems we face from our guardian angels that are in the astral dimension. These are guides whose ideas and tastes in the astral world resemble our own ideas and tastes while we live in the physical world.

Getting Started - a Meditation Exercise

Many meditation techniques are described. Of all the techniques described in this book, the seeker will choose parts that work best for him. There are essentially four components to every meditation: , entering the divine cave or altar of God in the brain and spinal cord, energising the physical body, watching the breath as you go deeper into the different sheaths, and listening to your inner sounds.

These different techniques will be introduced gradually. Starting with the first psychic-spiritual centre in the base of the spine, the seeker will be taken through the eight steps described by sage *Patanjali.* The five senses of the body will be analysed in order to sharpen every sense awareness beyond the influence of past habits, concepts, and likes-and-dislikes. .

The instructions given below are used by our Study Groups in Meditation.

Before Starting Meditation, Create a Protective Shield: To do this, there are various methods:

1. Non-denominational:

First sit in an the asana or posture of your choice. Make a protective shield by invoking the Divine Light of Awareness within and around oneself.

- *Mentally picture a cave in the brain and spinal cord and fill it with the Light of Awareness entering through* the *medulla (base of brain at hairline).*

"Feel" It go up to the sahasrahara (crown of head where prana or energy is stored) and then see it permeate down the spine;

- *Allow the awareness to radiate (within) to every tissue of the body of the practitioner. Now contract feet, calves, thighs, buttocks, back, abdominal wall, chest, hands, forearms, upper arms, shoulders, neck, face and head: this is to withdraw prana or life-force back into the divine cave. Now relax all the body parts and allow the energy or Light of Awareness to re-infuse the relaxed parts of the body. While focusing at the forehead (Kutastha) open the vision even further into this astral Infinity and enclose the stars and planets as well;*
- *Chant the following as you physically and mentally inhale the Light of Awareness:*

> ***"I bring the Cosmic Forces inside and around me***
> ***Give me strength, protection, and guidance. "***

- *Repeat this three times before starting meditation (for protection against disturbances from the physical, astral and heavenly worlds).*

2. Students of sanskrit may choose to invoke mantras in the order given below:

I. HARI AUM

AGAMA-ARTHAM TU DEVAA-NAAM GAMA-NAARTHAM TU RAKSHA-SAAM
KURVE GHANTAAR-VAM DEVA-TAA-HVAANA LAKSHA-NAM
Verily, the bounties (gains through sadhana) which are to be acquired and that which leave (those already acquired), may You protect them (from loss).

When the ringing of the bell is heard, be it known (that the bell represents Aum) - it is my calling out to the devas (in the astral dimension).

II. DIG-BANDH-AHA

AUM BHUR BHUVAH SWAHAA
ITI DIG-BANDHAHA
I now invoke the "Protective Shield".

I do so by also invoking (non-interference from the 3 worlds) the Cosmic Energy first which supports the three worlds (physical, astral and causal).
I reiterate that the protective shield is now established (kavach).

III. DHYAANAM

SHREE GANESH

EKA-DANTHAM CHATUR-HASTAM PAASHAM ANKUSHA DHAARI-NAM
RADAM CHA VARADAM HAS-TAIR BIBHRAA-NAM MUSHAKA DHVA-JAM
RAKTAM LAMBO-DARAM SHURPA KARNA-KAM RAKTA- VAASA-SAM
RAKTAM GAN-DHAANU LIPTAAN-GAM RAKTA PUSHPAI SUPU-JITAM
BHAKTAA-NU-KAM-PITAM DEVAM JAGAT KAARANAM ACHYU-TAM

AAVIR-BHUTAMCHA-SHRISH-TYAA-DAU PRAKRI-TEH PURUSHAAT-PARAM EVAM DHYAA-YATI YO NITYAM SA YOGI-NAM VARAN

Oh single tusked deva (sattva, free of raga dvesha), who in Your four arms hold and surround Yourself with reminders of self improvement. You are indeed fully ripened (red: rajas) with a large belly with the bounties of the universe (tamas); widely spaced are your ears (sattva in space and its power of hearing).

Red sandal-wood paste smears Your body (smell), red flowers are offered too (sight) - the offering is in the right attitude and conduct (mind/emotions). Worshipped are You as the First (father) deva and Cause of this world (as the unmanifest ideational Ishwara).

Matter and created beings, prakriti (life energy) and purusha (light of consciousness) - before all these; You were there as the Unmanifest Aum (as Ideational Ishwara). Thus, are You meditated upon, daily by yogis; truly, thus are You meditated upon, oh best among Yogis.

Ganesh is the Hindu deity to symbolise the divine-cave of the brain and spinal cord from which a living being is created. He is Cosmic Intelligence or *Purusha as Mahat* and Universal Intelligence at the *Kutastha,* located between the eyebrows at the *bhrumadhya* within the brain of the divine cave (brain and spinal cord).

Whether in the East or in the West, this is the Christ Centre or the Krishna Centre of Universal Intelligence. Christ referred to it as the 'door' through which you reach the 'kingdom of heaven'.

Tracing Ganesh's evolution in my own spiritual journey is fascinating:

1968 India: My four year old younger daughter returns from the Convent School to the Engineering Postgraduate Students' Residence in Roorkee. It was half-day at school. The Hindus were celebrating *Ganesh Chaturthi* [four aims and ages of world-cycle] and parading the images of the elephant-headed deity of the Hindus. The Catholics were parading Mother Mary with baby Jesus through the streets also.

She had had a bad day at school. Her clothes were covered in mud and her face was stained with tears. She must have had an altercation with a classmate "Why can't we have gods with human faces? Why does our god have an elephant's face"? she sobbed uncontrollably.

I had no answers. My own religious upbringing was very Protestant and image free.

1975 Canada: On a Sunday in St. John's, Newfoundland I told my daughters the following story borrowed from "God Symbolism" by Swami Chinmayananda: Ganesh is the first son of Lord Shiva. He is the Lord of Circumstances and

Remover of all Obstacles. Therefore no Hindu ritual is possible without invoking His Grace first. He is considered married to both *Lakshmi* and *Sarasvati* and therefore is Master of Wealth, Knowledge, and Achievements.

We all know that Westerners are shocked to see Hindus revere a divine Form so ridiculous and absurd. To the *vedantin* [seeker following the Path of Philosophy] he is the Path towards the Infinite. To the devotee, his large ears are for listening to the teachers. His large head harbours a massive intellect capable of embracing a world-vision. His trunk is representative of a special adaptive efficiency for both mechanical and scientific ingenuity: it is capable of plucking a blade of grass as efficiently as uprooting trees. He is able to discriminate and resolve world problems as efficiently as analysing the inner layers of his personality.

His one broken tusk is to remind seekers to go beyond judgements. His wide mouth indicates that a man of perfection must have an endless appetite for life and to experience Consciousness. His big belly is for stomaching all experiences of life peacefully. When this Master-Mind dangles one of his feet to the ground while folding the other under him, it is to symbolise that a man of wisdom integrates his emotional mind with the logical intellect.

He is surrounded by endless eatables to remind every seeker to enjoy the glories of his physical existence. There is always a mouse with folded front paws sitting in anticipation for permission to eat. He represents desire which must be mastered so that the urges of acquisition and pleasure are held in obedience to the will of the Master. His four arms represent four inner subtle equipment's used on a seeker's spiritual pilgrimage.

It had taken me seven years to answer her agonising question. She was now eleven years old.

1994 New Delhi: We were guests of a friend at their home. Joti my husband, was snoring and the fan above cranked its circumambulation in a rhythmic noise. The mosquitoes could be heard making valiant attempts to enter the shield made by the fast moving air, with little success. At 0400 hours I was trying very hard to enter myself in meditation. I felt irritated with the noise and my unfamiliar environment. I was quite surprised at myself when I entered the divine cave of the brain and spinal cord.

My next surprise was seeing a shockingly white image of the head and trunk of Ganesh in my divine cave. His head was my brain and his trunk was my spinal cord. Every time I straightened my slumping back, his trunk would move as well.

"So that's who you are. You represent the brain and the spinal cord" I said to myself. I saw the image revisit me every day for a about a week and then it disappeared. We were now formally introduced!

Meditation Used for Sadhana and Solving Personal Problems

First, **define meditative goal you wish to achieve**:

- Inner serenity;
- Spiritual serenity; or
- Getting answers to questions.

***If seeking answers to problems**:*

Enter problems and questions into the divine cave with its Light of Awareness and expect return answers, messages and impressions after intense concentration into the queries while meditating.

***If meditation is for sadhana or inner serenity**:*

- *Infuse the light of awareness into the "cave" of the brain and spinal cord through medulla at the base of the skull;*
- *With back straight, **lower abdomen pulled in**, shoulder blades pushed back and together, hands resting at the abdomen-thigh junction. Watch the breath intently rising and falling into the chest and through the nostrils. Feel the touch of the breath coursing in and out of the chest through the nostrils (normaly 16 times/minute);*
- *Push the head backwards (so the chin is parallel to the ground) and raise your eyes as if looking first at the ceiling and then directed backwards in **an inner gaze** inside the brain cave. This is looking at (with eyes shut) the Kutashta Chaitanya (also called the Krishna or Christ Centre) behind the eyebrows (centre for Universal Intelligence). Its characteristic is of an Infinite Cosmic Vision;*
- *Roll the tongue back to touch the back of the throat at the uvula. This opens the 'mouth of God' wider at the medulla.*
- *Next, arch backwards to further lengthen the spinal cord. Lift both arms and place the interlocked two hands over the 'mouth of God' at the back of the head above the level of the hair-line. Next **feel the divine cave arch** first backwards, then to the left and then to the right. Maintain awareness in the divine cave as you look at the dark hollow of the cave. The cave is the Altar of God.*
- *With **an inner feeling,** feel the in-coming breath of inspiration rising as a cool current from the lower end of the sternum to the base of the throat (felt as a "coolness" in the back the throat/spine);*
- *Now feel/visualise the out-going breath of expiration as a warm current (also felt at the back of the throat) descending from the base of the throat to the lower end of the sternum. Continue this normal breathing for five minutes. Bring the hands down to rest at the thighs.*
- *Watch the breath coursing in and out through the nostril for as long as it takes to get the answers*

- *Wait in silence for the answers without changing the position of the head and eyes. Leave hands relaxed palms open upwards and lying on the thighs.*
- *Always remember to roll your tongue backwards, turn your gaze back into the divine cave, watch and feel the breath pass the nostrils with inspiration and expiration.*

Continue to watch the physical breathing and experience the silence of thoughtlessness within oneself. This is concentration. Over time and serious efforts at concentration, there are fewer and fewer wandering-thoughts to disturb the awareness of the practitioner, until there are no more thoughts.

Now wait to receive messages without concentrating on anything. Messages are received visually or through any of the senses:
- *Responses come as sudden flashes of inspiration or the spiritual eye may be watching you and you can see vistas of images in the "third" eye;*
- *You may see a flash at the edge of your right vision indicating the Guide's presence (do not jerk or get frightened).*

Before getting out of the meditation, offer a short healing prayer to use up the built-up force in the cave-of-awareness, which should be seen to dissolve itself into oneself.
- *Direct any residual power to any specific person in need of help through the Kutastha;*
- *Close the infinite beam of awareness and let it enclose you.*

In the early stages of meditation, the seeker spends a great deal of his time in the seat of meditation dealing with wandering thoughts. These disturbances are necessary. The seeker will first watch the thoughts of his waking state; then he sees thoughts and images of his subconscious mind; lastly, he encounters thoughts of his causal state which have gurgled into the subconscious. They too need to be paraded on the stage of awareness. The Master always reassured us to remain a witness to all the 'dirt' that surfaced. "Watch them fade away into oblivion". This is purging the mind of its present, past, and previous births.

The Materialistic Man

Man has fought many inner and outer battles in innumerable incarnations. Battling within man are the competing forces of good and evil. The purpose of meditation is to align man's efforts on the side of righteousness.

The soul of a child is attracted into a family in which the "family heredity" is in conformance with the child's past *karmic* desires (*vasana* or causal state). *Within the mother's body*, the child struggles against disease, darkness, and the frustration of confinement. The mother's environment through the pregnancy adds vibratory influences on the unborn child.

After birth, the child struggles between the instinct of survival and the helplessness of an immature bodily instrument. *Childhood* is a battle between *karmic* instincts which brought the child into his new parental home and parental wishes for their new child. The child has an instinctive desire to play while the parental desire for the child is to learn. *As a youth*, the child is confronted with problems he has not been prepared to meet. Temptations of sex, greed, moneymaking, and social influences present themselves as invading armies of worldly experiences.

It always surprised me to hear the wisdom of the Master. In his frugal language, he admonished as well as lovingly directed the parents of young children. Young parents, he knew, had little logical training in child-rearing. He had the wisdom that children under the age of five (with inherent *vasanas* or desires) were struggling to become part of their new family who had their own agenda or *vasanas*. The Master first taught me and then my two daughters who later also became mothers:

> "For the first six years, treat him like a 'god' and allow for fearless growth. For the next six, treat him like a 'king' to learn the art of 'command'. For the third six years, treat him like a slave, to teach him 'obedience'. From eighteen onwards, consider him a 'friend'. He will be your faithful child to the end!"

Unless the youth is nurtured correctly, this *adult-youth* now spends his life cultivating the kingdom of his own body. He finds he is overrun by misery-making wrong desires, destructive habits, failures, ignorance, disease, and unhappiness. The psychological conflicts of health, prosperity, and self-control have to be addressed early and daily by the parents of children.

Introspection: A Prelude to Inner Awakening

Man, awakened through introspection, has a desire to meditate. He strives to establish himself in the soul's inner kingdom, which is located in the subtle centres of life force and consciousness in the spinal cord and the brain.

For meditation to come to fruition, the Conscious Principle (the "I" functioning through "Me") of Man must desire God to manifest His Love. The moment it is desired, this Conscious Principle's Energy and Force, becomes manifest within the body. His inner *guru* makes a demand and situations and persons make their appearance to get the seeker started.

In the Body are Physical and Metaphysical Fields of Energy

The **Mind** manifests in the grosser structures of the body as the **five senses**. The **forces of the soul** include: mood and feeling, will, intellect, insight, love, and awareness. These dwell in the *kutastha* or Christ-*Krishna* Centre of Universal

Awareness and also in the *ajnaa chakra* or sixth spiritual centre at the base of the brain.

The life-force or *prakriti* enters the brain and spinal cord through the medulla through the *ajnaa* as a*um shakti* or Energy or Life-force.

The **inner chambers of the soul** occupy several areas of the brain. The centre of Universal Energy and Life force is found in the medulla at the base of the brain:

- *Kutastha Chaitanya* in frontal lobe for Universal Intelligence which is physically located between and behind the two eyebrows (Christ or *Krishna* Centre); and,
- Individualised Awareness of the soul or *jiva* as superconsciousness, located in the *ajnaa,* at the base of the brain.

As the *jiva* or soul descends from the base of the brain, it enters the special senses and brain-stem and spinal cord plexuses. The descent is influenced by the vibrating energies of the seeker's past lives which determine his personality and the actions of his present life.

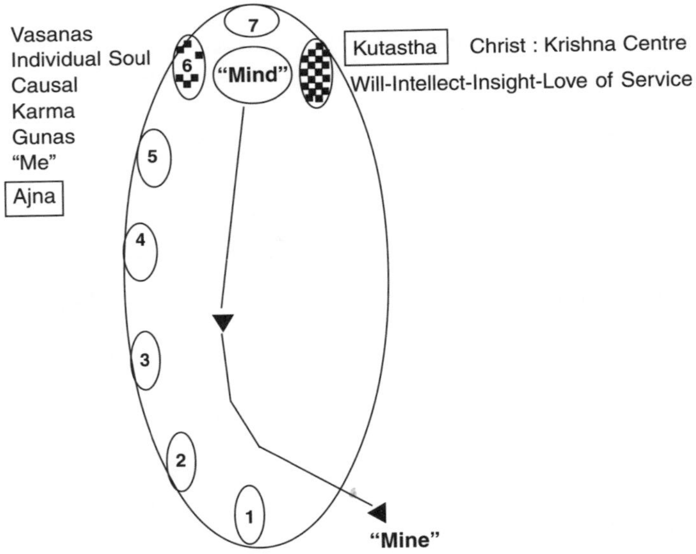

Figure 12. Location of the Causal Being ("Me") and "I" in the Ajnaa and Reflected in the Christ Centre

The influencing factors on any individual soul are:

- The law of qualities or gunas or *tamas* (inertia) - *rajas* (activity) - *sattva* (harmony of the two) causing Man to seek indulgences for pleasure;

- The law of relativities embedded in the causal "Me" the pseudo-soul or ego, expressing as *raaga-dvesha* or likes-and-dislikes;
- The law of karma or cause-and-effect leaving the causal body with traits of past *karmic* traits and habits.

The old causal being who shed his physical body at the end of his previous physical manifestation takes birth in a new physical body and locates himself in the *ajnaa* or sixth centre at the base of the brain of the newborn. Here he lives as the pseudo-soul or ego "Me". Through the Mind-Intellect he connects with the five senses and the five organs of action. His unique 'personality' is embedded in his autonomic nervous system (*ida)* and shines through the *kutastha* or Krishna-Christ Centre. As infant and child the "Me" in him manifests his unique personality, despite his parents and environment.

As youth and adult, he registers all new information into his sixth or "Me" centre which is permanently recorded (as deep as the DNA molecule of that part of the brain) in the *Kutastha* as 'observation' made by the *devata* or "I" who is at the service of "Me".

The result of this change is the release of specifically modified neurotransmitters and neurohormones from the master-glands: the hypothalamus and the pituitary organs.

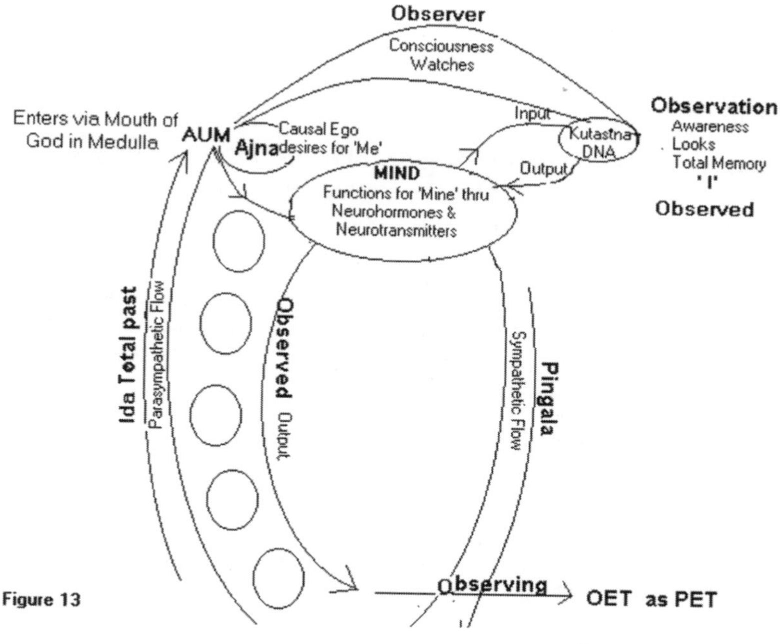

Figure 13

Figure 13. Old "Me" becoming the New "Me" in a new manifestation and a new environment

The Master glands respond to observed changes in the causal being where all changes are recorded in response to spiritual self-effort or *sadhana.* These are responses to the changes made in the *chitta* (mind-intellect-ego complex). The effect of these changes is felt by the body-mind-intellect (BMI) which is under the influence of the nervous and endocrine systems (sympathetic autonomic nervous system or *pingala)* of the body.

The new perceiver-feeler-thinker (PFT) now has a different view-of-life when he contacts and is observing the world of objects-emotions-thoughts (OET).

Therefore, the motives of visible action and audible speech are deeply embedded in the causal or desire of that individual. The Master cautioned all seekers to stop to think and ponder upon all actions and thought.

> and the Master defined motives of action:
>
> ". . Action is performed by three bodily instruments, namely *man-vak-kaya or* Mind-Speech-Body.
>
> "Noble thoughts of devotion, knowledge, dispassion, charity for spiritual evolution are mental *karmas.* Lustful thoughts pertaining to sense-enjoyment, for harming others, non-belief and disrespect are bad *karmas. . .*
>
> "Truthful noble talk, words of love and compassion is noble speech. Words of disrespect, fault-finding, engaging in verbal vulgarities is pain producing speech.
>
> "Bodily austerities, cleanliness, seeking company of the wise are noble bodily actions, while immoral acts causing injury to others are sinful *karmas. . .* "

The predominance of certain qualities or ***gunas*** (*sattva* or equanimity; *tamas* or sloth; *rajas* or activity), determine the effect of the power of *maya* on any one individual.

Maya is a 'magical' power of delusion (of Matter or *prakriti)* that leads one to believe that the mirage is real and one's materialistic aspirations are for keeps. *Maya's* power of delusion is part and parcel of Matter's Law of Qualities or *gunas.*

The deluded and tempted being begins to think he is the body (mind and senses) and identifies with "Me and Mine", the pseudo-soul or ego. He, the *jiva* or individualised pseudo-soul, therefore, remains circumscribed by the limitations and circumstances of the body, emotions, and logic.

To illustrate this, a wise visiting monk gave us this illustration at a lunch meeting:

> "There is an *'unconscious' knowledge* of *attachment* of how one must deal with objects-emotions-thoughts (OET). The *perception* of the Truth is different in different animals. Man is the only animal capable of *understanding* the difference between desire and greed, attachment and delusion. The power of *maya or* delusion or *avidya* is a function of causal awareness or *vasanas* or desires of past and present births. He has created habits of reaction to every cause-stimulus whether they be objects, circumstances or relationships.

"Thoughts preoccupied with *attachments* promote *avidya,* despite Man's ability to acquire understanding and wisdom. Worldly attachments to positions, persons and possessions ('Me' and 'Mine') are the root cause of troubling thoughts of greed and desire. The five sins of the extrovert are because of Man's indulgences which lead him to lust, anger, greed, attachments, and pride (*kama, krodha, lobha, moha, and mada).* They prevent pure intuitive perception of "I", and promote confusion, desecrate the body-mind-intellect, and create false attachments, despite good advice. In Truth, "Me" is none other than the pure perceiver-feeler-thinker (PFT), the "I".

** Anatomy of Man's Bodily Field of Activity

The nervous system in the divine cave (brain and spinal cord) is divided into three parts:

- **The physical bodily field inhabits the periphery of the body.**
  It consists of the peripheral five instruments of knowledge (skin, eyes, ears, tongue and nose) and five instruments of action (touching, seeing, hearing-speaking, excreting-procreating, and locomotion through hands and feet). In this field sensory and motor activity occur. Here, ***rajas** and* ***tamas*** reside as activity, sloth, and ignorance.
- **The second bodily field is in the cerebrospinal axis.**
  It consists of the five physiological centres of life-force and awareness physically, physiologically, and psychologically represented as five nerve plexuses (coccygeal, sacral, lumbar, thoracic, and cervical):
  - The **sensory mind** or *manas* pulls the centres outwards thereby keeping the motor and sensory functions of the body active on the body surface.
  - The **extrovert intellect** pulls the centres towards indulgences and desires. It responds to their demands of desires and executes actions through the *manas* pleasure. The **introvert intellect** or *buddhi* pulls the faculties inwards towards introspection.
  - The three lower centres are under the control of the desiring mind-intellect.
  - The two higher centres can be coaxed to fall under the control of the introspective intellect.
- **The third bodily field is in the brain - the brain-cave.**
  The pair of cerebral hemispheres are divided into four lobes covered on the surface with specific cells that are a few millimetres thick and

**The sections on "anatomy and physiology" would be of interest to those in the medical profession. Those not interested in these subjects should skip the previous two sections. This omission will not result in any loss of understanding of the philosophy. **

histologically distinct from each other. The four lobes are connected by association fibres which can achieve integration and unified awareness by sinking down through the six layers of neurones. (Please refer to Figure 20).

Deeper still lie the limbic cortex, and the subcortical structures which encircle the whole brainstem. This is where emotional and motivational transformation takes place. The basal ganglia has connections with all the other parts of the brain and is involved with cognition, orientation in space, behavioural patterns, and motivation. It receives input from the limbic cortex, regulates the autonomic nervous system, transmits emotions, controls functioning of the master glands for the secretion of neuro-hormones and neuro-transmitters, and gives awareness to the cortex.

The connections of the brain, coupled with the spinal cord, integrate with:

- The ego, intellect, and mind as the unenlightened *chitta* which resides in the medulla;
- The intellect, to channel progressive logical thought;
- The mind, to channel emotions through the senses;
- Involves the five *pranas* through the master organs (hypothalamus and pituitary) for physiological functions of the body.

These eight factors (ego, mind, intellect, *chitta,* five elements, five subtle elements or *pranas,* five senses, five organs of action) are products of *Prakriti* or Matter. Every individual neurone of a particular person has a memory bank of every exposure and action and perception endured through millions of incarnations.

The individualised awaring brain upholds the cause of Man's being.

- It allows the expressions of life and awareness to create and sustain man's physical, astral, and causal bodies.
- Through these three fields the soul enters new bodies or leaves the three bodies and returns to Spirit.
- *Sattva* or harmony predominates in this area of the brain *[kutastha]* as will, wisdom, insight, love, life-of-service, bliss, and vitality.

**Cellular Physiology of the Divine Cave

The central nervous system in the divine cave (brain and spinal cord) acts as a master clerk with the ability to organise and co-ordinate the activities required to integrate perfectly all the bodily functions. The individual neuronal cell contains the entire historical information (DNA) of the individual through the millions of reincarnations he has previously endured.

The neuronal cell also allows new changes to be constantly recorded as 'observations' which trigger appropriate changes in the DNA molecule of the causal body (also called the *devata or "I"*). Bodily changes are made through the medium of modified neuro-hormones and neurotransmitters released in the brainstem by the master organs: the pituitary gland and the hypothalamus. All changes now assume a *chhandas* or specific changed quality. All observing of the world of objects (OET) is directly related to the new information programmed into the causal body where "Me" (ego) and "I" (soul) reside.

The result of all this activity which one calls 'living' is a constantly evolving process of a combined observer-observation-observing individual. In this transaction, the *rishi* or observer who watches is the eternal witness; the *devata* or "I" makes all the changes demanded by the "Me" and records them as new observations - the *devata* merely looks on and makes the changes made by the practitioner's desires. The observed data now acquires a specifically changed or *chhandas* quality. Now all observings of the world of objects acquire a new quality, based upon new information which is acquired.

All bodily activities of *yoga* and the changing awareness are initiated through the entire central nervous system and recorded in the memory of the brain. Awareness looks at the input, makes the necessary changes in the DNA of the neuronal cell, and permanently records it as an observed-observation. All future action through the medium of neurotransmitters and neurohormones is now a modified observing, hearing, seeing and feeling – based upon 'new' information being logged into the causal body.

All these activities occur within the 'divine cave' of the brain and spinal cord. The changes are permanent for that time in Man's existence and are transported as the causal being into the next reincarnation.

A nurse working with me found it intolerable that Hinduism supported the Doctrine of Incarnation. She was alarmed that the Master wrote what follows. She could not discard the logic but also would not accept it!

> and the Master writes:
>
> "The Reincarnation Theory is not a mere dream of the philosophers, and the day is not far off when, with the fast-developing science of Psychology, the West will come to rewrite its Scriptures under the sheer weight of observed phenomenon. An uncompromising intellectual quest for understanding life cannot satisfy itself if it is thwarted at every corner by 'observed irregularities'. We cannot, for long, ignore them all as mere 'chances'. The prodigy Mozart is a spectacular instance which cannot be explained away; to be logical we must accept the idea of the continuity of the embodied souls. . . "

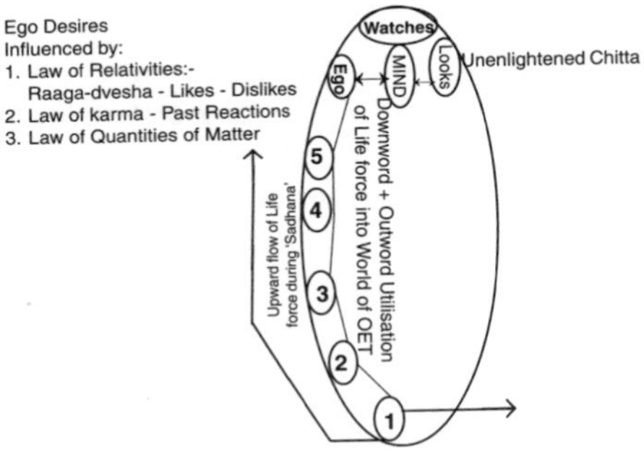

Figure 14. "Me" the pseudo-soul or Ego reflecting as the Unenlightened chitta (mind-intellect-ego) personality

Ego

Ego "Me" is the self-serving intellect: the pseudosoul, which is located in the *ajnaa* centre at the base of the brain cave. It imitates the soul "I" or *rishi-devata* and tries to dominate the bodily kingdom. Because it is the pseudo-soul or ego, it can never gain entrance into the chambers of superconsciousness. These centres of superconsciousness include the centre of Universal Consciousness in the *sahasrahara* or seventh spiritual centre. The other centre is at the *Kutastha (Krishna*-Christ Centre) at the *bhrumadhya* between the eyebrows in the forehead: this is the centre of Universal Intelligence where the enlightened *chitta* manifests as pure awareness.

The ego "Me" is the cause of all individualised existence. It is the template of form for a being. Through the medium of creative energy, *prakriti* or Mother Nature utilises Her elements *(tattvas*) to produce a specific body with specific sense-tendencies and perceptions as well as the organs of action. By mutual consent, *Prakriti* or Nature allows the "Me" to manifest. This individualistic ego fails to identify with the Spirit; instead, it identifies with the outgoing forces of Nature.

In this artificial make-believe state, "Me" the ego gives its own existence to all forms and sensory objects. Its individualised sense of 'beingness' as "Me" lacks discrimination. The inner-seeing ego in the astral plane identifies with the sense mind *(manas)*, thinking intellect *(buddhi*) and with feeling *(chitta)* or unenlightened mind-intellect-ego.

Ego can gain entrance into man's awareness (as awake state) and the subconsciousness (as dream state). At these levels, it is subjected to material desires, emotions, habits, and sense inclinations recorded in the template of his past births. Only the discriminative intellect *(buddhi)* can reveal the truth and be attracted to the Self or Spirit in the superconscious state.

The physical tracts of the lower three nerve plexuses are centres of *rajasic* or creative energy. They are constantly agitated, and their demands are honoured through the senses. This leads to body-identified pleasure-seekers, indulgent, and self-centred on "Me". Influenced by ignorance, "Me" falls into evil ways and bad habits. Thoughts, will, and feelings become negative, limited, jaded, and unhappy. The bodily cells become disorganised, inefficient, and debilitated with poor health and disease.

When ego expresses through the intuitive enlightened wisdom of the causal body, it becomes discriminative divine ego. The inner-seeing ego can become transcendent as the discriminating ego of the astral and causal bodies. Awakening "Me" or pseudo-soul, reaches the shores of pure individualised sense-of-being, the "I" - the soul. The purified enlightened *chitta* sits resplendent as "I" within the cave of the brain, near the *Kutastha.*

In a Western environment, a little ego is not normally considered unacceptable. As one brought up in the West, it was difficult to accept the Master's admonition. Here is an example of one of them:

> and the Master hammered:
>
> ". . You are drunk with the idea that you run the show, full of egoistic sense of importance", he scolded!
>
> I mentally protested that was not true and vowed to understand the ego over the ten days the Master was lecturing on meditation.
>
> ". . Ego is memories of the past, excitements of the present and anxiety for the future. . "
>
> Not yet clear, said my mind!
>
> ". . Ego is memory of the dead and decaying experiences which must necessarily stink. . "
>
> My instincts revolted and asked if that was the motivating force of all my efforts?
>
> "Work in a spirit of selfless duty and loving sacrifice, a *yagna* spirit. . " he lovingly concluded!"

Offer all actions at the feet of the Cosmic Mother in love and adoration, for Her sake, he seemed to be telling me! By doing this I no longer needed to take responsibility for the failures or the successes of all my actions. As long as my actions are sincere and an offering at the feet of the Cosmic Mother, I will not be rejoice nor will I lament at the results of a dedicated action. What a load off my shoulders!

Essence of Astral and Causal Bodies

The physical [*annamaya kosha* or food sheath] and mental-intellectual [*manomaya* and *gyanamaya koshas* - mind and intellectual sheaths] worlds of individual bodies are inert matter. The **life-force or *prana*** is the **creative energy** of **intelligent life-force** or *Aum,* stemming from subtle dimensions originating before manifestation of the astral and causal worlds. The essence of every manifestation is recorded in the Cosmic Intelligence of *Purusha or Mahat.* Symbolically, Cosmic and Universal Intelligence in the Cosmic Brain is represented by *Ganesha*, the beloved elephant-headed deity of the Hindus. The divine-cave of the brain and spinal cord is the individualised beloved *Ganapati (also Ganesha).*

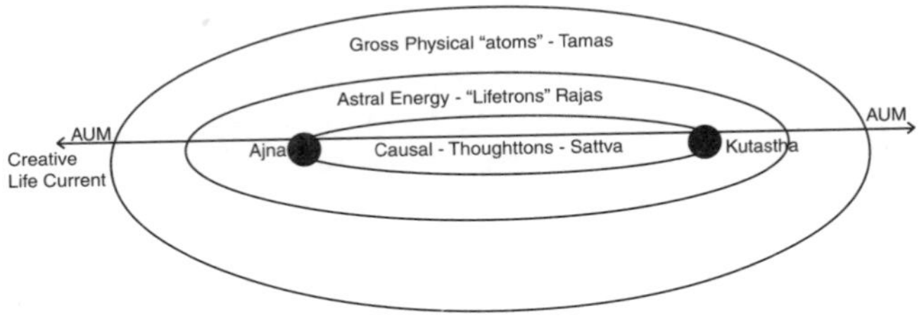

Figure 15. Quality or gunas of the three bodies or shariras

- The **physical world** is the least subtle of the vibrations of energy and manifests as matter. In its minutest state, it is the atom of matter. Since it is inert, it is *tamasic* or dense. It is composed of sixteen units.
- The **astral world** is pure energy. It is the energy in five subtle *(pranas)* elements, five senses, and five organs of action. It includes the energy of the mind, and intellect. With ego, mind and intellect or *chitta* plays the role of past existences within the universe in a present existence in this unique individual body. *Swami Yogananda* calls the energy of the astral body, lifetrons as opposed to physical atoms**.** The energy is active and therefore *rajasic.* It is composed of nineteen units.
- The **causal world** is characterised by the ideational essence of both the physical and the astral bodies **causal units** [35]**:** they are the essence of the physical body [16], and the essence of the astral body [19]. *Swami Yogananda* calls these units thought-trons because they are the essence of ideas.

The causal body of the individual resides as the ideational thought essence in the *ajnaa* centre within the mouth of God in the medulla. The centre of Universal Intelligence is located in the *Kutastha* behind and between the eyebrows**;** this is also called the *Krishna* or Christ Centre or the gaze-centre of the Third Eye between eyebrows or *bhrumadhya-drishti.*

Nerve Plexuses or Chakras

****Astral Body (Mind and Intellect):**
The Physiological-Psychological Body

The subtle body and its powers are principally those of life-current or ***prana**** or pure energy - Aum . **Life-current** is a mixture of awareness and electrons. The **creative** *or rajasic* **life-current**, present in an embryo (united sperm and ovum), descends into the physical body through seven subtle energy centres: two in the brain and five in the spinal cord. Here, it remains concentrated for the purpose of **outward expression** through the peripheral nervous system manifesting as the **senses** and the **motor functions** of the **organs of action**.

Just as the physical body consists of a physical brain, central nerve centres (cervical, thoracic, lumbar, sacral, and coccygeal) forming plexuses, and the peripheral nervous system, the inner astral nervous system is also represented here where it supports and nourishes the physical nervous system with life-energy.

The **astral body** controls and maintains the physiological and psychological functions of the physical body. Within the astral spinal cord and peripheral nervous system, reside **channels of light and energy** called ***nadis***.

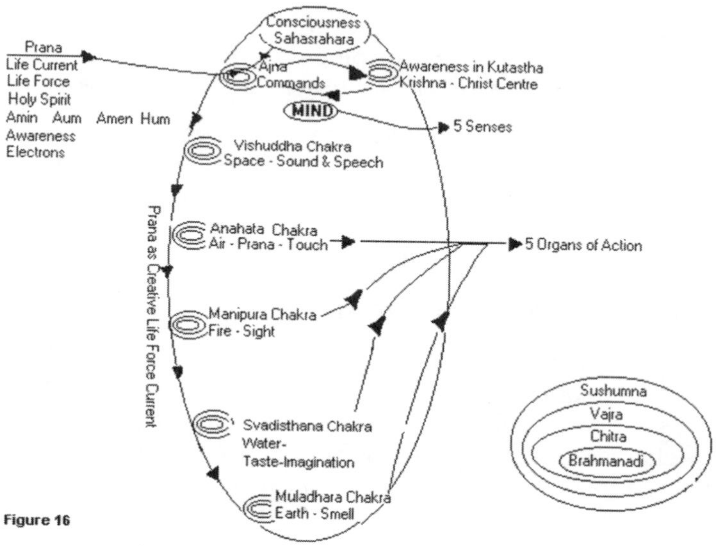

Figure 16. Spiritual Centres or Chakras

**prana* is used as a common name for all the functional divisions of this energy. It is also used to indicate breath of respiration

** The reader is also being introduced to the term *chakras* or spiritual centres of the spinal cord and brain. Each of these centres or *chakras* will be dealt with individually in separate chapters. The three envelopments (physical. astral, and causal) of the spinal cord are also being described briefly. Please feel free to ignore it at this stage if it disturbs your thought process.

*** For an image of what is to follow, please refer to Figure 16.

The **astral nervous system channels** the flow of life-force as energy or *prana** as five differentiated *pranas* for the purposes of crystallisation, circulation, assimilation, metabolism, and elimination. It manifests itself in the physical body as intelligent life-force and energy. **

The main **astral spine of light** is the ***sushumna.*** Within it are two other luminous coverings: the ***vajra*** and the ***chitra***. ***

- The ***sushumna*** or dura mater is the outermost covering of light and controls the gross functions of the seven astral centres and the five vibratory creative elements (earth, water, fire, air and space). It extends from the coccygeal plexus or *muladhara* to the base of the brain.
- Within the *sushumna* is the second astral spine - ***vajra*** or arachnoid mater. It provides the motor functions to the physical body through expansion and contraction. It extends from the sacral plexus or *svadhisthana* to the brain.
- Within the *vajra* is the third astral spine - ***chitra*** or pia mater. It extends from the lumbar plexus or *manipura* to the brain. It relates to spiritual activities towards greater consciousness.

The **activities of the three astral spines** are controlled by the **astral brain** or ***sahasrahara*** that emits specific rays of light and intelligence.

Varying degrees of **light** and **intelligence** are expressed through all the astral nerve plexuses or *chakras.* They manifest in the physical body as characteristic activities of the various physical nerve plexuses (coccygeal, sacral, lumbar, thoracic, and cervical).

Causal Body (vasanas or karana)

The physical body is made of flesh *(tamas)*, while the astral body is made of intelligent life-force or *prana* or energy or life-trons *(rajas).* The causal body is made up of the essence of thoughts and ideas of past births or thought-trons *(sattva)*; its characteristic is awareness. The presence of the causal body behind the physical and astral bodies sustains existence and makes man aware of one's desire to live.

This causal awareness lies within the three astral spines of the spinal cord. It courses through a separate channel, the ***brahmanadi.*** It is characterised by thought vibrations or **awareness**. The causal body serves as the reservoir for awareness which is expressed as the power behind all that **feels, thinks, wills and cognates** as **memory**.

- The **causal brain** is the ever-existing, ever-aware, ever-blissful essence of thoughts that express as the **Individualised "Me"** or unenlightened *chitta.* As this awareness descends down the causal nerve plexuses, it manifests as different characteristics of thought essence.

- In the **head** as ***sahasrahara*** *or padma chakra*, it is the seat of the *Purusha* or Spirit.
  Its seed symbol is ***aum*** and is the seat of the Self which guides all the energies or *prana* and the essence of thoughts (causal).

**On a physical level, it governs the autonomic nervous system and the endocrine glands through the pineal and pituitary glands. On a psychological level, it is the seat of pseudo-soul "Me" and soul "I".

- At the **causal *ajnaa*** or command-*chakra,* it expresses as wisdom, capable of guiding all other *chakras*. It has two petals and is the seat of the mind or *antakarana* in space. Its seed symbol is ***ksham*** for patience, fortitude, and peace. It rules through the mind: via the sense organs and the organs of action.

In the physical brain the causal body relates to the cerebellum and the brain-stem and governs the **autonomic nervous system through neurotransmitters of the pineal gland. In the endocrine system, it works through the *pituitary gland* through the medium of neurohormones. On a psychological level, the causal body not only resides here as the **ego** "Me"**,** but also expresses itself through the centre of **Universal Intelligence** between the eyebrows as "I", through which a seeker identifies himself as ***vishvatma*** or one with the Universal Self.]

- In the **cervical** or throat or ***vishuddha*** *chakra* the causal body expresses as subtle intuition with calmness. It has sixteen petals and is the seat of space. Its seed symbol is ***ham.*** It rules the organs of sound or ears and expression or mouth.

On a physical level, this causal body is related to the oropharynx or throat, the larynx or voice box, and the respiratory system. In the endocrine system, it works through the **thyroid gland. It is where clear expressions are made through the power of **intuition**.

- The **dorsal** or ***anhaata*** *or heart chakra* is located in the spine at the level of the heart. It is here that the natural inner music of the subtle body, the "unstruck sound" is heard. It has twelve petals and is the seat of air. Its seed symbol is ***yam.*** It rules the organ of skin as touch and the organs of action as grasping hands. It is here where **all *prana* or life-force** takes origin *(pranaya, apanaya, vyanaya, udanaya, and samanaya).*

On a physical level, the causal body also relates to the heart plexus and to the cardiovascular system. In the endocrine system, it functions through the **thymus which controls bodily immunity**.** On a psychological level it is the site of devotion and spiritual **aspiration**.

- The **lumbar** or ***manipura*** *or navel chakra* is the <u>City-of-Gems</u> acquired through he power of **self-control** in this seat of fire. It has ten petals and its seed symbol is ***ram.*** The causal body here rules the organs of sight and the organs of action of the feet for movement.

On a physical level, the causal body is connected to the digestive system through the solar plexus and is especially related to the functions of the small intestines and the liver. Endocrinologically, it governs the functions of the **pancreas. On a psychological level, it relates to the power of personal will and ego or **my-will**.

- The **sacral** or ***svadhisthana*** *or pelvic chakra* is also called the sex centre and is located just above the root chakra in the coccyx. It signifies self-abode, where spiritual energy lies dormant and hidden. It has six petals and is the seat of water. Its seed symbol is ***vam.*** It rules the organs of taste, tongue and the organs of action of the reproductive system manifested as emissions of the essence of the physical body *(ojas).* It can be controlled by the **power of adherence** to restraints.

On a physical level, the causal body is further related to the sacral plexus for control of the urogenital system. In the endocrine system, it relates to the **testes and the **ovaries.** On a psychological level, it is the seat of desire and the **desiring mind**.

- The **coccygeal** or ***muladhara*** *or root chakra* is located in the base of the spine and is the root-foundation of all the *chakras.* It has four petals and is the seat of earth. Its seed symbol is ***lam.*** It rules the organs of smell in the nose and the organ of action as elimination in the rectum, anus and bladder.

On a physical level, the causal body also relates to the coccygeal plexus as an organ of the **excretory-secretory system. In the endocrine system it works through the **adrenal** glands. On a psychological level, it is the site of ignorance and fear. On a spiritual level, it is where the power of **restraint** is harnessed.

Awareness Flowing Outwards

When awareness flows outwards from causal to astral and to physical bodies, it is drawn by the magnetic pull of sense attachments to matter. The distance in awareness away from the divine cave is a measure of man's ignorance of the Self.

The original fine essence of the soul becomes increasingly deluded *(maya)* by memories of past *karmas*, habits, inclinations (individualised delusions), and *raaga-dvesha* or likes- and-dislikes. *Maya's* inherent qualities (the triune *gunas* of matter) further complicate actions as automatic expressions sieve through the various bodies and sheaths of the individualised being.

The **outward expressions** of awareness filtered through the unenlightened *vasana*-empowered physical/astral bodies are:

- ***Kama*** or lust (coccygeal) - the compelling desire is action for sense indulgences and coerced by desire;

** Of medical interest. May be ignored by seekers of pure spirituality and meditation.

- ***Krodha*** or anger (sacral) - born of frustrated desires and manifesting as paroxysms of anger from past habits in different births; often parading as righteous-anger;
- ***Lobha*** or greed (lumbar) - enslaving the ego according to whims and fancies ingrained in the individual's judgement as *raaga-dvesha* or likes-and-dislikes;
- ***Moha*** or attachment (dorsal) - expressing as suppression of evolution of the pseudo-soul or ego who imagines delusively that he is the soul with his possessions;
- ***Mada*** or pride (cervical) - expressing as arrogance, conceit, haughtiness and passionate behaviour as regards "me and mine";
- ***Matsarya*** or envy (medullary) - expressing as a very private internalised ego-dissatisfaction despite the presence of materialistic accomplishments.

In sum, ego-consciousness or pseudo-soul "Me" parading as "I" has six faults which compel a person to forget one's Self or soul.

Spiritual Centres

In the world of opposites, the two forces exert a centripetal versus a centrifugal force so that there is harmony of life-on-earth and energy-provided. Both are necessary to maintain equilibrium. There can be no *sattva* or harmony between the two unless *tamas or* inertia balances the forces of agitation or *rajas.*

For every evil inclination, desire or bad habit, there is a corresponding divine discriminative quality that can be employed to defeat the enemy. This dichotomy was illustrated in the *Mahabharata,* the more voluminous of the two epics: *Itihasas* (of Heroes and their Heroic Pursuits), and the *Mahabharata.* It is about the war of Inertia versus Agitation represented by *Kauravas* (one-hundred greedy sons) *and Pandavas* (five good sons and cousins of the hundred brothers). The *Pandavas* are symbolically represented in the spiritual centres or *chakras.* The one hundred cousins are symbolically the one hundred tendencies for indulgences through the five senses and five organs of action. Their force is ten times ten or one hundred. In the *Mahabharata,* the War of *Kurukshetra* is likened to the efforts made at making one fit for meditation. The body-mind-intellect is the 'war zone'. The physical body itself is to be retrained, and restrained. This is the inert or *tamasic* zone.

> and the Master explained:
>
> "The heroes of the War, the *Pandavas (Yudhisthira, Bhima, Arjuna, Sahadev and Nakul)* were made to live amidst the unjust tyranny of their Machiavellian one hundred cousins, the evil *Kauravas. Arjuna*, the greatest archer and hero of those times, became a despondent, bewildered, and a neurotic due to the intervening layers of egocentric assumptions and desire-prompted anxieties. He decided not to fight evil (training and redirecting himself towards meditation). *Krishna*, his charioteer (the "I"), cures *Arjuna* of his psychological derangement (that he is

"Me") and ends his delusions. Through the Bhagavad Geeta, *Krishna* defines the means and the way (of *sadhana* and meditation). "

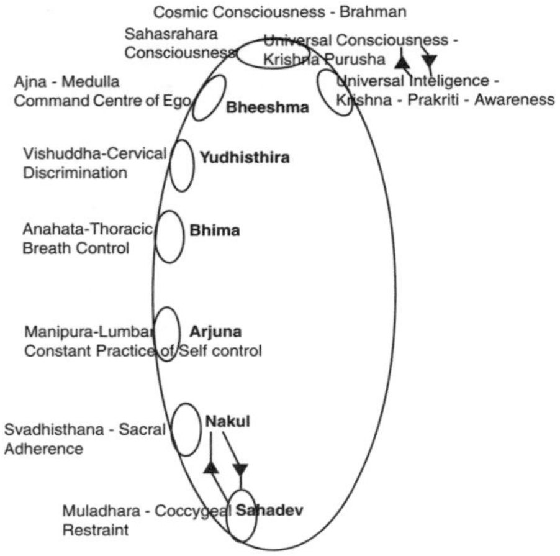

Figure 17. Symbolic representations of the Pandavas with the Spiritual Centres or *chakras*

The five outgoing desiring senses and the mind are *tamasic* tendencies of the physical body. The lower three *chakras, muladhara* (coccygeal)*, svadhisthana* (sacral)*, and manipura* (lumbar) are the *rajasic* areas of the divine cave (brain and spinal cord) where maximum self-control and training is necessary. The next two centres, *anhaata* (thoracic) and *vishuddha* (cervical), are considered *sattvic,* where the body-mind-intellect are harmonised from previous efforts and is ready for the next flight!

As illustrated in Figure 17, Man has seven spiritual centres.

1. ***Sahadev* for Restraint** (*muladhara* or coccygeal or earth centre) It has the power of restraint against negative rules of morality. It is signified by *yama* or 'Thou-shalt-not. . . ' rules.
2. ***Nakul* for Adherence** (*svadhisthana* or sacral or water centre) has the power to follow the prescribed positive spiritual rules. It is signified by the *niyama* or

'Thou-shalt. . . ' rules of non-injury.

3. ***Arjun* for Self Control** *(manipura* or lumbar or fire power centre); it has the power of patience during efforts in self-control.
4. ***Bhima* for Life-force and Breath control** *(anahata* or dorsal or air centre). The withdrawal of the senses makes this centre enter a state similar to animal hibernation. In deep meditation the breath may drop to 4/minute and the pulse to a basal level of 40 or less per minute.
5. ***Yudhishtira* for Calmness** *(vishuddha* or cervical or space centre). It is the centre of discrimination.

*Of interest to practitioners of reiki, ayurveda, and other health sciences. May be ignored by others.

6. ***Bheeshma for* Partial union *(samadhi)* in astral and causal planes for intellectual-Intuitive Ego knowing about "Me" and "I"** - (*ajnaa* in the medulla). The *ajnaa chakra* and the *Kutastha Chaitanya* or the Christ Centre for Universal Intelligence, reside in the *ajnaa chakra.* It reflects in the *bhrumadhya* in between the eyebrows as **Awareness**.
7. **Complete *samadhi*** *in Sahasrahara* **for Realisation that the Self is All and All is Self**. This is Universal Consciousness within the cup of ***Krishna* or Spirit**. Here, the practitioner finally erases the difference between Universal Intelligence or awareness in *prakriti* and Universal Consciousness or *purusha* and merges in the ecstasy of *yoga* as Cosmic Consciousness or *Brahman* or God. The *sahasrahara* is located in the parietal lobe of the brain, but the ecstasy is "mindless" and resides in the heart *chakra (chinnamasta).*

**Srotas (physical) and Nadis (astral) or Channels:

***Srotas* are channels in the physical body that interconnect with *nadis* or channels of the subtle body for the supply of energy or *prana.* Seventy-two thousand *nadis* are said to exist: only fourteen of these will be referred to since they are involved both with spiritual aspirations and good physical health, both necessary for meditation.

The **three chief *nadis*** are the subtle channels of ***sushumna*** (in the spinal cord)***, ida*** (parasympathetic and ancient) *and* ***pingala*** (sympathetic and controlling). These subdivide into fourteen *nadis*, which in turn divide into many thousands of *nadis* located all over the body.

The **parasympathetic nervous system** is related to the *sushumna, ida, pingala, and varuni* which act as carriers of life's vital energy - *prana.* The *sushumna* is the most important of these channels *(pranavaha)* because it deals with the body's physiological functions. Acupuncture meridians correspond with the *pranavaha channels*, without which it would be impossible to function through the parasympathetic and the sympathetic nervous systems. It would also be impossible to utilise the mind for the creation of impressions.

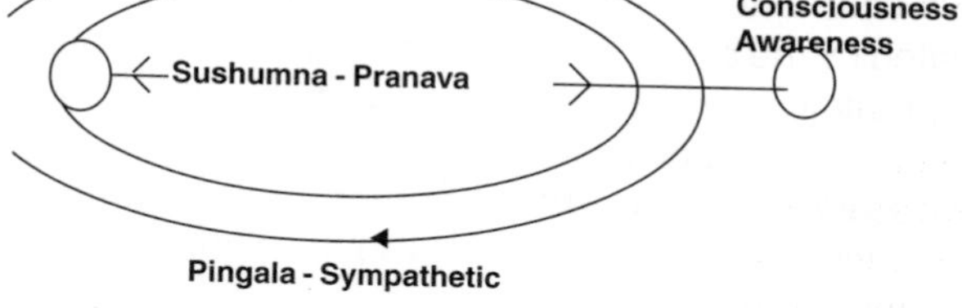

Figure 18. The parasympathetic or *ida* and sympathetic *pingala* connect to the main nervous system

The **sympathetic nervous system** involves the *manovaha nadi* which carries the mental and psychological energies. *Ten nadis* belong to the *manovaha nadi group* and are interconnected with the *ida, pingala, pranavaha* and the *varuni* channels. (fourteen in all.)

The ***sushumna*** is the most important of the *nadis*. It begins in the pelvic plexus and ends at the cerebro-spinal axis, between the two cerebral hemispheres. Running through the centre of the astral spine, it controls all the functions of the body and the *chakras* and corresponding to the central spinal canal in the physical cord of the spine. It controls all the other energy-requiring functions of the body and the seven *chakras.* It has the nature of space and is balanced in terms of *ayurvedic* humours (*kapha,* ***pitta****, and vata*). It is activated by ***prana shakti*** (life-force *aum*) and is ***sattvic*** in quality. It is related to the essence of the lustre of **fire** as the ***tejas*** of awareness.

Auxiliary to the astral spinal cord and the brain, and on each side of the physical spine, are two major *nadis* whose movement intertwines in figures of eight, one on top of the other: the **astral sympathetic and astral parasympathetic nervous system.**

The **left *nadi*** is the ***ida*** or the chief **parasympathetic channel** reflecting lunar energy, and the **right *nadi*** is ***pingala*** or the chief **sympathetic channel** reflecting solar energy**.** These are the primary channels or *nadis* of the astral autonomic nervous system that control the physical autonomic and endocrine systems of the body. Their pervasiveness of effect is through the release of neurotransmitters and neurohormones.

The ***ida nadi*** runs from the left genital to the left nostril. All yogic practices of breathing or ***pranayama*** begin in the left nostril to promote longevity, creativity, visualisation and the nurturing of higher emotions of calmness of nerves and silence of the mind.

- ***Gandhari*** *and* ***hastajiva*** *nadis* are companions to the *ida nadi. Gandhari nadi* starts at the lower corner of the left eye and ends at the left big toe. *Hastajiva nadi* begins at the lower corner of the right eye and ends at the left big toe also. Ascending psychic energy travels through these nadis from the lower half of the body to the *ajnaa chakra* within the medulla.

The **right *nadi*** is the ***pingala*** or the chief **sympathetic channel** reflecting the aggressive solar energy. It runs from the right genitals to the right nostril. It is also activated by the breath through the right nostril for the promotion of stamina, vigour, and vitality by reviving the body's dynamic energy. It stimulates the aggressive rational practical self.

- ***Yashasvini*** *and* **pusha** *nadis* are companions of the *pingala nadi. Yashasvini* runs from the left ear to the right big toe, the *pusha nadi* from the right ear to the left big toe.
- The ***alambusha nadi*** that begins in the mouth and ends in the anus

provides *prana* for the assimilation and evacuation of food and water as well as for assimilation of ideas and thoughts.

- The ***kuhu nadi*** begins in the throat and ends in the genitals and is used in tantric worship to master the senses.
- The ***shankini nadi*** begins in the throat and ends at the anus and lies to the right of the *sushumna*. It is activated for *vata* disorders when cleansing the colon in *ayurvedic* treatments.
- The ***sarasvati nadi*** begins in the tongue and ends in the vocal chords. It is responsible for speech and the dissemination of knowledge. It accompanies the *sushumna* and has the lunar nature and energy of the female principle.
- The ***pashyavini nadi*** is located in the right ear lobe and connects with the cranial nerves. It is used in *ayurveda* (body-piercing with specific metals and gems) to reduce stress and addictive behaviours.
- The ***varuni nadi*** helps in the purification of bodily wastes and toxins. It originates in the throat and left ear and ends in the anus. It works with the *apana-vayu (pranic* energy) in the large colon and prevents stagnation, characteristic of *vata* disorders of the body. It runs parallel to the *alambusha nadi* but in the opposite direction.
- The ***vishvodhara nadi*** is the last of the thirteen auxiliary nadis located in the navel chakra. It stimulates the adrenals and pancreas and distributes *prana* throughout the body. It is the body's central energy source and is referred to as the *Ki or chi*. *Pranayama* serves to strengthen this pivotal *nadi*. Martial art practices (*Tai chi, quigong*) as well as *yoga* practices are efforts to strengthen this *nadi*.

According to ***ayurveda,*** the Indian Medical Science of Life and Health, the body is made up of seven *dhatus* (body systems) that sustain the body. They are chyle or *rasa*, blood or *rakta*, flesh or *maamsa,* fat or *meda,* bones or *asthi,* marrow or *majjaa,* and semen or *shukra.* These systems keep the body immune from infection and diseases. They are churned together in *pranayama* or breathing for the production of the nectar of life *(amrit).*

Meru is the spinal column. Energy in the parasympathetic *ida* controls the upward ingoing breath while the sympathetic *pingala* energises the outgoing breath. Together with the *sushumna*, they churn the in-breath and the out-breath to create energy stored in the seven chambers or *chakras* of the spine. *Chakras* act as transformers. The vital energy thus generated is *prana* or life-force.

Nadis govern the five senses and the five organs of action and are also connected to the *chakras.*

By seeing how these channels connect with the spiritual centres, the seeker will understand that without *yama and niyama*, he will be unable to overcome obstacles on his spiritual path.

- The head centre or the *sahasrahara* [where all pranic energy is stored] is connected to one central channel — the *sushumna;*
- The medulla has the third eye or *ajnaa centre* (reflected as the *Kutastha*) which is connected to six channels: sensory apertures of the eyes, ears and nose, *ida and pingala* (autonomic), *pusha* and *gandhari, payasvini and shankhini;*
- The throat or *vishuddha* centre is connected to only one channel: the tongue channel of *Sarasvati;*
- The heart centre or the *anahata* is connected to three channels: a general channel *(varuna*) and the two hands *(yashasvati and hastajiva*);
- The navel centre or the *manipura* is connected with three channels: *vishvodhara* to the navel area and the *yashasvati* and *hastajiva* for the lower limbs;
- The sex centre or *svadhisthana* is connected to one channel: the *kuhu* for reproduction;
- The root centre or *muladhara* is also connected to one channel: *alambusha* for elimination.

Prana or life-force emits radiance or auras as it moves in and out of the body through channels. Aura is a function of *ojas,* the essence of the physical body. When the flow is intact and balanced, the energy field of the astral body (physiological-psychological) is clear. If flawed, the energy field is weak and the person shows evidence of:

- Impaired immune system;
- Emotional integrity that is easily unbalanced by unwanted extraneous situations, emotions, and contacts: the whole character is weakened; and
- The *apana vayu* motivates the forces of decay and disease.

Healing begins by restoring the energy field of the subtle body through the increase of *ojas* and reversing the processes of *apana vayu.* Changes in life-style, eating habits, and exposure to external stimuli and environment are needed. Moral issues must be taken into consideration. Finally, efforts must be made to still and silence the mind by reflection and meditation. **

Balancing Nadis

The *nadis* or channels help balance the **three mental energy essences** of the three bodies of a mortal. The energy essence of the **physical** body is the ***ojas;*** the energy essence of the **sensory mind** is the ***prana;*** and, the energy essence of the **intellect** is the ***tejas.***

**Of interest to practitioners of health sciences and may be ignored

These essences flow through the *nadis* or subtle bodily channels. Balancing them requires patience, sensitivity and the gentle persuasion of the will. *Yama* or restraint *and niyamas* or observances of restraints are pre-requisites. *Asana* correct posture at meditation, *pranayama* or regulation of breath, *and dharana* or concentration, lead one to meditation and finally, to *samadhi* or tranquillity in oneness. Until the seeker succeeds in his *sadhana* or spiritual practice, he will make mistakes and must not be judged while trying!.

> and the Master wrote:
>
> ". . Never judge the man; judge his actions. If a man is immoral, a cheat, a gruesome murderer, it is only because of low values, false education, wrong thoughts, and baser goals in life. These you judge and keep away from.
>
> "A patient suffering from typhoid is judged or diagnosed; hate not the patient, hate the disease germ".

Indulgences and Diseases of the Body

The sensitivity of *chakras* is dulled when hammered by indulgences and irresponsible behaviour. Ordinarily, the physiological and psychological control systems nurture the physical body throughout life and try to negate the impacts of wrong actions against it.

- Energy rises to clear paths of ascent and also regulates effects on glands and bodily processes.
- Both the sympathetic and parasympathetic nervous systems act on the plexuses but in opposite directions (constricting and relaxing respectively).
- The parasympathetic fills the body with vitality, supported by cosmic energy - *aum,* while the sympathetic consumes it.
- The *chakras* are transformers for the creation of energy or life force. Sexual energy as *ojas* is the most basic expression of this life-force. Control of life-force does not mean one must not enjoy the pleasures of the senses. For many mortals pleasure of all senses is the only motivating force of their endeavours.
- Continence is the control of life-force and is expected of all mortals. It provides the energy that carries us to goals other than indulgences that are thoughtless or promiscuous. Adolescence is a period of intense studentship or *brahmacharya.* It is also characterised by an enormous outburst of energy which is released by puberty and which needs to be contained and channelled for the child's all-round growth. If the youth-child indulges in sexual activity at this age, a large part of his human potential is thrown away.

The youth-child needs to study and apply his idealistic motivation to achieve. If youthful energy is squandered instead of conserved, the youth-child will discover the life-force in later life only with enormous difficulty. Lack of control leads to despair, dejection and depression in the life of a growing youth. If energy, however is conserved and controlled, he discovers hope and confidence and his mind automatically turns to higher thoughts

As the Master once wrote to one my adolescent children:

> "Such a dull state of mind would visit all of us during growth and maturity. Keep clean thoughts and give yourself a schedule of work for the hands and mind. It will come only in waves; it will never remain permanently. Try fasting - say one day a month and every Sunday drop dinner. . . during such mental inner restlessness and lack of sleep. "

This is not necessarily easy. Nonetheless, the rewards are immeasurable. Steady living without a surplus of possessions in the child's life nurtures lack of greed. With his idealism, he discovers the true meaning of life which graces him by unfolding right before him. The child-youth must be first taught the basics of meditation through focusing on **a thought**. In adolescence, he must be taught the Science of Yoga in greater detail. He must be shown the triggers of desires and their ability to lead him to indulgences and taught how to resist them.

Mind-Altering Drugs and Environments

When the **life-force is balanced**, the energy in the sympathetic or *pingala* and the parasympathetic or *ida* autonomic systems are equal. This happens during meditation. In this state of 'beingness', there is a higher state of mind and perception.

A healthy astral body also has a **balanced flow** through the body's subtle channels. **Excess flow** through the channels manifests as hyperactivity, hysterical behaviour, dizziness, insomnia, hallucinations, and disturbing dreams. **Deficient flows** through the *nadis* are characterised by the opposite which take the form of apathy, fatigue, dulled senses, dulled mind and emotions. **Blocked *nadis*** manifest as severe emotional blockage and pain with difficulty in self-expression, leading to inappropriate emotional outbursts, neurosis, and even insanity.

Mind-altering drugs cause excessive flow through the *nadis or channels, which become* overstimulated and eventually burn out. ***Nadis*** can be similarly **deranged** by wrong attitudes, and impressions, and a poor environment, negative emotions, egoism, poor upbringing, incorrect diet, lack of exercise, and sexual indulgence.

Emotional Disorders

Weakness in the left lunar channels or *ida* cause dramatic swings of emotional outbursts varying from elation to depression.

- These are reactions from conditioned-beings with tendencies of lethargy, self-obsession, and negativity.
- They become prone to senile decay because of chronic pressures on the left sided channels and right brain.

To implement desires, the *pingala* or solar channels activate motor activity through the *sushumna* as well as the intellect. Motor activity triggered by desires registered in the right brain become a by-product of ego in the left brain.

Brain Hemispheres

The two hemispheres of the brain perform complementary but opposite functions.

The **left brain** monitors the right side of the body.

- It specialises in linear thinking (planning, analysis, language, and investigative memory processing).

The **right brain** monitors the left side of the body.

- It is concerned with memory, insight, sex drive, foresight, logical thinking, and past desires, emotions and anger.

The left hemispheric brain has the ability to transform and transcend itself and the mind's conditioning from many previous births. It can lose its preoccupation with sense involvement and emotions.

- It expresses itself as learning and development.
- Creativity expresses here in newer structuring, behaviour patterns, conceptual thinking, symbolic language, abstract thinking and painting.
- Its development requires a delicate link through the *chitrini* in the fifth *chakra*.
- Inspired creativity operates through the *chitrini* that has connections with the Infinite Collective Consciousness.

When there is channel-overload in the *ida or pingala*, there is constant irritation which blurs the normal sensitivity and weakens the stabilising effects of the life-force energy.

- Because the nervous system is unable to decode the messages in the autonomic nervous system, bodily cells malfunction causing disease, fatigue, and exhaustion.
- All bodily diseases are, therefore, the result of senseless indulgences for the sake of pleasure.

The acting man, in his ignorance, thinks he is the doer: the body is him. This false assumption of the ego strengthens excessive activity in the right-sided channels *(pingala)* and the left side of the brain: both of these swell until there is no more room to expand.

The energy overflow spills into the right brain at the super-ego or *vasana* personality centre and submits the left channels to overload. A person experiencing this becomes calculating, aggressive, cunning, absurd, and lacking in spontaneity.

Physical Expressions of the Astral Autonomic Nervous System

The conscious principle or "I" functioning as "Me", must desire "I" (God) to manifest His Love. The moment it is desired, the Life-Force Energy become more manifest in the body.

The physical and metaphysical fields of energy exist as **the desiring force**:

- The metaphysical fields of energy exist on the left side in the **lunar channels** of the ***Ida.*** With them, come the awareness of past memories to assist and modify present actions, both in the waking or conscious and dream or subconscious states.

  These memories are unconscious conditions, beliefs, and concepts which influence and colour all actions in this life.

  As long as there is desire to live, this channel is active.

  This channel awakens conditioned emotions and past habits.

  It manifests as the super-ego on the right side of the brain.

  The super-ego (with vanities, beliefs, righteous indignation) is the personality of feelings - the psyche of the individual, the unique *vasanas.*
- **To satiate and implement desires**, the life-force assumes moods for action down the **right side** of the spine in the ***pingala*** through the **solar channels**.
  The activating force is the desire to act or the will which requires "me" to function through a logical mind to execute the willed act.
  The act is therefore a by-product of the Ego or "Me" which resides more on the left side of the brain.
- Both **right and left autonomic channels** express subtle energies. This energy becomes manifest as physical activities, supported by **physiological and psychological life-forces.** This is an expression of the combined working of the *ida* or parasympathetic, *pingala* or sympathetic and the *sushumna* or the connection to central nervous systems.
- While the desiring-force converts all desires into action, the **"Me" must sustain itself by enjoying and experiencing pleasure.**
  This **pleasurable experience** is the power-of-sustenance and **connects the astral *sushuma*** with the **pituitary and pineal glands** (source of neurotransmitters and neurohormones)**,** and **the limbic cortex** (where the mind records emotions and addictions) **near the spiritual eye.** The sustenance of the subtle body functions and the evolution of man are

executed through the central spine - *sushumna* via the *brahmanadi.* Through this channel, man or **object** links with its source or **subject**.

aum - pranava: the Ultimate Support of Manifestations

The voluntary and the autonomic nervous systems are incapable of decoding messages presented to them as essences of thought [thought-trons], energy [lifetrons], and atomic units [electrons].

It is *aum*, the all comprehensive, sacred, mystical symbol, which stands for the Infinite, Indefinable, mysterious power that pervades everything, known as *Brahman* or God in Hindu philosophical thought. It is the *pranava* or <u>Word-God</u>, the <u>all</u> in each of the three bodies of the mortal:

- As **Awaring Principle** in the **causal state** of each cell, *aum* is vibrant and alive as its thought-essence in each atom and cell in the *sattvic* body;
- As **life-force energy**, this vibrating force is the Life-Force, *aum* which enters the cord and brain or divine cave, through the Mouth-of-God or medulla as *prana* into the *rajasic* body;
- In the divine cave, a*um* **enlivens the subtle astral or spiritual centres** of the spine and brain. At all these centres, *aum* can be heard" in different tones, as *aum*-Awareness or God-Awareness. In the *Sahasrahara* it is "heard" as *aum* of many oceans!

At one of our meetings, my wonderful Master of few words nudged my thoughts as I languished in the thought of how this 'meeting' with the Self would be like. As usual he had picked my thoughts:

the Master roared:

". . *"aham brahma asmi:"* Every human being can attain to the knowledge of this truth and make his whole life an expression of It. Perfection is not only open to all, but is in every one already. It only has to unfold. There is no such thing as 'spiritual death' apart from a refusal to evolve. All humanity is an expression of the divine. ."

I suddenly realised I was 'That'! Why was I looking for It outside myself? What meeting? With whom was I to meet? Why did I need to erase myself? Why does it take so long for me to be convinced that I was divine?

The Chakras or Spiritual Centres

The psycho-spiritual plexuses or *chakras* are not ordinarily open because they are dominated by *tamas* or inertia of the physical *and rajas* or activity of the subtle envelopment of the divine cave. Their opening is a reflection of the person's *sadhana* or spiritual practices and signify the attainment of *sattva* of inner harmony. Even to merely awaken or spiritualise the lower three *chakras* requires *yogic* discipline and effort. Only when pure *sattva* dominates a *sadhak* or seeker do the *chakras* undergo awakening and spontaneous opening.

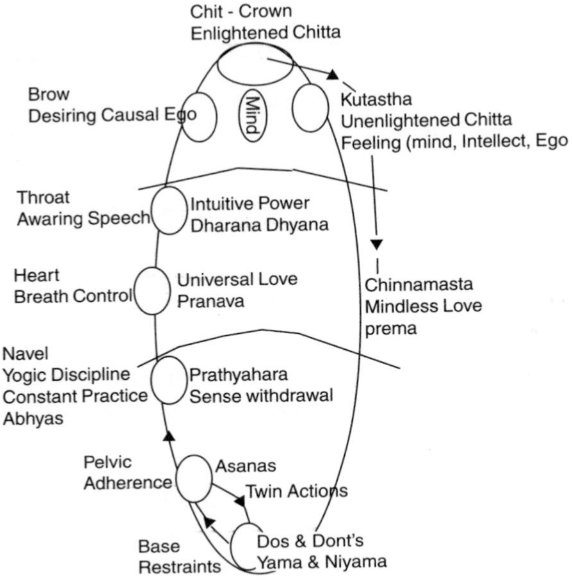

Figure 19. Chakras, "Me" & "I"- Disciplines of *sadhana*

All work done to spiritually open the *chakras* are mental in nature *(yama* or restraints, *niyama* or observances, *asana* or correct posture, *dharana* or concentration, *pranayama* or regulation of breath, and *pratyahara* or wilful withdrawal from the senses*)*. They can be opened with drugs as well as with the use of powerful mental techniques. **I**

In *yoga*, no one sets out to physically "open" *chakras*, especially not the lower three *chakras*, which involve in indulgences, anger, and greed). *Yoga* only aims at stilling the mind and silencing it.

Disarming the mind results in the triggering of finer emotions in the heart and throat *chakras.* The involvement of the *ajnaa chakra* harmonises the causal body as *chitta* with the self or *chit.*

Spiritual knowledge is gained through the heart *chakra,* by negating the ego and superego.

A meditative experience of a *void* is a sign that the seeker is in the *sushumna* and must now enter the various *chakras* for further evolution. There is a gap in the ***sushumna*** at the navel point near the ***manipura chakra***, and is where seekers encounter a "hurdle." The rising awareness achieved during meditation, meets an obstruction at the navel point and efforts at intended meditation slip. **Activity in the *chakras* can be experienced, during meditation, as vibrations**

in different parts of the left hand, as well as, the left foot):

- base chakra or *muladhara* at the left wrist = **coccyx**
- pelvic chakra or *svadhisthana* at the left thumb = **sacral**
- navel chakra or *manipura* at third finger = **lumbar**
- heart chakra or *anahata* in palm periphery of hand = **thoracic**
- throat chakra or *vishuddha* at fifth finger = **cervical**
- brow-aligned or *ajna*a at index finger = **medulla**
- crown chakra or *sahasrahara* at palm centre = **parietal lobe**

There are *seven chakras* or spiritual centres in the divine cave, in *three groups of evolution*:

- Group 1: the first five *"mundane" chakras* that serve "Me";
- Group 2: the *ajnaa chakra of "thought" and life-force* that serves unevolved *chitta* or "Me" masquerading as "I";
- Group 3: the *sahasrahara chakra* of the "beyond" or *chitta* becoming the *chit.*

I. Mundane Chakras

i. The mundane *chakras* are the *chakras* of the five senses and the five organs of action.

ii. They are concerned with five vital airs or physiological life-forces and psychological (emotions, mind/intellect) makeup. **They motivate all the functions of the endocrine systems through the medium of neurohormones and neurotransmitters.
   - Adrenals through the *muladhara* or base *chakra*;
   - Ovaries and testicles through the *svadhishana* or second sacral *chakra*;
   - Pancreas, spleen, and liver (small intestine) through the *manipura* or navel *chakra;*
   - Thymus and heart through the *anahata* or heart *chakra;*
   - Thyroid and parathyroid through the *vishuddha* or throat *chakra;*
   - Pituitary and pineal glands through the *ajnaa chakra;*
   - The *sahasrahara chakra* controls all the previous *chakras.*

According to ***Ayurvedic* classification of disease**,

- Most *vata disorders* originate as dysfunction in the *muladhara chakra*, involving the metabolism of earth and *apana vayu* in the colon.
- Most *kapha disorders* originate as dysfunction in the *svadhisthana chakra* involving the reproductive centre of indulgences and water metabolism.
- Most *pitta disorders* originate as dysfunction of the navel or *manipura chakra* involving the fire of digestion in the small intestine and the liver.
- Most psychological problems originate as dysfunction of the heart or *anahata chakra* where all negative emotions are stored.

**The next two paragraphs are for readers interested in the ancient healing sciences of the East. Those not interested in the subject should skip it.

These are physical, physiological, psychological diseases of the anatomical 'physical' centres. **Spiritual awakening** of the *astral chakras* involve **mastering *pranas*** or the elemental essence of the elements: **they are processes** that occur at different levels of spiritual effort.

iii. Five observances are required in *sadhana* during self-improvement of the five *mundane chakras.* The restraints are *yamas* or universal moral commandments are rules of self-purification to be achieved. They are "Thou shalt" commandments of:
   - cleanliness;
   - contentment;
   - self perfection of body and senses;
   - self analysis; and
   - attentiveness.

iv. Five observances or *niyamas* are moral rules to be observed are. They are the "Thou shalt not" commandments of:
   - non-injury to others;
   - truthfulness;
   - no theft;
   - spiritual conduct; and
   - absence of greed.

II. Thought Chakra at Ajnaa for Chitta

This is the point where the *Ida* or parasympathetic *and Pingala* or sympathetic nerve channels join the central channel in the *sushumna* to end in front of the *ajnaa chakra* in the medulla oblongata. It (the central nexus) is in alignment with the *Kutastha Chaitanya* or the Krishna-Christ Centre [in front] behind and between the two eyebrows, in the region of the pineal and pituitary glands. The *ajnaa* is the "home" of the *chitta* or the complex mood-feeling of the mind-intellect-ego, combined.

- Awareness enters here, into the abode of "Me" (pseudo-soul) the causal or desiring or *vasanic.* Sage *Patanjali* describes the enlightened *chitta* as "consciousness of," without the encumbrance of "Me" (unenlightened *chitta)* when it is purified.
- This is also the location of the "third eye".
- When control has reached this level, "I" reigns increasingly supreme because "It" has understood and appreciated the pleasures of the five mundane *chakras* catering to "Me".
- Transcendence of this *chakra* leads to the 1000 petalled lotus of the secret *chakra* in the *sahasrahara.* The *chitta* becomes *chit.* Awareness of Universal Intelligence now becomes Universal Consciousness.

III. Crown or "secret" Chakra (Sahasrahara)

The comprehension of this *chakra* is beyond intuition.

- In its centre is the Void beyond space of Universal Consciousness or *chit:* the Ultimate that is served in secret even by all *devas* or divine beings.
- Its experience is beyond the mind-intellect-ego or *chitta* and thus beyond thought. It is experienced in the spiritual heart.

Patanjali says that although the mind-intellect-ego as *chitta* is necessary to get to the sixth *chakra*, the mind (thought) must be erased, in order to merge into the Universal Consciousness of the seventh *chakra*. The soul or *chitta* or awareness or *shakti or prakriti,* now stands temporarily apart from the eternal witness or *chit* or *shakta or purusha,* and merges as "One" Universal Consciousness that becomes the Cosmic Consciousness or *Brahman* or God.

Swami Chinmayananda was always a 'master' at describing the un-describable, so here he goes again:

> and the Master wrote:
>
> ". . When the Self shines forth absolutely free from all limiting adjuncts, brilliant, as a homogeneous mass of consciousness in its nature as pure intelligence, independent, then it is spoken of as *pratyag-atman,* the inner Self. . "
>
> "This is the Self of the *jivan mukta* (enlightened soul). This is *"tat twam asi"*: the indicative or implied 'Thou' in 'Thou are That' is addressed to the Pure Consciousness, the Self which is free from all identifications or *upadhis. . . "*

An illustrative designation of the bodily kingdom was devised by *Paramahansa Yogananda* (author of 'Autobiography of a Yogi'), who describes the bodily kingdom affected by rulers and inhabitants. The Palace is the brain, where rulers reside in the domains of superconsciousness. It is Centre of Universal Consciousness for Bliss; Centre of Universal Intelligence at the *Kutastha* in the Krishna-Christ Centre between and behind the eyebrows; and, Centre of Life Force or Aum in the medullary *ajnaa chakra*; here, the causal or *vasanic body* is buried as the *unenlightened chitta* (mind-intellect-ego complex) for sense existence, or as the *enlightened chitta* for emancipation.

The enlightened *chitta* discovers that self is the Self. This can be conceptualised but needs to become part of the seeker's psyche. It requires constant introspection and assimilation.

Yogananda says the rulers have loyal subjects influenced by the enlightened intellect or intelligence or *buddhi:*

- Medulla where the *unenlightened ego* resides in the *ajnaa*;
- Cervical or *vishuddha chakra* for intuition or dishonest speech and pride; and
- Dorsal or *anahata chakra* for peace or sensuousness.

There are as well, common subjects who suffer the vagaries of the sensory mind or *manas* when ruled by the ignorant ego. They are obedient only under the influence of a wise discriminative intellect or *buddhi* and the *enlightened chitta*:

- Lumbar or *manipura chakra* for self-control and constant practice of spiritual practices or *sadhana*;
- Sacral or *svadhisthana chakra* for observances or adherence to restraints; and
- Coccygeal or *muladhara chakra* for restraints

The Master never tired of reminding me that my pragmatic mind cannot intellectualise God. Even to this day, I regret that my intellectual arrogance came in the way of the Master's teachings. I am convinced I was a difficult student to handle! Yet, he never tired of coaxing me on! Lovingly and gently, he prodded me into the direction that would be of most benefit to me! A perfect Master, he never tired of the same question in different apparels:

> and the Master wrote:
>
> ". . Because Brahman or God cannot be conceived by the Intellect, It cannot be defined. Still, to convey some idea at the intellectual level, some sort of "remote control" method of describing and pointing is depended upon:
>
> "*Yato vacho nivartante aprapya mansa: saha*" from *taiittreeya Upanishad* II: 4 - "Whence all the speech turns back with the mind without reaching It: that is the Eternal Truth, the Brahman" or . . .
>
> *"Satyam jnaanam anantam anandam-Brahma"* or 'That which is Reality, Knowledge, Bliss, is *Brahman'.* The Reality is the indestructible. . .
>
> "That which, when name, space, time, substance, and causation are destroyed, dies not is the indestructible *satya,* the Reality. The essence of Intelligence that has no beginning and no end, Knowledge or *jnana. Ananta* or Bliss, the Infinite is that which remains the same as does clay, gold or cotton in all their modifications like pots, ornaments and cloth respectively, the antecedent all-pervading Consciousness that is in all phenomenon of creation beginning with the Unmanifested. . . " Tat Tvam Asi". . **That You Are**"

Patanjali's Yoga Sutra

Sage *Patanjali* lived between 500 to 2000 BC. Much of what is known about him comes from legends. . His writings on music, dance-form, *ayurveda* or Indian medicine, *sanskrit* grammar, and the *yoga sutras* (yoga of meditation described in 196 sentences) survive him.

I. Moral training

Man has been moulded and remoulded in accordance with the predominating order of the three intermingling characteristics of the three fundamental bodies *or shariras* (gross *or sthula*, subtle *or sukshma,* and causal *or karana*) and their qualities or *gunas (tamas* or inertia*, rajas* or agitation*, and sattva* or harmony*).*

Man is endowed with mind or *manas*, intellect or *manas-buddhi*, and ego or *hanker* - collectively called *"chitta"* or a mood-feeling of self-awareness. The *chitta* is the source of all feeling, thinking, understanding, and acting. As the wheel-of-life turns, the *chitta* experiences five types of miseries:

- *Avidya* or ignorance;
- *Asmita* or selfishness;
- *Raaga* or attachment;
- *Dvesha* or aversion; and
- *Abhinivesha* or love of extrovert life.

The *chitta* is like fire. Fuelled by desires or *vasanas*, it burns until the end of the cycle- of-life. Without desires, the *chitta* becomes without-fire. In this pure state, the *chitta* becomes a source of enlightenment, from the pinnacle of awareness.

Patanjali devised eight stages on the path of realisation. *Chitta,* at first in a stage of dullness is purified through the processes of ***yama*** or restraints***, niyama*** or observances *and* ***asana*** or right posture***. Asana*** and ***pranayama*** or regulation of breath bring the wavering mind to a state of stability. The disciplines of *pranayama and* ***pratyahara*** or withdrawal from the senses at will, and ***dharana*** or concentration make the *chitta* attentive and allows it to focus its energy. It is then restrained enough to reach the state ***dhyana*** or meditation *and* ***samadhi*** or state of oneness**.**

The Master commented on *Patanjali's* prescription of chastening the unenlightened *chitta:*

> and the Master wrote:
>
> ". . . There are three stages of moral and intellectual discipline. ***Shravana*** or listening with faith and acceptance of moral traditions, ***Manana*** or logical reflection to discover the Truth, arrived at by reasoning with oneself, and ***Nidhidhyasan*** or contemplation of your logical reasoning by your own spiritual experience. "

As it progresses, the higher stages of *yoga* become predominant. The preceding stages, however, lay the foundation for this progress and cannot be ignored or neglected. Before exploring the unknown, the seeker must learn about the *chitta.* If he knows the known in its totality, mind-intellect-ego or *chitta* can merge with the unknown, like a river merges with the sea. At that moment, the seeker experiences the highest state of joy or *ananda.*

First, *yoga* deals with health, strength and conquest of the body through the energising of body parts with Life-Force *(pratyahara).* Next, it lifts the veil of difference between the body or matter and mind as energy through regulation of the breath *(pranayama).* Lastly, it leads the seeker to the light of peace and purity by listening to *(dharana-dhyana)* and merging *(samadhi)* with the sound of the AUM or the Holy Spirit. These exercises are efforts at controlling the will.

Yoga systematically teaches man to search for the divinity within himself. He unravels himself from the exterior towards the within. From the nerves of the bodily senses, he enters the mind that controls all emotions. From the mind, he penetrates the intellect, which guides reason and logic. From the intellect, his path takes him to Will and from there to *chitta* the awareness of "Me", the pseudo-soul. The last stage is from Awareness-of-Me to I-Consciousness. It is here that "Me" or self merges with "I" or the a*tma* or Self.

To clarify this further, The Master repeated the need for restraint and observances in spiritual practices:

> "Religion only asks us to live in knowledge, in discriminative understanding of things and beings, and of the correct values of life. There is a lot of difference between facing a situation with the nerve-shattering befouling spectacles of I-ness and My-ness, and facing it in utter dedication to God's will. When attachment oversteps its limits, there is danger of pain at every moment. Religion only wants us to understand ourselves and the world around us, and then to correct the relationship between ourselves and the world. . . "

The purpose of *Yoga* Meditation, therefore, is the unification of "Me", the *chitta* or object with "I", the Self, the subject. It is a journey of the **individual soul** or ***chitta*** or self with the Universal Soul or Self **or *chit*.** This is the quest for the subject and ultimately for God the Spirit.

Before *chitta* can be negated, one must make great effort and endure self-imposed hardship. The aim is to "cast off the extrovert body and the mind" and become a "temple" of the soul. When this happens, the *chitta* leaps into a higher dimension of identification. Doing this repeatedly over time, allows the meditator to achieve union or *samadhi.*

In this state of oneness or *samadhi,* there is neither subject ("I" or *chit)* nor object ("Me" or *chitta).* There is only unification of soul with Spirit, or *chit with chidakasha*, the state of superconsciousness.

The subject ("I") and the object ("Me) stand in opposition. The subjective knowledge ("I") requires the object (Me") to recognise this knowledge. The knowledge is not about the object. To understand the object, one needs to unite the object with the subject. This unification offers the seeker an intuitive understanding of the essence of matter and phenomenon.

To attain *Yoga,* one can follow *Patanjali's* eight-stage cultivation process for the purpose of integration. According to the sage *Adi Shankara* who lived about 1500 years ago, there are fifteen steps involved in the *sadhana*, or spiritual efforts. Both are commentaries on the *Yoga Sutras.* To both these, the Master had this to say:

> "While *Patanjali* prescribed eight steps, the sage *Shankaracharya*, who lived fifteen hundred years ago, advised fifteen steps every seeker must pursue. This is prescribed in the text *"Aparokshanubhuti "*

This text has been taught to the Master's audience in different cities of the world. The Master commented that the message is the same! All seekers start with moral training.

Moral Training involves cultivating attitudes of behaviour and character so that the organs of perception and the organs of action are freed from impediments. Many have wondered why seekers make no progress despite years of meditation practices; others have asked why they "fall" by the wayside during spiritual efforts. The answer to this is that we repeatedly ignore the *yamas* or restraints *and niyamas* or observances of ordinary living; unless these are reasserted every day of our lives, no gains can be made. At the end of the day, one needs to carefully review his daily activities:

Things to Ponder:

and as a wise one said:
"Does my work harm others in any way?
Do I steal from my employer in small ways?
Does my choice of work reflect my spiritual values?
Do I bring a generous heart to my work?"

1. ***Yama* or Restraints or 'do no evil'** is a collective name for universal commandments. Great vows (*mahavratas)* are made of non-violence *(ahimsa*), truth *(satya)*, non-stealing *(asteya),* continence or self-control *(brahmacharya*), and non-covetousness *(aparigraha*).

The seeker practices non-violence by withdrawing from injury in thought, mind, and deed. There is now instead a *residual characteristic of an all-embracing love for everything and everyone.* The seeker is ruthlessly truthful and honest with himself. Whatever he thinks or speaks turns out to be true. He controls his wants and things come to him without asking. Temperance or self-restraint or *yama* is enjoined in imagination and in fact.

> and the Master wrote on *Yama:*
> "... to intellectually appreciate the insistence of the scriptures that "All is Brahman" and sincerely try to turn our attention entirely away from the sense-world is *yama*. This natural sense control that is effortlessly gained by an ardent seeker when he practices to turn his attention to the Divine Self within is true and enduring *yama*.

2. ***Niyama* or Adherence to restraints or rules of self-purification** include purity *(saucha),* contentment *(santosha),* austerity *(tapas),* study of scriptures (*svadhyaaya),* and surrender of all actions at the feet of the Lord *(ishvara pranidhaana).*

The seeker knows that his body and senses are susceptible to desires which prejudice the mind. He starts by rooting out the six evils: passion *(kama),* anger (*krodha),* greed *(lobha)*, infatuation *(moha)*, pride *(mada),* and envy *(matsarya).*

> and the Master commented:
> ". . . To maintain in our mind an unbroken flow of similar thoughts about the Changeless, Infinite Self by effectively stopping all dissimilar thoughts - thoughts of the pluralistic world, rushing to disturb the existing rhythm of the quietened mind at peaceful rest in the Self is *niyama*: a state of dynamic quietude at the manual level. When a seeker's mind has come steadily to get lost in the contemplation of the Nature of the self, it is said to be established in *niyama*.

This eradication is possible by occupying the mind with thoughts leading to divinity. Contentment reduces desires; austerity disciplines body to endure hardships and adversity and directs the mind towards the self within; study leads to self-education in search for the truth. Surrender unto the Lord of Actions leads to a life abiding in His Will. *Niyamas*, therefore, are virtues that calm the mind.

The ability to calm and elevate the mind and control desires and emotions should start in childhood. *Yama and niyama* should be **nurtured in childhood by parents and teachers** who must start by teaching children to distinguish between right and wrong. Wrong should be punished sufficiently to allow for its permanent deterrent. Right should receive praise as reinforcement. These real-life **lessons work unconsciously and maintain a balance between their conscious and unconscious states**.

According to *Shakaracharya* in the text *"Saundari Lahari",* the only way for adults to enter the spiritual journey is to invoke the "housewife" of the creator of the universe or *Sarasvat*; the consort of the preserver or *Lakshmi*); and companion of the dissolver of the universe or *Parvati*. *Kali* is the first and phenomenon-form of the *Devi* or Mother Nature. The *Devi's* nine functional-forms combined is *Durga,* the *Mahamaya or Mahashakti* - the Holy Spirit or Mother Mary.

Once, after meeting the Master, my daughters had a discussion about adoring Mother Nature. Both girls refused to adore Her, and the Master advised that the ancestral deity *Kali* should be worshipped, explaining,

> "She represents how Mother Divine becomes angry when anyone troubles Her devotees. It is the expression of Mother's Love. . And She protects all Her children through their evolution. "
>
> "She is the Eternal Physical Universe. As **phenomenon,** She manifests in many ways, both pleasing and terrible, as a serene benefactress and also as the destructive forces of lightning, typhoons, and earthquakes. "
>
> "In an ocean there are many waves, but all the waves are just different manifestations of the same ocean water. There is only One God, one Infinite power and the deities are different manifestations of that one power . . of Mother Nature. "

The, *Mahamaya or Durga or Mahashakti* represents knowledge, wisdom, and the three *vedas* for the three faculties of speech, mind and breath. Worship begins with Knowledge which is Her real form. Inner worship is meditation.

The Master's comment reminded me of my study of the Bible. The Master's teachings clarified my study of this text also:

> "In the beginning was the Word, and the Word was with God. . All things were made by him; and without him was not any thing made". . John 1: 1,3
>
> "I am Alpha and Omega, the beginning and the ending, saith the Lord, which is, and which was, and which is to come, the Almighty". . Revelation 1: 8

The Master confirmed that all inner search must lead to the discovery of the "Word" - the Cosmic Sound: *aum*. This discovery is both a teaching and an understanding. It is mysterious and causes us to lose interest in the mind. She, the *Mahamaya,* takes us beyond time and space into the secrets of Eternity and Infinity.

> And now to digress with a personal experience of Western misunderstanding of Eastern thought My father was never one for the "luxury" of "boredom and self-pity". . **'write down what bothers you'** he admonished repeatedly:
>
> "Whatever it is that bothers you, vomit it up on paper with your pen! When you have finished with your self-indulgence, forget whatever it is that happened".

In the nineties, a "Fisherman's Club" sent me a copy of " The Traitor, the *Kali-Ma* of India!" I was incensed with the material! As urged by my father, I penned a research paper on *Kali* which I was going to send in 'retaliation'!

The research material was beautiful and informative even for the likes of me. What follows is to introduce the *devi* worship practised by Hindus. They adore Mother Nature in all Her functional forms.

How can anyone fathom the Holy Spirit? It is Mother Nature who inspires, guides, unfolds and leads to the comprehension of Her Energy and Power, and of Herself as Creation: the ultimate manifestation and embodiment of Motherhood! May we meet Her in all Her Forms in our journey into ourselves.

Also, allow me to share with you what I found in the Bible about adoring God and the Cosmic Mother in every form imaginable:

> "In whatever way people are devoted to Me, in that measure I manifest Myself to them" . . Mathew 10: 29.

Yoga techniques involve the awakening of this Energy of the physiological-psychological or subtle body residing in the seven *chakras*. Each *chakra* governs a single element, sense organ, organ of action, life-force or *prana*, and a function of the mind. Each has a physical counterpart through a physiological system, nerve plexus and an endocrine gland:

- *Muladhara* or coccygeal plexus is governed by *Shakhini*. It is related to earth and bones and rules smell, nose, organs of reproduction and lower organs of action and governs mind as ego and **downward moving energy** or *apana vayu;*

- *Svadhisthana* or sacral plexus is governed by *Kakini.* It is related to water and water tissues of fat. It rules taste, tongue, and organs of elimination and governs the sensate mind as emotion; it is an **upward moving energy or** *prana vayu;*
- Manipura or lumbar plexus is governed by *Lakini.* It is related to fire and fires of digestion in the small intestine, liver, pancreas, sense of sight and the lower organs of action. It governs the reasoning mind or intellect and **upward moving energy** or *udana vayu;*
- *Anahata* or thoracic plexus is governed by *Rakini.* It is related to air, blood tissue, and upper organs of action and rules sense of touch and skin. It governs conditioned awareness as *chitta* and is the **seat of diffusive energy** as *vyanaya vayu*, governing all the other *pranas*
- *Vishuddha* or cervical plexus is governed by *Dakini.* It is related to ether, plasma, and rules sound in ears and vocal cords and is where individual soul resides. It is source of inspiration, and **balances air or *pranic* energy** through *samana vayu*;
- *Ajnaa* in the medulla is governed by *Hakini.* It is the centre of command of the previous five *chakras* and is related to the nerve connection with the seven tissues *(dhatus)*. It rules the mind as organ of senses and organ of action and is the **seat of all the *pranas*, intellect, and ego as *chitta*.** As well it is the seat of Universal intelligence or *chit* and is in contact with Universal Consciousness or *chidakasha* as *Ishvara, or Purusha.*
- The *Sahasrahara* in the parietal lobe is the seat of pure Universal Consciousness, the seat of *Purusha* and the latent *aum.* It is governed by *Yakini,* **the essence** of mental and physical ethers and the essence of life itself as *ojas, tejas and prana.* It is physically related to the cerebrum and the motor nervous system. Its essence controls the endocrine system through the pineal and pituitary glands.

Raja Yoga

Meditation is a subject that must be learned. To make progress, loving attention must be given to the subject. One must have an intense desire to learn and an earnest spirit of inquiry. Finally, there must also be steadfastness until the desire is attained. The Bible confirms the same truth:

> "I am the way [Universal Consciousness of Christ or Krishna], the truth, and the life: no man cometh unto the Father [merging of the Spirit beyond Creation], but by me" John 14. 6
>
> "Faith is the substance of things hoped for; the evidence of things not seen". . Hebrews 11: 1

Most of us spend our best efforts and time securing our worldly existence or indulging in intellectual controversies over theories, but seldom think it worthwhile to realise and patiently experience life's truths. Others spend their misguided efforts flitting from one organization to another or from one teacher to another seeking satisfaction: this only leads to spiritual indigestion. Whatever the faith of the seeker, there has to be both trust and faith in the teachings of their scriptures. This creates a single-pointedness of intent: "I want God!"

> "Trust in the Lord with all thine heart. . . In all thy ways acknowledge Him, and He shall direct thy paths" . . . Proverbs 3: 5-6.

One must understand that all spiritual ignorance is the result of bondage to the body over millions of births. Bondage cannot be freed in one day nor during short practices at meditation. To reach the supreme state of happiness and bliss, one must practice for a very long time, until the inner organs can be wilfully controlled.

The brain works through the seven spiritual centres: energy currents flow through these centres to the outer sensory organs as well as through the internal organs, keeping them vibrating with "life". The brain is the supreme power-house and the highest centre. It sends intelligent sub-atomic energy or *pranic* current to connect all the centres with the senses and organs of action. Therefore, the brain has the power to shut off these thought creating currents from the senses, the internal organs, and the motor system. It does that automatically in <u>unconscious sleep</u> and can be made to do the same in <u>conscious-sleep</u> or meditation.

The Bible confirms the same with:

> "Neither shall they say, Lo here! or lo there! for, behold, the kingdom of God is within you". . Luke 17: 21
>
> "Know ye not that ye are the temple of God, and that the Spirit of God dwelleth in you?" Corinthians 3: 16

As with sleep, the rest resulting from meditation revitalises the internal organs and their working power, thereby prolonging life. Just as we are not afraid to sleep, there is no need to fear to practice <u>conscious death</u>, which gives rest to the internal organs of the body, especially the heart and the lungs. Death, then, is under our own control: when we think the body is unfit, we are able to leave it of our own accord.

The Master simplified this subject by alluding to the BMI Chart. He wrote to me on physical and 'death' in meditation:

> ". . When you die, you leave the gross-body (B) and it is only your subtle-body (M and I) and the causal-body (V) that leaves. Even when you live as a mortal or in meditation, how can your children or their father "see" your (M and I)?

Raja Yoga then, is a scientific method to draw the life current from the periphery into our central part: into the Acave of awareness" in the spinal cord and the brain. Over time, this area is magnetised and can be withdrawn through the seven star-like astral cerebro-spinal centres. Each opening of the *chakra* reveals the mystery of an ascending understanding of the Spirit.

Attractive sensations are felt in the course of the magnetising of the spine. Continued practice brings conscious Bliss that counteracts the excitement of body-consciousness. We experience a real expansion of our real selves. Our narrow individuality falls away, and a state of Universality is reached. We gradually leave the world of senses and wandering thoughts and come to the region of heavenly Bliss.

When by constant practice, the consciousness of this blissful state becomes real, we find we are always in the presence of the inner Bliss. We discharge our duties better, paying attention to duty rather than for ego. We have solved the mystery of existence and the real meaning of life. This is also confirmed in the Bible:

> "But seek ye first the kingdom of God, and His righteousness: and all these things shall be added unto you". . Mathew 5: 33.

Harnessing Life Force

Ordinarily, our normal existence binds us to our own narrow individuality through the **life force** that is directed outwards, keeping our body and mind disturbed with our bodily sensations and passing thoughts. *Raja Yoga* turns this very same life-force inwards towards our own Awareness of the Self. All religions enjoin the control of the life force so that the seeker can transcend the body and the mind. However, one must know how to reverse the life force at will.

Knowledge is based upon perception, inference and intuition.

- The senses receive stimuli from the world of objects and the mind connects their influence as impressions. If the storage of these impressions is haphazard, they remain confused and disconnected. If the discriminative intellect takes in the impressions and has them codified against distinct associations (memory, likes and dislikes, and habits), the *buddhi* interprets them and projects them to the various parts of the brain as stored "knowledge". This is **knowledge through perception.**

  When *buddhi* or intellect turns back upon itself to know the ultimate knowledge of Truth, it remains confined within its own past associations with the senses. The intellect cannot see beyond itself into the pre-sensuous knowledge of knowing, the blissful state of beingness.

  In response to the following complaint: "The Hindu Scriptures are designed to confuse and blast all intelligent thought!"

  and the Master responds:

  "When the bell in the temple is rung, some recognise it as the friction of two metals: others hear the lingering resonance of the warble. This applies to Scriptural statements and their unending re-echoing suggestiveness". . . .

- **Knowledge through inference,** whether through deduction or induction, is also based upon distinct past associations of a knowledge base ("there is no smoke without fire"). Once more, the intellect cannot go beyond itself to experience the mystery of the Truth. Meditation and devotional prayers can still the thoughts, but our old habits of many previous lives do not allow us to penetrate into the pre-sensuous blissful state.
- **Intuition** is the only way to know the pre-sensuous world; here, there are no senses and no thoughts. This is where all knowledge of things and beings and laws of Nature reside, sealed away from mankind. Man can only hope to reach its threshold through intuition. Through an intuitive experience and a realisation we can reach the Truth.

Intuitive understanding was discussed by the Master. Guests at a gathering were discussing the poetry of a series of misunderstood poets of yore, such *as Omar Khayam, Rabindranath Tagore, and Khalil Gibran.* A recently translated Persian manuscript on the mystic-poet *Nassrudin,* led to the following discussion:

> and the Master said:
>
> ". . . *Nassrudin* while riding a donkey, suddenly lost control of the animal who ran helter skelter. A passer-by, who was watching the ride cried out: '*Nassrudin*, where are you going in such a hurry?" Precariously holding on to the mad donkey, *Nassrudin* screamed back. . " Please ask my donkey. '. "

The power of intuition is held hostage by the frailties of the human form. The body and mind are subject to physical diseases that are the result of indulgences, mental incapacity, indolence, doubts, false beliefs, instability of the mind, and identification with the world of objects and aspirations. These frailties are inherent as *samskaras* (natural tendencies from previous births) or because of our association with persons and situations that prevent such inquiry. Only will power and association with the right persons and environments allow the spirit of inquiry to grow.

The Bible clearly identifies all that has been discussed in the introduction. The spiritual centres in the divine cave is the ladder that must be ascended during spiritual practice. The sound of the 'Word' must be followed to its destination in the brain area of the divine cave.

> "I was in the Spirit on the Lord's day [Oneness *in samadhi*], and heard behind me (*ajnaa chakra*) a great voice, as of a trumpet [Cosmic Sound *Aum*]. . and I turned to see the voice that spake with me. And being turned [inside in meditation], I saw seven golden candlesticks [seven *chakras*];
>
> and in the midst of the seven candlesticks one [seven spiritual centres in astral body of divine cave] like unto the man [physical body]. . and his voice as the sound of many waters [vibrating *Aum* sounds of different tones emanating from the seven astral centres]" Revelation 1: 10, 12, 13, 15.

Conclusion

We are told constantly: "God is everywhere" and that "He is in you". None of us see Him because none of us were told that He is both Spirit and matter combined. "I am in God". God is not relegated somewhere in the Infinity to an antiseptic corner dictating what is and is not to happen. Rather, each individual soul, from the level of a stone to the highest evolved being, exists in the Universe by virtue of the "total desires".

It is difficult for some to conceive of God as Spirit, as both Light of Consciousness and Energy of Matter. We are unconscious of the existence of the Cosmic Energy, *Aum* ("the Word". *Amen, Amin, Hum*) which is the substratum of even the most minute atom. The macrocosmic vibrating universe is transcribed in man who has been made in His/Her image. What follows in the coming sections will give meaning to what Christ said to humanity:

> "No man cometh unto the Father [Cosmic Consciousness], but by me [the Son or Christ or Krishna Consciousness at the *kutastha* between the eyebrows]" John 14: 6

SECTION ONE

Topics in Section One

The Holy Trinity

"I cannot understand the Trinity nor can I fit this into what you talk of *Purusha and Prakriti"* complained my older daughter.
"Let's talk about a one child family" I explained.
"In a single Family Unit, there is a Mum, a Dad, and a Child"
"I accept your proposal" she replied.
"The Family Unit is God or *Brahman* who is and was there before the Trinity came into being in the Cycle of Creation"
"Go on"
"The Dad is *Purusha,* Mum is *Prakriti,* and you are the Child" I replied.
"Keep going" she said.
"Purusha is God-the-Father who is the eternal witness and 'watches' His household. *Prakriti* is the Mother. She is the Energy and the Spirit or Life-force who 'looks' to the needs of Her Family Unit. Her family, ofcourse is the whole Universe. You are the Child", I replied.

"Not yet clear, Mummy" she said in exasperation.

"Purusha is God-the-Father. His characteristic is Consciousness".
"Who then is the Holy Ghost " she replied.

"Prakriti is the Holy Spirit. The Holy Spirit is a She and we Hindus call Her *Devi.* Power and Energy are Her ultimate characteristics and therefore we call Her *Shakti.* She supports all Her children on a substratum of Her eternal Song. This Song of 'Aum' or 'Amen' or 'Amin' or 'Hum' fills the void with different tones and frequencies of sound. With this hum She energises every atom, molecule, and manifestation, both visible and invisible with Awareness. "

"You mean a stone has Awareness too"? she said incredulously.
"Yes, a stone's manifestation is also supported by Her will" I replied.
"Where does the Son or Daughter or Child fit into all this?" was her next question.

"Both *Purusha* and *Prakriti* are manifested completely in a son. The *y* and *x* chromosomes unite as a perfect replica of the Mother and Father. Herein lies the seed for of regeneration in Her Universe"
"Is that why every culture values a male child"? she asked.

"Little do they know that without Her, there would be no male child. Your parents love and adore their two little girls. We need no male child to carry the family name. Do His and Her work and sustain Their Name" was my answer.

Years later, we see them doing His work in sincerity, love, devotion, and pride.
I was in my early thirties when the Master had predicted in Montreal that we will require no sons!

Muladhara Chakra

Preamble

Chakras are spiritual centres, as well as physiological centres controlling the entire body, mind, and intellect. Each ascending *chakra* represents the five elements: earth, water, fire, air and space. Each of the elements also has a sensory connection with smell, taste, sight, touch, and sound.

The study of yoga meditation involves at least eight injunctions. The first two centres prescribe "Do's" and "Do Not's" (*yama and niyama*) which restrain the desire for indulgences. This involves the first two *chakras.* The third ascending *chakra* calls for constant practice of the first two, through the control of sensory desires and of speech.

All actions that begin in the mind as thoughts must be chastened by constant analysis. In thought, word, and deed the seeker cannot be influenced by *raaga-dvesha* or likes-and-dislikes.

All likes-and-dislikes nurtured in every human bosom take their birth from past habits, concepts and desires. Their influences have been imprinted in the causal body through millions of past births. They manifest as personality and play the role of the ego. This ego or pseudo-soul must be stripped of all its ignorant qualities that manifest through man's body, mind, and intellect (BMI) as the extrovert perceiver, feeler, and thinker (PFT). The aim of yoga is to create an introspective creative (PFT).

Muladhara Chakra
First or Base Chakra (coccygeal plexus)

Muladhara Chakra is the first of five "mundane" *chakras,* so called because they instinctively make connections with the world of objects, emotions and thoughts (OET). The *muladhara chakra* possesses the Creative Energy *(Shakti)* of Mother Nature.

In this *chakra*, the foundations are laid for moral training. Acquiring self-control requires one to carefully and gradually analyse and assimilate the material presented in this text. The *sadhak* or seeker must work with it through the process of logic.

Each living thing possesses a mind. Even the Earth is a living organism. It has a Mind and is Aware. Awareness is consciousness of and requires Consciousness as its substratum for manifestation.

This first *chakra* as an energy centre manifests as awareness coupled with a sense of direction. Here, is embedded the earliest foundation of *feeling* or psyche. This *grounding* supports all higher *chakras.*

The *physical* centre of this chakra is the coccygeal plexus which governs retention and excretion. It also determines and regulates reproduction through the desire for sustenance, in accordance with the laws of collective-sanctions or *dharma.* This centre controls the sense of smell and is related to *elemental earth.*

The five senses pull the body in ten (negative and positive for each sense) different directions. Their power is awesome and, unless the Mind is controlled, the seeker will be pulled in too many directions also.

Symbolically, this chakra is the centre of *kama* or the desire for indulgences through the five senses and the five organs of action. Self-improvement begins with *restraint* of the senses *(*symbolically represented by the twin *Sahadev of the Pandavas in the Bhagavad Geeta),* beginning with speech.

In ordinary human activities, Sound through Speech is used for self-expression and communication. At this stage of self-effort, however, the Power of Speech is not understood**:** *rather in order to hear, one must be silent in speech and mind.*

To hear the Voice of Conscience, all verbal and mental chattering must cease. In the silence which results from deep meditation, the *sabda aum* or Cosmic Sound, emanating from this first *spiritual* centre, is heard as the humming of a bee. This inner hearing is an astral hum emanating from the astral element of earth which this centre represents. The *hearing is an awareness,* a definite *presence* in one's own beingness, often, however, it is ignored as inconsequential.

This is the 'inner sound' my father taught me to hear when I was seven years old. He also roused in me an exciting sense of expectation that I would be hearing newer inner tones to this 'buzzing of the bee', if I tried harder and for longer periods! Today, we teach this to our grandchildren. The four grandchildren are normal but quiet! They play an inner game all within themselves when not interacting with each other.

The Bible also alludes to the substratum sound of "Amen" as the first witness of all Creation

> "These things saith the Amen, the faithful and true witness, the beginning of the creation of God. " Revelation 3: 14.

Man's preoccupation with the world of an unenlightened perceiver-feeler-thinker (PFT), leads him to conceive his standard-of-living as a birth right. Man uses his body-mind-intellect (BMI), in the pursuit of objects-emotions-thoughts (OET), only to discover that his inner awareness is disturbed by the outer world.

All religions advise that he must learn to *listen* to the messages in his own awareness. Only faith allows the seeker to hear the "Word":

"Faith commeth by hearing, and hearing by the word of God" . . Roman 19: 17

Different levels of *awareness* exist in the Spinal Cord, wherever the Life-force or Aum which has entered the chakras through the medulla, exerts dominance.

To listen to the Voice of Awareness:

Discrimination must be clear. Essentials and non-essentials about living and life itself must be recognised and sorted out against the background of an awakening awareness.

Realisation is like the light that shines in the darkness of man's awareness. It must be embraced and assimilated, until the *enlightened awareness* merges with *consciousness* through intuitive thinking and feeling.

"And the light shineth in darkness; and the darkness comprehended it not" . . John 1: 5.

The Voice of Awareness

Sound is the first manifestation of Absolute Reality. We know nothing about Nature as it exists except the It is! All scriptures have tried to tell us all about Creation and how it emerged from the Absolute. They say *brahman or* God was one and non-dual. They say It caused a vibration. The vibration was a Sound and that Sound was *aum.* It was from this Sound that all manifestation came.

As long as the force of desire to remain manifested lasts, the Cosmic Vibration and the Sound exists. When the Cosmic Desire to Exist ceases, the Cosmic Vibration and the Sound ceases. They both then disappear into the transcendental Being. The world disappears into Sound and the Sound disappears into *brahman or God.*

The Master was explaining this to me when he suddenly said:

"Before the sound in you gets involved [in worldly activities], know the substratum *Aum.* Plug your ears and listen to your within. The sound emanates from your heart"

He was indicating to me that there exists a certain sound within me supporting all my activities. He was informing my extrovert nature that when this sound gets involved into its cause the "Me" who is the pseudo-ego, my earthly life will take a turn towards the "I" the Self or soul.

Sound forms the basis in all the six *chakras* in the divine cave of the brain and spinal cord. In the lower three *chakras,* it is not heard too clearly since they are controlled by the *tattvas* or elements earth, water, and fire. The element air or *vayu* in the fourth or heart or *anahata chakra* allows the sound to be heard more distinctly. The nature of the Sound differs according to the disturbance caused by the vibrating element. At the heart centre, we hear a combined vibration of the gross physical *(sthula)* and subtle *(sukshma)* physiological-psychological sounds. The hearing of this voice of awareness depends upon the intensity of our concentration and the quietude of the element or *tattva.*

Anahata sounds are melodious mystical sounds heard by the sincere seeker who progresses in his efforts at meditation. The sound can be heard through the right ear with or without the plugging of the ears. The right ear is suggested as the better side because the solar *nadi* or *pingala* ends on the right side. The *anahata sound* is also called *antardhvani* or the inner sound. It is due to *prana* or vibration of life-force *aum* in the heart centre. It is also called *nada.*

The Power of Speech - Shakti

Speech, in the form of *Shakti Devi*, is present in every one of the *chakras* as *pranava* or Cosmic Sound, also referred to in the Bible as the Comforter, the Holy Ghost or the Holy Spirit. Following It leads the seeker to all possible knowledge.

> "But the Comforter, which is the Holy Ghost . . . shall teach you all things, and bring all things to your remembrance, whatsoever I have said unto you" . . John 14: 26

Unknown to most of us, control of speech is the basic and most important part of self-development. It evolves as the practitioner gains progress through self-effort.

The Power of Speech is connected to Spirit. If divorced from emotion and mental activity, it can lift Man, through its *creative energy,* to the highest stage of *beingness.* There are three stages to the evolution of speech:

1. Mind-emotion desires improvement based upon a *concept* of purity.
2. The *mind* is given the *creative energy to will* an action for improvement. The *will* for improvement is empowered by *awareness aum* - to become a Power for both individual and collective consciousness.

Even as just a youngster, one of my daughters has always been quick on the defensive with her tongue. She is also very introspective and quick to retract with an appropriate correction. The reflexive responses originate from her past births and the Master is responsible for her introspective retractions. The Master once wrote to her about the connection of mood, thought, speech, and action. His letter was a gentle reprimand that only one with high ideals and controlled tendencies has the right to lead another.

> ". . . You must score high. . . Then and only then can you lead the children. Be sweet to everyone. You may be sad or even angry or tired. But nothing is an excuse for you to behave badly to others. If you can't be sweet to others always, then go to bed and don't come out! You are sweet. I want you to be sweeter still. . . "

Speech has two aspects; the audible and the inaudible.

- **Inaudible Speech** is intuitive speech, the *language of the heart;* it is not a mere chattering in the mind.
- **Audible Speech**, when cultivated and refined, eventually becomes intuitive: Its objective is to transmit the *power of the mind*, thereby gaining *divine insights* for a collective good.

The power of speech should be coupled with a desire to create words in the *service of others*, for a collective good.

If the mind is a collection of thoughts and if thoughts crystallise to become speech, then mind-power can be increased through the use of a single potent word or *mantra* in focused meditation. This type of *sadhana* or self-effort in mind-control, activates and amplifies the latent Cosmic Forces within each one of us.

Practising Speech Control

Man expresses himself with audible speech. It is the barometer of his emotions and of his mind. Audible speech is expressed with the voice. Control of audible speech is necessary to reduce restlessness and to negate the urge to talk.

The urge or *desire* to talk originates from:

- fear of silence; or
- a feeling of loneliness; or
- the desire to show off what one knows; or
- an inclination to give advice, whether help is needed or not; or
- the tendency to contribute one's "two cents worth".

Before these urges can be controlled, one must be aware of the characteristics of speech.

Analysis of Speech

The following group discussion outlines the different ways man speaks *automatically*. The aim of the discussion is to create an awareness as to why we speak. We must analyse why we use certain *tones of voice* when we speak **and** identify the *emotions* behind the speech. Preconceived *concepts* of our assertions must also be deeply considered as well as the *body language* of the speaker.

A. To **control the act** of talking:
Keep a ring, pebble, or coin under the tongue or in the cheek. This will

provide enough time for the practitioner to ask:

- What do I want to say?
- Why do I need to speak?

B. Identify the **urges to speak**:

- Am I speaking to kill time?
- Am I trying to justify my actions?
- Am I avoiding listening to others?
- Am I trying to be self-important?
- Do I want to be noticed?
- Am I trying to avoid listening to myself?
- Am I trying to impose my beliefs or attract pity?
- Am I afraid to listen to what others are saying?

C. Observe the **tones of voice** used in speaking:
Are these tones:

- arrogant;
- badgering;
- confrontational;
- emotional;
- fearful, joyful and happy.

Do they express doubt?

D. Can one be silent despite the urge to speak: ***(Mauna)***?

- All urges must be controlled;
- Determine the length of time of *mauna* or silence to be observed, beforehand;
- Enforce discipline and record results.

Man is endowed with the instinct of speaking. His thoughts originate from the intellectual sheath or *gyanamaya kosha*. His emotions originate from his emotional sheath or *manomaya kosha*, and his concepts arise from his bliss sheath or *anandamaya kosha*.

All the three bodies (*shariras)* or the five sheaths or *koshas,* collectively express themselves through the organ of speech. The energy is derived from the *pranamaya kosha* which is a sheath of pure energy. The body language is derived from the energy in the food sheath or *annamaya kosha*. The above is diagramatically expressed in Figure 7.

The *Bhagavad Geeta* says, to invoke speech, care must be taken that it is *satya* or truthful, *heeth* or useful to the listener, *priya* or loving to the listener, and *meetha* or sweet in intonation. Unless all these four elements are present, speech should not be invoked. Refined speech is a Song used to glorify a Power greater than the seeker.

Speech

Coarse or *literal speech* is audible. It manifests at the level of conventional words and relates to our senses in the waking state as *audible speech originating in the throat.*

When thinking deeply, we begin to *ponder* and speech acquires a creative force of beauty. It acquires dream-state of thoughts originating from the *emotions of the heart.*

When speech acquires the power of *illumination and perception*, it does so in the light of underlying universal truths which underlie all events and things. These are experienced in deep-sleep as the essence-of-thought, sensed in the gut at the level of the navel.

When *speech becomes a revelation* of the forces behind all works in creation, *speech is experienced as an experience and a realisation.* This is *transcendent speech* of the super-conscious state. In this state, thoughts and words are eradicated, and there is only the silence of the *aum.*

In the beginning of any spiritual journey, the power of speech must be investigated from the level of the first or root *chakra.* With maturity in understanding through introspection, the seeker allows the energy of awareness or life-force to ascend gradually. Restraint and adherence to speech-control allows the seeker to awaken to her higher potentials. She begins to hear the inner sound emanating from the divine cave in the brain and spinal cord.

The music of the inner sound takes the seeker to listening and watching the breath. Over time, the inner sound of an inner *mantra* along with that of the breath, takes the practitioner to different levels in the seven *chakras* of the divine cave of the brain and spinal cord. Here, speech can be gradually harmonised with the Divine Cosmic Word.

But first, there is the issue of refined audible speech. That is where the seeker starts. Our tendencies may be coarse, but our efforts can correct all reflexive responses ingrained in our causal beingness!

The Master was a man of few words. When he spoke, seekers made notes for future reference. All his letters are teachings for prosterity. Volunteers continue to collect letters he wrote to the thousands of seekers. In one of his many letters, he wrote on speech:

> and the Master wrote:
> ". . . Six most important words: I admit I made a mistake
> Five most important words: You did a good job.
> Four most important words: What is your opinion?
> Three most important words: If you please.
> Two most important words: Thank you.
> Most important word: We.
> Least important word: "I. "

Muladhara and Smell

The physical body composed of the five senses and five organs of action is inherently inert, gross, and therefore, *tamasic*. The psychological-physiological or astral body is energetic and therefore *rajasic*. The intellectual personality desire-filled causal body is the subtlest. It is composed of a *balanced essence of both the physical and the astral body*, and is therefore *sattvic* or in harmony with the rest of the bodily sheaths.

Each *chakra* controls one of the five senses. The wave-density of each of these centres matches one of the primary elements (earth, water, fire, air, and space). The first *chakra* known as the *Muladhara*, controls the sense of smell (earth). This sense may or may not be developed.

Lack of development indicates predominance of inertia or *tamas*. The sense of smell must be developed at least to the level of healthy activity so one can assess aromas, their source, and man's connection of the smell with the external world. When aware, man becomes aware for example, that an attraction for a particular person of the opposite sex is perhaps because of the physical sense of smell alone. This is the *rajasic* characteristic of smell which initiates desire for indulgence.

When harmony sets in with spiritual effort, the sense of smell manifests as a presence as well. This self-effort in *yoga*-meditation begins to manifest as benevolence from the inner teacher or *rishi or guru* who is experienced by some seekers as a delicate fragrance of violets or of sandalwood. Similarly, when groups who meditate together for long periods transcend their individual personalities, this *sattvic* sense of smell can be experienced as a certain fragrance or as a definite *Presence*.

Swami Yogi Satyam had a seven day meditation *yagna* [spiritual training] at our home recently. Some days after he had left, my younger daughter who was alone at her mother's home, was surprised by a police officer knocking at our door. The security alarm had asked for a police presence. She became very concerned. They both decided to investigate both the home and the grounds. Once he had finished checking the ground floor, he said: "There is an incredible vibration of peace in this home. I have never experienced that feeling before. What is it"?

"You are sensing the recent meditation sessions held in the home, Sir. We had a saint live here for a few days. You are feeling his presence" she replied.

This fact was also emphasised by the Master when this same daughter who had asked him, many years earlier: what do people mean when they told her that the 'vibrations in your home are those of a presence of peace'?

> and the Master wrote to one of my children:
> ". . . When many come together in devotion and perform a ritual. . . somehow, somewhere, a unique atmosphere arrives to tickle us into an inner Joy and Poise."

Analysis of the Sense of Smell:

Smell different items. Identify the smell. Observe if and how it is stimulating.

- Does smell tempt me to eat or drink?
- Can I eat what smells bad? Will I eat what tastes bad but smells good?
- Do I enjoy the taste of coffee or tea?

Note how body odours and bad breath smell different:

- Smell your own clothes and perfumes and those of others.
- Do these blend with my own body odours?

Does my body odour alter with changes in diet consumed or through fasting?

- Can illness be identified through odour?

Increase respiration to blow off unpleasant odours of sickness.

Both *tamasic* and *rajasic* states of smell are facets of one smell. An alert mind has the ability to analyse the emotion displayed by himself when contacting the object of his smell. The seeker is able to identify the play of the mind motivating an action triggered by the sense of smell.

The intellect makes a logical decision and the seeker harmonises the two tendencies. In this *sattvic* state, the seeker's intelligence has analysed smell and refined the mind. He is not motivated by habits and past tendencies. He is able to give the sense of smell its real value base. He realises that there is neither good nor bad in the sense of smell. There is only an emotional attraction or repulsion tendency towards a particular smell.

The mind-intellect or awareness resides in the *cave* of the brain and spinal cord. Life-force radiates from the *divine cave* to all the senses of the body. The *distance* away from the mind-intellect leads man towards *mindless* indulgences. A seeker must make every effort to remove the ignorance about his senses by analysing all facets of each sense faculty.

Muladhara in Health and Sex

The Creative Energy, which resides in the *muladhara chakra* or coccygeal plexus, is neutral; consequently, one needs to be responsible concerning how it is used. Creative Energy is expressed most powerfully through sexual activity. Most often, this energy is expressed on a mental *(rajas)* and a physical *(tamas)* level while the spiritual *(sattvic)* level is neglected.

On a physical level, exercise and proper food are necessary to ensure a healthy body. A healthy *temple* of the soul is of importance if man is to pursue a life of *yoga* and meditation. Healthy eating habits must be taught from childhood.

Early meditation techniques can be taught to children. They will be able to hear their own inner sounds through introspection and inner hearing. The tendency for over-indulgence is naturally curbed when children are able to *listen* to their own body. In later years, this discipline and self-restraint is required for a better understanding of the creative life-force.

The natural physical or *tamasic* tendencies and instinctive physiological-psychological creative urges or *rajasic* tendencies of the maturing body have to addressed by knowledgeable teachers and insightful parents.

In the early years of their adolescence, I agonised about how I would be able to cope with the adolescence of my two daughters. We had to address the issue of peer pressure. We knew there was a cultural difference which could trigger an identity crisis. We had to be sure that the value system they would be exposed to would have a universal application. We as parents were very fortunate that we had the Master to bear the brunt of their early years physical instability and emotional insecurity. He gently led them through the ups and downs of adolescence. There were 'secret' letters between them. One of them is reproduced here:

> and the Master wrote to one of my daughters going through adolescence :
>
> ". . . Do not waste your time worrying about what others are saying or thinking [about bodily and emotional changes]. So long as you are honest and pure, you go ahead. Dogs bark, the caravan moves on. Later on, in your success with your *dharma* (value based living), they will rediscover your worth and between us, there is nothing wrong if you fall in love. What has the public got to do with it? But let not this distraction disturb your studies. . "
>
> ". . but never give up your *japa* (reciting the mantra) and a short but sweet meditation. This will help you to be quiet, self-confident, and effortlessly consistent".

The need for a healthy body and mind is important for spiritual journeys. Adults who practice more advanced meditation similarly require a very healthy body and mind. On a biological level, adults too must inquire if sex is just for procreation or for pleasure or perhaps for a *bonding* of two unknowns.

Analysis of the Muladhara Chakra and Marriage

Is sexual union an expression of tenderness and respect between two persons?

Answer these questions:

- Have I control over sex and its power?
- Do I obey its instincts and if so, why?
- Is marriage just a social institution?
- Is it because of sex that marriage is socially acceptable?

Why did I marry this person?

- What were my hopes then?
- What are they now?

Did I want a life partner I could trust, one who would be endowed with character? Was I seeking mutual companionship?

Is sex the search for a "higher value" in the life of two persons - an expression of a new aspect of Love?

Do I use sex to punish and reward?

- If I am indulging in self pity, do I use sex for compensation?
- Was there any ideal to start with?
- If so, is there quality in the relationship?

If one is disappointed in the relationship, is divorce a solution?

- Can separation or divorce erase the disappointment?
- Should I feel responsible for the failures of my partner?
- Should they feel responsible for my failures?

Man adapts continuously to the processes of external environment, operating through the brain and reflecting through the contents of the mind and emotions. Bodily health is a function of the brain's connection to the body through neurotransmitters, neurohormones, including endorphines, the immune system, and the like. What goes on in our awareness, affects our body, emotions and thoughts - each leave an imprint on the other.

Our memories are scars on the soul, and they need positive re-programming through analysis. Personal interpretations are adaptations to disruptions in mind, emotions and thoughts. These remain imprinted in our causal being as anger, resentment, shame, guilt, and even a desire to criticise.

Both happy and sad relationships in marriage and sex create thoughts that are individually characteristic. These shape our lives and experiences through the process of repetition and habit. Situational wrongs precipitate emotional and mental orientation which grind the body one way or the other.

Troublesome marriages also take their origin from causal concepts and tendencies, habitual reflexive responses to conflict, and a desire to be in control at all times. Possessiveness and the need to mould the other partner is the mill through which marriages are subjected to. Many tolerate the indignity. Others choose to change partners. Some wise ones analyse the situation and become witnesses of the shenanigans of the controlling element! The Master addressed this issue at one of the *satsangs* or meetings with the wise.

> the Master subtly reprimanded both husbands and wives:
>
> ". . . There can never be 'her fifth and his sixth marriage' for a Hindu wife! Even in modern days, 'the man of the house is likened to a 'cave-man'. *Rejuvenated* after a night's sleep *at her expense*, he roars for breakfast, and she better stay out of his way at this time of the day. He storms out of the cave, club in hand in search for the next 'kill' which he brings back to his hungry family. He *rudely* flings this through the door and disappears until the meal is ready according to *"his" unasked specifications!*

> "He *expects* the meal to be ready; while he fills himself, the cave-man *expects his wife to hear his tales of woe and trepidations.* She must soothe him, heal his wounds, and allow him to sleep! Rejuvenated at *her* expense, he starts the *ritual again every morning!*
>
> "The wife feels wounded and may even erupt, but *she must control herself until he leaves for the day.* She can now break as many dishes as she wishes after he leaves. . . " Swamiji laughed.

The Master never made judgements. I will leave it to the reader to decide whether such behaviour is to be advocated or decried. My own feeling is that he was reprimanding both the husbands and the wives.

Marriage - Masculinity - Femininity

Morality is like a chameleon: it assumes the colour of its society and family beliefs. In spite of this, however, the Laws of Nature remain unaltered and resplendent in their own Truth. These inscrutable laws [*dharma*] uphold Creation. The Master alluded to the *dharma* of marriage in one of his potent statements to seekers of Truth:

> and the Master said:
>
> ". . . Love is more than a 'convulsion' in the bed!"

Yoga asserts that Man is Nature's highest achievement because of his brain and spinal cord. Here in the skull and spine lies the altar of God. Here is where spiritual efforts take you to: in the presence of God. It is here that the brain cell [neurone] has all records of his past births, habits, concepts, and likes-and-dislikes. Man, consequently must respect procreation as a sacred testimony to his own creation: it cannot be abused.

Every being contains the essence of a soul: which is neither masculine nor feminine, but combine both natures. Masculinity has Nature's characteristics of the intellect or *buddhi*: self-control, discrimination and exacting judgement. Femininity has Nature's characteristics of emotion or *manas*: love, sympathy, kindness, all feelings of the mind.

These two aspects of Nature are united and harmonised for spiritual procreation. When balanced, the seeker finds contentment *because he has achieved the perfect union of mind and intellect.* Conversely, imbalance makes the seeker dissatisfied and restless. It is the *karmic* patterns of past actions that determine if a person will be born male or female.

The objective of marriage between man and woman is to up-lift each partner in a commitment of divine friendship, love, and loyalty in the process moving both parties back to their true Nature - to their innate divinity. Marriage is a commitment of sharing in this incarnation. It is a promise between two people to provide a home and environment for other souls seeking birth. Whether one seeks soul-harmony through right marriage or celibacy, the final culmination of

Man, whether male or female, is the reunification of that soul with God!

A definite exchange of Energy occurs between two persons in the act of *sex*. The mechanics of this exchange are not understood, but the dynamics can be grasped when the purpose of sex is investigated.

Creative Energy expressed through the physical act of *sex* is the most precious Energy. It is That *(aum)* which brings a new person into this physical manifestation as a mortal.

The *individualised* being enters the mother's womb where the fertile *matter* (sperm and ovum) have already united with the help of the *creative energy*, the life-force or *aum*. At around the twelfth week of pregnancy, the *essence* of the individualised causal being of thirty-five *tattvas* enters the fertile matter. *Tattva* is a reality-principle resulting from a combination of the physical and astral bodies of an individual, existing as ideas.

This individualised essence of *ideas-principle* enters the matter-foetus through the *kutastha* or Christ/Krishna Centre of the forming embryo. It spreads its special identity through the mind into the senses and into the spiritual centres in the cave of the brain and spinal cord. This is done with the help of *prana,* the primal energy - *aum,* which enters through the mouth of God in the medulla at the base of the brain.

Externalisation of the individual results in the creation of the senses and the organs of action, again with the help of a*um,* the Holy Spirit.

Therefore, this Energy or the *prana* or the Holy Spirit is not for senseless scattering or for pleasure alone. The energy is *prakriti.* She is the basis and cause of all manifestation. She is also the unmanifest energy before manifestation.

Accidents of conception produce children lacking dignity and love. Parents with spiritual values produce children in harmony with Divine Laws.

Spiritual Marriage

Spiritual marriage is possible when two persons have equivalent *dharmic* or righteous values. Such *dharmic* or duty-bound individuals bond together in a spiritual marriage and sex, then, is a spontaneous physical communication between two person who truly love each other.

On higher levels, people do become *soul mates* and, together they strive for the Most Highest even when faced with a family and career responsibilities. In a wholesome family, it is the introspective mother who silently observes all actions and their effects on the family. She ensures righteous activities are adhered to and she puts right all negative forces. It is a true statement of fact that the first *guru* [teacher] of a child is the Mother. No mater how dysfunctional a father and therefore a family, it is the mother who holds the home together.

The following story illustrates this:

the Master was invited to a wedding anniversary party. The couple had been married for over 70 years. Both the husband's and the wife's facial creases clearly showed that these two people were a very aged couple. *Swamiji* had known the old man for over thirty years as a cross crusty old man!

> ". . How did you ever put up with his nonsense all these years?"
>
> She let out her secret.
>
> With a toothless smile, she spoke to *Swamiji* in confidence:
>
> ". . I allowed him to rant and rave and disrupt the peace in the house. When he was gone, I would do exactly what I wanted to do. He never knew the difference."

The Ecstasy of the Ultimate Union in Death

Once one comes to terms with sex, one must acknowledge the *mystery* that sex has a beginning with *birth* and an end in *death*. The wise say both are inter-related.

Although, sex has a function in bonding two individuals together, it must *die* for the sake of Love. The *mystery* is that sex, birth, and death are one unit, not separate incidents in the life of a seeker.

From a spiritual point of view, the Creative Energy or *shakti of aum* must rise or be born to meet with the Awareness at the *ajnaa* or sixth chakra. As refined *chitta* (the combined *feeling* of mind-intellect-ego) in the *ajnaa chakra, the chitta* is enlightened at the *Kutastha* with Universal Intelligence. The "Me" or ego or pseudo-soul, becomes progressively more refined and intuitively intelligent:

> The mortal *realises* that the "I" (the subject of my search) in "Me" (the pseudo-soul or object or ego) are one and the same. "Me" must become the enlightened soul "I" or Self as Awareness. The refined *chitta* (awareness) realises he is the *chit* (consciousness) in essence and must merge in It.

Finally, the seeker (enlightened awareness or *chitta)* must erase himself (or *die*) in the seventh *chakra* or *sahasrahara* in order to merge with Universal Consciousness *(chit).*

Self ("I" the subject) realises that he is one with the Universal Self (ultimate subject of the search). He knows intuitively that this Self is the Self in All and the All is the Self. In the final *death* of individuality, the soul "I" or Self, the Universal Self, and the Cosmic Self become One.

> Even the Bible asserts that man must rise towards this ultimate secret place in the Christ or Krishna Centre, under the shadow of the Centre of Universal Consciousness in the *sahasrahara*, the seventh *chakra.*
>
> "He that dwelleth in the secret place of the Most High [*ajnaa*] shall abide under the shadow of the Almighty [*sahasrahara*]". . Psalms 91: 1

Analysis of Sex

Nature maintains itself through the search for food and the impulse to propagate. Both are powerful driving forces which are expressed more prominently in the human than in the animal. The animal eats only what he must and procreates during definite seasons or biological changes.

A spiritual way to assess sex is to ask the following questions:

- What does sex mean to me?
- Is it an automated biological functioning?
- Is it for procreation?

How do I use sex?

- For enjoyment and pleasure?
- To have children?
- As compensation, punishment, reward? or
- Do I accept "free" sex without responsibility or bondage?

Is sex outside marriage a sin?

- How did I arrive at my conclusion? Through cultural precepts, my upbringing, or a concept? Is sex a sin?

If sex is love, why does it inspire so many the conflicts?

- Why is bad language often associated with sex?

Why are children, the products of sexual activity, often rejected or half-heartedly accepted?

Is there energy exchange in sex?

- Is there any psychic power exchanged?
- Is love a factor in sex?

Can sex be a part of a spiritual marriage or must it be excluded?

Is there such a thing as soul mate?

- How does one know?
- Is there such a thing as a mystical marriage?
- Is sex part of it?

Why is celibacy important to some?

- What do I think of it?
- Would the world disappear if everyone was celibates?

Is Universal - Cosmic Consciousness, through the practices of meditation, only for celibates? Is sex a responsibility of the attachment in marriage or bonding of love?

- Is sex a "force"?
- What is Her (*Prakriti's)* expression?
- Does She manifest as "creative energy"?

Intense emotional situations activate neurohormones and neurotransmitters which include endorphines for pleasure. The experience of pleasure demands a need for repetition. The *experience is of universal happiness* and cannot be possessed and re-created on demand. A blissful relationship in friendship and in marriage are gifts of *Prakriti* or Mother Nature or Holy Spirit and must be acknowledged as an *awareness, in Her Awareness.*

Educating Children about Creative Energy

My children were pre-adolescents when they innocently asked the Master if he would be their *guru.* They had found in him a friend. I had found in him the perfect 'godfather and godmother'. Within two weeks of this incident, he called me back to be with him for another ten days in Montreal. He knew that I was one of those isolated units known as the urban 'nuclear family' with little if any, support from live-in elders in a culturally intact joint family system. What follows is what he taught me, who was already a parent but a very young one.

Children must be taught a healthy life-style. An ideal diet of fruit, vegetables, grain and milk should be started very early in life. Overeating and unhealthy eating habits are indulgences of the senses and should be discouraged. Lack of exercise, absence of fresh air and sunshine, and exposure to loud music and noise should be guarded against. Cleanliness of body, mind, and intellect should be stressed. Children should be watched for habitual worry, nervousness, and emotional outbursts. The burst of sexual energy in adolescence should be channelled into sports, martial arts, and dance.

> During a gathering of parents and children in an auditorium at a school, the Master said:
>
> ". . . Children do not learn from books. Higher values cannot be taught by institutions, society, community or committee. They imitate their parents. Unfortunately, if the parents are vulgar, the child will strive to be vulgar!
>
> "What pre-natal education are the mothers giving to their children today? Cinema, vulgar movies, bars, hotels. . . these are the ideals you are feeding your children and when they come out as *rakshasas* (monsters), you say 'The children have gone astray! We do not understand what is happening to the world'. . .
>
> "It is our mistake. Your children are your future and mothers are the moulders of your children. . .
>
> "Monsters or angels, what is the future going to be? To remould and recast the future, supply the children with a 'vision' between the ages of 6 to 12. Next change the pattern of their thoughts with a moral education. Expose them to the correct attitudes to things and beings.
>
> "The father's abilities are usually centred around ideals in ambition, greatness and success. The mother imparts ideals of charity, goodness, tenderness, affection, and forgiveness. She does this by living them herself and the ideas become embedded in the child. . .
>
> "When mothers themselves have lost touch with spiritual values, their children who have now become young adults, find that the values imparted to them are all hollow and empty. Their dissatisfaction takes them to drink, drugs, self-ruination and suicide. . .

"There is no need for children to grow up as unnecessary by-products of parents who do not know what to do with them. Breast feeding has stopped. But this is a time when mother intensively contemplates while looking into the eyes of her child and becomes mentally intimate with her child. The child looks devotedly at his mother while suckling. This habit of devotion remains ingrained in the psyche of the child. . .

"Lastly, it is not sufficient that the children be trained in the higher values of life. We must teach them the courage and heroism to live up to their convictions! . . ."

Children should be taught to tap the creative energy as oxygen-laden *prana* or life- force. They should be taught to invoke the life-force to combat stresses. They must first be taught to watch the breath and hear it coursing up and down the chest. The restlessness of the breath will be seen to recede when the child listens to his inner sounds at the same time. Stresses of growing are silenced when the bosom breathes harmoniously! They learn to become introspective with these first steps.

With the advent of adolescence, they should be taught to consciously recharge the body with the life-giving *prana* or energy. Recharging exercises will be shown in section four of this text. In the beginning, slow breathing exercises are sufficient, while the mind focuses on the *prana* permeating the entire body: from cell to cell.

It cannot be over-emphasised the children should be trained in the basics of introspection by learning to *hear* their own *inner sounds* emitting from their astral body. It is the only way I know to empower our children with a secret to successful living! (This will be covered in meditation techniques later.)

A parent was heard making this comment:

". . . Gone are the days when children were considered ignorant of the ways of the world. . Today, their thirst for knowledge, their indomitable curiosity, and their eagerness to express their feelings leave present day elders baffled. Their environment fills these young ones with confidence. "

Said one youth who had overheard the comment and pondered upon it. In his opinion:

". . There is an elaborate pattern behind every apparent 'flaw' and nothing is purposeless. . . all ideas of perfection find expression in Him. Evil, then is a distracter, an option we must scrupulously avoid, and sweep our avenues clear to find our way more easily towards God. . . "

The most difficult time for children is during adolescence. They discover their parents are not infallible. Their imagined perfect world comes crashing down! They are looking for a perfect parent and none is to be found. Perhaps the Western tradition of god-parents and the Eastern tradition of connecting adolescents to a spiritual master or *guru* stems from a critical need for a perfect parent at this time of their lives.

Changes in the body of a growing child manifest as he approaches adolescence. Unless the child is trained in introspection through meditation and exercising the body through will power, he loses his chance of understanding himself. He has to be awakened to the presence of this surge of *energy* which can be channelled into *excellence* in all his actions.

> the Master wrote in of his letters to my daughters:
>
> "Now that you are older and in High School, you have a larger responsibility towards yourself, your younger sister and towards society. Be regular with your *japa* (using prayer beads to chant a given mantra). Bring your mind to the joyous stillness: in such inner silence you gather your divine experience. In contemplation, gather wisdom and in joyous love, pour it all out to the world. . "

This basic education keeps the child's body performing efficiently. It is continually replenished and nourished by good habits, positive thoughts, right living, and the ability to heal itself whenever discouraged, tired, in pain, or unsure due to the stresses of an ever-changing environment and the child's own bodily metamorphosis.

The Master made it very clear that the moral training given by him would be upheld by we, the parents. His instructions would be from one who is the infallible perfect parent and teacher. For this grace and precious gift, I will always honour the Master!

> "You both parents have been assigned the task to feed and clothe them. Educate them in school and University. They are my children. I will bring them up myself. They will be with me every summer holiday. That is all that you both must do".

The *muladhara chakra* or coccygeal plexus is where automatic responses to pain, pleasure, involuntary speech, competition, aggression, birth, fear of death, and motives of action are recorded as 'automatic reflex action". Each of these need self-analysis. The aim of the exercises is to reach the core of my being, free of all such preconceived encumbrances.

Analysis of Pain

Pain and pleasure are the result of contact of senses with name and form. A decision that something gives pleasure or pain is based upon the individual's past habits, concepts, and likes-and-dislikes. They can therefore be made to appear and fade away at will. It is not wrong to protect oneself from pain but it is better to accept both pain and pleasure with indifference. Untouched by sensations, the seeker acquires peace of mind.

It is not unusual for me to come across young persons in my practice who are pained for many reasons and react with actions that are noisy and disruptive. These young persons demand that a local anaesthetic not be used, while treating them for their cuts and bruises! Because they are usually inebriated, it is often better to heed to their demands. Observations made during the treatment are both intriguing and logical. The young ones are usually smiling silently during the procedure. They leave the department happier than when they were first seen.

Let us analyse the sense of touch. A light touch is a mere sensation. A gentle massage is soothing and pleasurably relaxing. A harder painful squeezing of the same area of the body induces uncomfortable physical pain. A mental pain can be forgotten with the induction of physical pain. It therefore stands to reason that pain and pleasure are two extremes of the one sensation: touch. A logical approach to pain and pleasure allows the mind to function without emotion. The intellect also functions in the light of logical understanding.

Pain is the greatest Teacher.

- But what is Pain?
- How when and where do I experience pain?
- Is it self-created?

Discuss the meaning of the words "pain" and "hurt" and how these words are used:

- Investigate the ideas associated with these words;
- Study **the power** these words convey to the mind.

Analyse physical pain and emotional pain:

- Enter pain and experience it deeply - then let it go.

Yogis or the wise, say pain is self-created:

- When I am hurt, what and why are there self-created repercussions?
- Am I hurt because my plans have been thwarted?
- Am I attached to the plans?
- Do I dislike changes made to my plans?

Is the hurt felt because my own "inner balance" has been inconvenienced?

- Where do I feel the hurt?
- Does this "hurt" have a shape and form?
- Perhaps I am angry *("krodh")* because I am inconvenienced?

Can I hold my emotions and recognise the difference between hurt and being inconvenienced?

- Can I learn from my mistakes and allow them to fade away?
- Will they fade if emotions are kept alive?
- Is this discrimination by intellect?

How much energy have I locked in the hurt in me?

- Can I forgive and forget the hurt?
- When the energy is freed, where can I use it?

The urge to retaliate when hurt is a reflexive response of the "Me" who is the ego. The hurt may remain hidden in the causal memory and determine all future actions. The reflexive response is often thought to be righteous, as the next parable shows:

> "Then came Peter to him, and said, Lord, how oft shall my brother sin against me, and I forgive him? till seven times?
>
> "Jesus saith unto him, I say not unto thee, Until seven times: but, Until seventy times seven" Mathew 18: 21, 22.

We create notions about who we are and what we are. Our mind creates images of ourselves within the limited concepts of personal expression and freedom of movement. We handicap ourselves with beliefs of opposites or *raaga-dvesha* and distort our representations in beliefs about ourselves.

Pain occurs when our mind exceeds the margin of our conceptualized body tolerance. In order to decapitate our tolerance, we learn bodily postures that are compromises. These too, are new pains at the cost of adaptive atrophy, because we are too weak to carry our normal, natural *karmic* load. The body will adapt to whatever it needs to keep functioning. With an optimal state of adaptation, a *sadhak* or seeker increases the bodily options by negating excessive internal demands, negative thoughts, and distorted images.

Being non-judgmental and un-involved, witnessing rather than participating, is the key to dealing with the pushes and pulls and imbalances of world situations, emotional undulations and mental opinions.

Pain and Pleasure

We are consciously aware that we are perceiving, feeling, and thinking (PFT) whenever we use our body and mind and intellect (BMI). Underlying all this awareness, is a common denominator: the *ego*.

The ego thinks it governs all actions; never does it occur to this little self, the "Me", that it is a mere reflection of the bliss-filled Self, the Spirit. The self remains forever separated from the one Universal Self. This is the cause of Man's physical and mental suffering, which he calls "pain". This identification with the transient body and the restless mind is the ultimate cause of our pain: where we separate the "self" from the "Self".

Desires seek fulfillment. Some desires are natural and take the form of habits; others are created tendencies for continued new wants. "New wants" eventually become "natural habits" and become ingrained in the personality.

The more the wants, the greater are the possibilities of pain, because wants are difficult to fulfill, especially if the demand is for immediate fulfillment. Wants becomes a permanent mental agitation or desire, which will continue to amplify in the physiological-psychological body as pain, until they are satisfied. Pain however may be emotionally 'justified' as is shown in the next illustration:

the Master wrote to one of my daughters when she was 'suffering' a mother's pain:

"... The Lord gives not only sorrows but also the power to endure them. In life we must learn to endure such sudden calamities and yet live graciously.

"Fortunate are the parents, chosen by the Lord, deemed fit to care for such a delicate piece of His Creation. "

Just as desire leads to pain, it can also lead to pleasure. The experience of pleasure has a habit of dying away. Whether pleasure or pain, they both have a tendency for retaining the experience in the memory-bank of what gave the mind pleasure or pain. Both pain and pleasure therefore are conditions of the mind which is emotion. Pleasure is a satisfaction and pain is a dissatisfaction; both are feelings and emotions of the mind.

There is nothing wrong with desires and wants. It is wrong, however, to continually hanker after new wants for the sake of pleasure. This will lead to pain. To lessen this, the mind must be weaned off attachments, habitual wanting, and desiring.

Man has duties in life. He comes to his present manifestation with an agenda of unfulfilled desires from his previous lives and it is duty or *dharma* to fulfill them. Some of these duties map out the direction of his life until the desires are fulfilled. Once this desire is accomplished, whether through a profession, or wealth, or position, Man experiences both pleasure and satisfaction.

He concentrates his energy in perpetuating the pleasure, constantly seeking more - better education, higher social position, higher public office, or fame. In doing so, he continues to suffer the vagaries of both pleasure and pain, until exhausted he dies dissatisfied.

Luke also affirmed what the Master admonished repeatedly: "When your desires are done, hurry home - *hari aum*" [salutations]!

"And seek not ye what ye shall eat, or what ye shall drink, neither be ye of doubtful mind. For all these things do the nations of the world seek after: and your Father knoweth that ye have need for these things. But rather seek ye the kingdom of God; and all these things shall be added unto you" . . Luke 12: 29-31.

Desire is the root cause of Man's misery. It is caused by sense identification of the "I" with the "Me". Such suffering can be cured by first intensely playing the part of desire satisfaction. Having played it with the whole of his body and mind, the discriminating intellect should walk away from the stage-of-life, unaffected and unruffled by the successes and the failures of the stage actor.

and the Master wrote:

" . . . Looking back into our past, we are helpless victims of our own past actions but looking ahead of us, we become the architects of our own future. Let us never look back for a moment, but dynamically march forward creating a glorious future of magnificent achievements by rightly exercising the independent self-effort, which is man's prerogative."

Through dispassion and severing off identification with emotions, the mind is freed to desire for higher ideals. When this happens, the calm inner self disowns all petty desiring and focuses instead on working for the world family. Here, there is no pain or pleasure: there is only perfect tranquillity, because there is no connection with the disturbances of the mind and body. Instead the connection is with the Universal Body of *Prakriti,* a transcendental state of healthy expansion. Man does his duty to this Universal Body for the purpose of a Collective Good.

Pain Raises Level of Awareness

Man cannot be master of his own destiny while engaged in a battle with indulgence, temptation, desire, and habits. He must transcend identifications with his body and emotions, and eliminate restlessness caused by his doubts and complexes and, above all, his soul-ignorance or *avidya.*

His perceptions are limited to his sensations and physiological needs. His psychological demands are based on fears of poverty, disease, insecurity, and death. He remains attached to his own name, fame, social standing, race, family, and possessions. In short, he is only aware of his body, his mind, and his connections with the world outside. Hypnotized as he is, he believes he is a finite being, the "Me".

In later years, he identifies with the limitations of aging and the natural imperfections of decay and disease. He now begins to believe in the duality of his body and mind and suffers the pain of his own ignorance. He must learn to sail his boat (body and mind) on the stormy seas of his life (time and space).

If man had the wisdom of "I" and "Me", he would know that "I", the soul, is independent of the pseudosoul, the "Me". He would have cared for the *health* of the body and rejected the demands of "Me" for pleasure through indulgences. With this wisdom, he would have nurtured the body against ill-health and decay and sailed across the sea of controlled "beingness". He would have anchored his boat to the lighthouse of the Self and allowed the boat to rock gently despite the storms of life's ocean. When Man discovers the changeless Self, he realizes the superficiality of the flux of health and disease, pleasure and pain, and happiness and disappointment.

My husband travels outside Canada for almost six months in the year. When the children were not as yet married, it was a simple matter to remain occupied with their needs. When they left for their own nests, I knew I needed to enter my own inner-being. I required motherly nurturing for my own inner growth and maturity. It was time to grow up and become self-sufficient. I give credit to my husband for this part of my spiritual journey. He left me to myself to find myself.

He is the half that makes me a complete whole. His actions force me to search what is missing in me. That is the purpose of a spiritual marriage. Pain and pleasure, birth and death, and separation and togetherness are the natural polarities of Man's life. They must be harmonized for the sake of a spiritual existence.

Birth and Death

Medical science claims that a normal person's brain changes substantially every eight years. This means that man is reborn eight times in one lifetime of sixty-four years. People with good *samskara* or upbringing can, therefore, hasten their evolution through meditation and living in harmony with the laws of Nature.

To illustrate this fact, the Master wrote about the imperative need to harmonize the seeker's health with that of the Cosmic Mother.

> "... Our life of harmony with the ampler scheme of the cosmos brings to our heart an inward peace and poise. When poise is maintained within us, problems and challenges vanish like mist before the rising sun. . "

An illumined *sadhak* or seeker does not have to undergo many mortal births and deaths. In the superconscious state he can condense the *karmic* experiences of many lives into dreams of the present.

Only a deluded individual considers his body, his family, and his position in life as invulnerable. Therefore when death strikes his family, he is shocked and bewildered. He is consumed with grief and horror when he confronts death or sees himself nearing it. He cannot maintain his mental balance. No matter what wisdom is offered, he grieves when a much-loved body must be given up.

During sleep, man forsakes his body and attachments to his mind for a restful state. From this joyful state, Man is born: for joy he lives; in joy he melts at death. Death is ecstasy which removes the burden of the body and the mind. It frees the soul of all bodily pain and of its false identifications.

> and the Master wrote:
>
> "Mankind stands between two worlds: one dying and the other struggling to be born. We are the makers of our own world. . and if today the world is an ugly place, it is because we ourselves are ugly. If we cleanse our hearts, we will find that the brilliance in the world is but a reflection of the brilliance within us!"

Analysis of Birth and Death

Enormous efforts are made to avoid birth and death; but *Yogis* recognize sex, birth and death as one unit. Thus, it is necessary to understand the meaning of birth and death - whether that of ourself or of our loved ones.

Physical death may be known in advance, through intuition or a voice in meditation. For a *yogi,* it means passing into another realm of existence. For the seeker, physical form will be reassumed if strong desires are left unfulfilled.

What does it mean when we say that if the "affairs" are in order, death results in little anxiety?

Will Divine Invocations of Aum or "life force" or Light of Awareness, make a difference in meditations and in death and if so, how?

- Is the cycle of "sex-birth-death" a "cause-effect cycle" to hasten a new rebirth?
- Will mortals do anything to keep fulfilling their desires?
- How does one choose their "next birth"?

Where do I want a rebirth or next physical manifestation?

How does an individual choose a particular family to be born in?

- What about upbringing or *samskars* of previous lives, which manifest during childhood and youth?
- Is my desire for a new birth environment to fulfill specific unfulfilled desire: such as an exposure to unmet career possibilities?
- Do I require a spiritual environment in my next life?
- How can I be sure I will get exposed to a spiritual master *Guru?*
- Is the new birth for a physical and a biological evolution?
- How long do I want to live and why?

What is the goal of my present life?

- What is this mystery of "my" ideals, ethics and standards established for myself in my causal beingness?
- How do these determine what I want for my next existence?

Does evolution go on in spite of "suffering"?

- Can suffering be minimized by spiritual "knowledge"?
- Does practicing what is learnt give a new meaning to life?
- Does knowledge and wisdom or *gyana and vigyana,* influence my present life, the time of my death or my next birth?

Do we play love and death games?

- Science prolongs and preserves life but can also prevent life.
- Some people sacrifice the lives of others for greed and power;

Emotional statements like those which follow reflect feeling of hatred and death:

- I could kill. . . ;
- I would die if. . . . ;
- I hate this color; or
- I hate going to work.

If my **words** had power (and they do: they remain as unmanifest "ideas" in time and space):

- How would I feel if I knew that I wished someone dead?

One must stop being careless with their choice of words and instead use precise language, saying exactly what is meant and avoiding needless exaggeration.

Does the word "love" trigger emotional reactions of sex and possessiveness?

- When I control my emotions, do I kill love?

In regard to "habitual" reactions of possessiveness *("moha"* or attachments):

- Is love-sex considered "alive" when controlling another?
- Does my soul feel more alive because I control another soul?
- Does my soul feel dead when I am not in control of situations and not possessing my "loved-one"?
- Is my soul still undiscovered in my understanding?
- Is the impending death of my present existence real or do I feel a sense of possessiveness and fear of "loss"?

All ideas relating to death must be investigated:

- What emotional responses do the notion of death generate in me?
- Can I accept responsibility if my ideas and wishes of death and dying materialize in "reality"?

Killing, whether physically or in thought, is a violent act and is linked to competition for power, riots, and revolutions. We use the word "kill" in many contexts, like speaking of killing:

- Someone's joy;
- Someone's reputation;
- The law;
- Someone's expectations; and
- Goodwill?
- In what contexts do I use the word "kill"?

When "words" express inner thought, is the mind exerting a power?

- Is the word existing in my Imagination?
- Are my emotions involved?
- Are my reactions to sex-birth-death issues, "wishes" to escape intolerable situations?

A killer may exert "violence" towards man, animal, vegetable or situation:

- On what emotional level does a "killer" act?

What of the emotions of the victim? Are they ones of:

- Sacrifice?
- Martyrdom?
- Suicide?
- Terror?

Automatic Reactions have Roots

All **words** used in our daily transactions have roots. The type of *language* we employ hints at what is hidden in the recesses of the mind, from past experiences and births. Difficult situations in life are secretly processed in the mind; they remain as scars in his personality. Man comes to terms with these situations through a series of adaptive reactions. He begins by indulging in self-pity, in an attempt to strike a blow against an actual cruelty or an imagined injustice. This reaction may stem from vanity of his own self-worth, or a sense of self-importance existing in Man's imagination. Consequently, one must ask if all actions have a hidden motive.

Do all these motives play a part in urges of "striking back"?

Undesirable characteristics found in the garden of the mind must be first cultivated for a better understanding and then weeded out forever. The Law of *Karma* applies to negative and destructive thoughts and characteristics, as well as to positive ones.

Until we look at our ugly tendencies and accept our negative impulses, we cannot begin to recognize and appreciate the positive. By postponing *weeding the garden* we allow it to be overrun. And because of procrastination or denial, the next time may never come. Each of us must ask :

- Do I really know myself?
- How do I regard my own life?

Physical symptoms and negative thought patterns characteristically are very individualistic. They shape our lives and experiences through constant repetition. Our childhood centers around core themes, involving being safe, getting love, belonging, self-support, the need for validation, knowing through understanding, mutual support, perfection, the ability to give love, commitments to community and culture, attention, abandonment, and Cosmic connection.

Our illnesses are linked to our beliefs about ourselves and our relationships with others, but especially to our relationship with the Universe. Much of this is determined by our past lives and present life experiences.

With the loss of an extended family, there is a loss of the social unit. The nuclear family is socially unstable and lacks the resources to deal with urban stress. There are failed ambitions and expectations, loneliness and conflicting signals about crucial matters from all directions.

Much of this is comparable to the experience of a child when he enters school where he faces unexpected threats, frustrations, compulsive behaviour, and unresolved issues stemming from infancy.

This devaluation and alienation are issues that lead to victimization, learned helplessness, feelings of weakness, the inability to control issues and situations, and alienation from the Cosmic Energy. Negative thought patterns create emotions of pride, unforgiveness, hostility, despair, cruelty, and thoughts of self-destruction. All adult experiences must be analysed in this context.

Sense Demands for My Pleasure

Man lives in the realm of ignorance or *avidya*. He believes "Me" is "I". "My" demands or *kama,* reign supreme. The pseudo-soul or ego, the "Me" has opinions about everything and imposes its will in ugly scenes of conflict, sense-rousing art and music, sensuous indulgences, and materialistic suggestions. It rejects all intelligent thoughts of good taste. "Me" pretends it is "I" and indignantly justifies to give importance to his own thought processes, both intelligent and profane.

> As long as thoughts are about "My pleasure" it is deemed "My right". A little silencing of the mind would allow the "I" to make the right decisions about "Me's" desires.
>
> and the Master wrote about 'thoughts':
>
> ". . . A change in thoughts can be effected by three methods namely, by reducing the quantity of thought, by improving the quality of thoughts, and by giving different direction to the thoughts. . "

Ego, the pseudo-soul "Me" resents all voices of beneficial truth and wisdom, wanting to hear only the artificially sweetened, poisonous untruths of flattery. This leads Man's intellect to a false awareness of self-importance or pride or *ahamkar* and his own self-sufficiency. Man [most] is convinced that his actions and evil deeds carry no inherent punishment. He denies all analysis of his misbehaviour and prefers to criticize others.

His sense of *smell* is a slave to his attachment to odours of meat, denatured prepared foods, and rich desserts, all of which are injurious to the body. Greed and gluttony or *lobh* eventually lead man to ill-health and an absence of mental peace. Greed or *lobh* creates unnatural cravings for overcooked, revitalized and injurious foods, leading to indigestion. Greed tempts Man to eat more food than is necessary for health. Each time greed defeats Man, it leaves a slight mark of damage which over time accumulates, becomes irreparable, and ends in death. Children entrenched in poor eating habits become victims of greed and gluttony in later life. Parents must become aware of a child's uncontrolled eating habits, hasty swallowing, and incorrect selection of food choices.

Man's sense of *touch* loves moderation in climate, food, and the real necessities of life. Healthy and wholesome bodily habits of necessity result in bodily and mental peace. Under the sway of the ego, the body becomes attached to comforts and luxuries, and to the sensuous feelings that rouse sexual desires. Friction of the rough world trigger thoughts of agitation, fear of pain, and terror of the need for exertion. The body becomes used to idleness, lethargy, and prefers to remain inert in too much sleep.

Unbridled passions in adolescence result in *slavery to the senses*, moodiness, irritability and lethargy. Years later, adults who have spent a life of excitable restlessness suffer from debility, ill health and premature old age.

If conduct was left to ego the "Me", Man instinctively grasps to possess, steal, and strike out in revenge with anger or *krodh*. Instead, the organs of action should be used constructively by pursuing community service and performing helpful deeds. Man should seek our places of inspiration and undertake wholesome exercises. The creative impulse and sex inclinations can be channelled into a positive direction, including forms of art such as painting, dancing, and the martial arts.

Analysis of Competition

In *Yoga* of meditation there is NO competition; rather, begin where I am. To carry competition into spiritual life is a disaster.

Do I compete, and if so, with whom? For what am I competing?

Yoga makes great demands on discipline. Any work worth doing must be done well, with perseverance and sincerity and not out of a sense of competition.

Keep a daily diary of how you follow instructions:

- It is important to record how much time is spent in chanting and meditation.

Competition is an intense emotional urge demanding a quick intervention. It is a stress producing emotional orientation patterns that grind the body, mind, and intellect. It frequently is an unconscious urge, beyond conscious control, continuously directing and influencing our lives. It reflects an aspect of our life that is self-threatening. It takes birth in our formative years when we have had to repress our functions. Unconscious motivations have to be analyzed from the standpoint of Awareness.

Manifestations of the Creative Vibration in Yoga

Restlessness is the identification of awareness with constantly changing thoughts (sensory mind and ego's thoughts). In contrast, calmness is the identification of awareness with the soul's tranquillity as enlightened *chitta or* beingness.

The *chitta* is the mind-intellect-ego complex. It is restless when ignorant and calm when the soul is enlightened in an individualized causal state. According to *Paramahansa Yogananda,* the victory of the soul's calmness over the ego's restlessness advances through four stages:

- Ego (thoughts) are always restless and the ignorant soul *(chitta)* is never calm;
- Ego is restless some of the time and awakening soul is calm some of the time;

- Ego is calm most of the time while the enlightening soul is occasionally restless;
- Ego is always calm, and the enlightened soul is never restless.

Under the control of the ego or thoughts, the bodily kingdom is restless and eclipses the discriminative intellect or *buddhi*. The emotional sensory mind is completely under the control of desires and ego (thoughts) of the causal state. The individual suffers from continuous restlessness, inefficiency, and ignorance.

In the second stage of this psychological victory, the soul wins at times but there is a great deal of self-ignorance must be eradicated through study and introspection. Months of deep meditation help with the attainment of calmness in thinking and the restfulness of the *chitta* or soul.

In the third stage of this psychological battle, deeper and continuous meditation destroys the ego's thoughts and there is calmness. The *chitta* or soul also acquires restfulness, experiencing prolonged periods of peace, despite the demands of outer circumstances at home, at work, or internal conflicts.

The fourth stage of this psychological battle occurs when the ego's demands are transmuted towards higher ideals and the *chitta* or soul is enlightened. The enemies of spiritual efforts (ego, fear, lust for desires, anger, greed, attachment, pride, envy, habits, and temptations) are vanquished with thoughts of discrimination. This body no longer fears, bodily decay, disease, or death. The enlightened soul reigns supreme.

This process is evolutionary and directly proportional to the efforts of *sadhana* and meditation. Individuals must not compete for attainments; success should be your private assessment.

> Study Groups are part of the Master's training for seekers who must be able to express themselves as they evolve in inner understanding. Often these sessions leave a leader of the group with a self-aggrandizing ego To them the Master wrote about Study-group *sevaks* [volunteers]:
>
> "The secret of giving the mysterious 'Touch of Life' to ideas, lies in practice. Live morality before you talk of it. Practice meditation before you preach it. Taste goodness before you recommend it. Gain bliss before you offer it to others"

Motives of Action

All of Man's actions are premised on the desire to *avoid pain and to attain happiness*. Some people avoid pain by adopting dispassion for living. These individuals often end up committing suicide.

All successful human endeavours, victories, discoveries, are efforts at overcoming limitations imposed by man, environment, or Nature. Teachers of all faiths and religions hold that spiritual seekers must also overcome the enigma of how he or she views social and human outlooks as it pertains to things.

Everything has a dual nature. Everything is bipolar. There is the positive and the negative pole. Without polarities, there would be no existence in between. Everything between the sun and earth exists because the earth revolves around the sun. The revolving is because of centripetal and centrifugal forces polarity. Ignorance of this fact in Man's life causes divisiveness and decay.

Man must learn the science of his own immortality. Manifestation is God's dream. It is a dream delusion of God. If God is loved, than Man must learn to love His shadow also. Meditation is the means to make an eternal link with this collective Love of Creation.

Ignorance or *avidya* of this wisdom is the cause of separation from God. Reversing the flow of life in an upward thirst for oneness with God in the divine altar is what is meant by 'twice born'. Man must know the Truth that every atom has life.

Until Man accepts that God is the Power behind all manifestation and activity, he will not succeed in seeing Him inside or outside himself.

Meditative efforts condition the mind to see the power of God. It allows for unity in all things and beings. The coming together of two forces, is a viewing of *Shiva and Shakti* or Spirit and Matter coming together. Although the behaviour of these two forces gives mortals an false sense of duality, all action is a unified effort and for the two-in-one Universal Being.

Meditative wisdom encourages the formation of eternal friendships with persons and people he encounters while on his spiritual journey. His old pain in every cell of the body undergo a definite change. There is a re-birth and self-healing in the brain cells as well as in every bodily cell. He begins to feel that his body is the Kingdom of God. He now has the confidence that God exists in me and that I exist in Him.

There is now no distance between God and me. I can harness the life-force and energise every cell in every part of the body. This spiritual journey is what is known as 'Seeking God'. It is the highest science known - after all, He wrote every other science known to Man!

Once this is intuitively understood, all love-hate situations disappear. Happiness becomes the mortal's perennial experience.

and the Master said about Life's Search for Happiness [God]:

". . . Life is a continuity of experiences. When it ceases, it is considered dead and decay sets in. There is a constant yearning to achieve a greater and better happiness, a fuller and deeper peace. To gain this experience, man must make contact with the world of objects and adjust his relationship with them for maximum satisfaction. . .

"A wrong estimation of the world, superimposition of false values to things and beings, result in imperfect experiences. Learn to reorient your views of the world of objects and beings. . . "

Those with the *habit* of indulging themselves often leap from one *desire* to the next, all for the sake of experiencing pleasure which can never be satisfied. *Pleasure-seeking* is a dangerous game because it can motivate future actions and cause pain. Such actions are based upon a lack of true understanding. It causes in man a sense of separation and confusion. Until he understands that every atom in manifestation is God, Man cannot experience this omniscient energy.

Once man has learnt the art of quieting the mind, the mind finds it unnecessary to pursue objects of the world for gaining peace and happiness. Once a person has achieved this state, he stands out as a beacon-light for others.

This is because what man is really *seeking* for in all his actions is a permanent pleasure or *bliss*, a universal and highest necessity. This Bliss or *ananda* is God. Man also seeks permanent Existence or *sat* which is God. He looks for this Existence in Consciousness or *chit*, which is also God. He therefore seeks *Sat-Chit-Anand* (Existence-Consciousness-Bliss) or God, in all his actions! He has found the common thread that courses through every name and form. He now sings His glory and works in the world for a Collective Good.

Analysis on Mechanicalness

There is a danger that the practitioner of *Yoga* may become mechanical and automatic in his practice. To avoid this, it is necessary to ponder the following questions:

What do I **physically do**, but in a mechanical way:

- Eating?
- Driving? and
- Sleeping?

What are my mechanical **emotional** reactions?

- Anger?
- Headache?
- Fear of the dark?
- Dislike of my own company?

What are my mechanical **mental** reactions?

- Do I suffer from a restless mind when I am not busy?
- Do I drift when things go wrong or become boring?

Everything in our lives exists because there is a <u>need</u> for it, whether this be from our environment or from our causal level. The symptoms, reactions, and conditions presenting themselves are outward expressions of the inner condition of the individual. A specific, natural reflexive physical reaction is the result of a specific thought pattern and/or emotional disequilibrium. What happens and what needs to happen expands us, moves us forward, or allows us to stop and heed the messages of our bodily actions.

What is God?

God is a vague, indistinct theoretical concept lying somewhere *within* us. For many, God remains a theory or idea which fails to convince, because we refuse to change our lives, or conduct our actions to get to know Him.

> the Master told my wide-eyed very young children the following story on how one finds God:
>
> ". . . Once upon a time there was this King who was in search of God. He asked his Minister three questions and told him that if he did not have the answers in ten days he would be beheaded.
>
> " The questions were: 'What is God? Who is God? Where Is God?' The Minister's cook overheard the conversation and became concerned. Five days had gone by and he knew the Minister was no nearer to the answers. "On the tenth day, the Minister decided to sleep-in and go late to the King's Court!
>
> "The cook became even more alarmed, disguised himself as the Minister, and appeared before the King and said:
>
> 'Sire, in answer to Who is God?**:** He is One who makes a black cow eat green grass to make white milk;
>
> 'In answer to Where is God?**:** He is everywhere just like a light of a candle that fills a dark room; 'In answer to What does He do?**:** He helps those who have faith in him'
>
> "Just then the Minister walked into the Court. The King was confused.
>
> 'Who then is this person who is answering on your behalf?'
>
> The cook owned up.
>
> And the Minister said: ' I had faith that I would not be beheaded!'"

Although vaguely there in us, yet, the sense that He exists within us as an *inner experience*, manifesting during meditation and in intense prayer, is not pursued. To those who pursue the search, He takes the form of bliss and inner tranquillity which wells up in the spiritual heart as *calm contentment*. These periods of contentment are enjoyed in the "thoughtlessness" of an inner calm.

During such moments in meditation, we rise to the Cause of this inner Bliss when intuitive realization dawns. Through the power of intuition, Man knows that his body is the Kingdom of God, but the blind Mind is the ruler of the kingdom. Without meditation, he cannot master the wisdom of this truth.

Man remains preoccupied with a need for his own immortality. There is too much distance between him and God. This space in separation shortens in time and distance in meditation. Matter becomes condensed into Consciousness. There is synthesis between matter and energy.

The Awareness which was once vague, is now an intense feeling of divinity and is felt right here in the cave of the brain and spinal cord, where Awareness and Consciousness merge as One. Once the nucleus of the body in the *ajnaa chakra* transforms, the centre of Universal Intelligence at the *kutastha* or Christ Centre heals and protects the rest of the body. The seven spiritual centres are magnetised with increased awareness within the altar of God.

This experience is *intuitive*. The intellect takes no part in its *realization*. When we *experience* bliss-consciousness in ourselves, our narrow individuality, the "Me", is transformed and rises above the duality of pain and pleasure, love and hate, and "Me" becomes "I". We are consumed by an all-embracing sympathy for the pains of the world. Imperfections dissolve and we see in that unifying vision a blinding realization, that this perfect Universe runs automatically, as it should - as *Sat-Chit-Anand.*

This experience pervades our every mood and action from now on. We are now convinced that the ultimate goal of man, his *growth,* within the limits-of-desires he came with, from his previous births. Man knows he must work single-pointedly to fulfill himself, and ultimately for the Common Good of the Universe or *Prakriti.* Having fulfilled these desires, he must now *unearth the mystery of our existence* as Man. The final fulfillment is the discovery of God in us as Existence-Consciousness-Bliss or *Sat-Chit-Anand,* in our transcendental state of "beingness", as "I".

Man's duty or *dharma* to his work, family, friends, and himself must be implicitly obeyed. Man must *mechanically* work outside while actively centered in his own spiritual self as a dispassionate seer of all actions. He lives immersed in His Bliss, in accordance with His will. He now plays the appointed part on the stage-of-life, without becoming inwardly affected by the loves and hates, or the pain and pleasures, of the actors on the stage.

Act he must. That is his duty and therefore his *dharma.* Man must fulfill the desires that prompted his present manifestation. That too is his *dharma.* He also has a duty towards his family and to the world he lives in. When he has found harmony in the midst of opposing poles of man's existence, he will be able to ride his inward journey and at the same time, serving the Cosmic Mother.

and the Master wrote about the *dharma of action*:

". . There is no word to convey all that it stands for, in any other language! It is the 'law of being'. The essential property of characteristic of a thing shorn of which it cannot remain as that thing any more, is its *'dharma'*; like the luminosity of the Sun, the heat of a fire, the coolness of the water, the sweetness of sugar, and the divine spark of Existence in man.

"Dharma is at two levels: the individual and the cosmic level. At the individual level, one's *swadharma* is one's own *vasanas.* At the Cosmic level, it is *Sanatana Dharma*; it is eternal and common to all individuals at all times. It stands for all ideals, purposes, influences, institutions, and ways of life and conduct which shape the character and evolution of Man, both as individual and as society.
It is the law of right living and observances which secure happiness in life and liberation from all bondage because it is ethics and religion combined. . ."

The world's complexities must be viewed as plays on the world stage of life. Man often makes the mistake of identifying with the play and thus feels disgust, pain, sorrow, pleasure, and attachment. Instead, he must learn to distance himself from the play, never identifying with it or coveting the part of another player.

> He must act as the Eternal Witness, defined by the Master as:
>
> ". . He who is the cogniser of manifestations of names and forms and the disappearance of the knower, knowledge, and knowing, but is Himself devoid of manifestation and disappearance. Because He is unmodified and unaffected, He is *saakshi*, the Witness. . "

Attaining Victory over Thoughts

Gradually, Man learns that victory in *sadhana* (self-effort) is achieved through consistency in right thoughts and actions *(yama* or restraints *and niyama* or adherence to pledged restraints*)* which are in harmony with divine laws. This is the only way that Man can ascend the ladder of evolution.

Each man is automatically positioned on the evolutionary spiral of "natural evolution". The *sadhak* or seeker and the *yogi* or advanced seeker, use a scientific method of meditation for their evolution. *A yogi willfully reverses the flow of awareness from Matter to Spirit.*

The *yogi* employs the same channels of the brain and spinal cord which were used to descend the soul into the body. The *yogi* directs the life-force from body into the cave of awareness in the spinal cord and the brain.

The more adept he becomes, the greater he is under the divine influence of the *enlightened chitta* (mind-intellect-ego complex). In even deeper meditation, the *yogi* develops an awakening discrimination. He is able to free himself from his egoistic attachments and earthly possessions and the circle of friends he kept for his indulgences and pleasures. He progressively becomes a renunciate.

> and the Master commented:
>
> ". . Just physically abandoning wealth, home, job, woman, or children is not true renunciation or *tyaga*. On awakening from a dream, when one realizes that all he had experienced is nothing but a dream, the waker's attitude is of disinterest. This is renunciation. On 'realizing' that all this perceiving, feeling, thinking of objects, emotions and thoughts is only a 'play' in our awareness, then the individual loses all interest in the 'non-existent world of unreal perceptions'. He experiences true renunciation. . . "

His motive is not that of *denial.* He is undergoing a *natural expansion* towards his own *self-inclusiveness*, through self-effort and study. He severs attachments and achieves his *goal in life*. Having achieved it, his love includes not only his own family *(tamasic or* self-centered giving and loving*)* and community of friends *(rajasic* or sharing with a larger family*)*, but all of mankind *(sattvic* or expansive sharing of oneself*)*. None of these gains are through mindless automatic mechanicalness.

> and the Master wrote on this natural expansion and self-inclusiveness:
>
> ". . Give! The greatest joy in life is in giving, in loving, and in sacrificing. To give we must have the abundance in ourselves. We can't give what we have not. Therefore, first create fullness: good health, good emotions in plenty, and great knowledge. Then, give physical help to all. Give love and sympathy to those who deserve them. Give knowledge to all who need it. Give! To give is life. . . to take is death. "

Analysis on Mind in Awareness and Consciousness

What do I mean when I speak of "consciousness" versus the "mind"?
- Are the two interchangeable?
- If yes, when or why do I use them as same or dissimilar ideation?

What characteristics does the mind exhibit?
- thinking;
- memorizing;
- concentrating;
- observing;
- daydreaming;
- learning; or
- procrastinating.

How do we account for insight, inspiration, sixth sense, and telepathy?
- Is this the mind or consciousness at play?
- Are there levels of mind and if so, what are these levels?

Understand the mysteries and functions of the mind and consciousness. Become aware of the awesome power of the mind because the mind is the interpreter of all experiences. It is the mind that co-ordinates the senses. It interprets, coloured and conditioned by past memories and concepts. Consciousness lends it an Awareness or a "consciousness of" faculty.

The ultimate reality is that self-healing can only take place by first developing Awareness of the existence of the causal being who is the essence of all previous lives lived. Tuning in to that *personality* involves taking it seriously. It implies, vigorous changes have to be made and acknowledged through corrective efforts, so that the underlying source of all human problem is addressed.

A neutral recognition of likes-and-dislikes leads to non-performance of aggressive reactions to thoughts, situations, and experiences. What is essential is that the seeker correct all habits and tendencies.

Love

The aim of human life is to realize happiness. The root cause of unhappiness is the suffering and unhappiness Man senses when he feels he is not loved. In this mental state of turmoil, Man views Creation as a source of diversion to keep his body and mind preoccupied with names-and-forms, likes-and-dislikes, old habits, and indulgences.

He has become anaesthetized by the charm of *conditional love or sneha*. He is unaware of the *unconditional love or prema,* that envelops and transforms him all the time while he breathes, sleeps, and digests food and air. It only requires a *still body and a silent mind* for man to come face to face with his *Eternal Lover.*

Man and woman, instead of seeking soul-emancipation through soul-unity, pursue the pleasures of the flesh through the sense of **touch** or "sex". Man's soul engages in a constant battle with the ever-present temptation of sexual indulgence. This magnetic impulse drags the soul away from the Spirit in the cave of the brain down towards the coccygeal plexus or *muladhara chakra* and into matter or flesh. The earth-bound conditions are impediments to the early seeker or *sadhak.* Even if married, he is advised moderation. He is advised to seek *love, respect for his partner, and above all with friendship* predominating in his relationship. Similarly, unmarried seekers or *sadhaks,* on the other hand, are advised the practice of celibacy or *brahmacharya.*

The seeker is urged to immerse in wholesome foods, the company of the good and wise, literature expressing uplifting thoughts, regular exercise, and creative activities. These activities make him tranquil and at peace with the *all fulfilling thoughts of Love for God and guru.* This *peaceful pleasure* is transmuted into divine Love and Ecstasy experienced in deep meditation.

The *thirst of affection* is predicated upon a sense of duality between the lover and the beloved. The lover should be able to see the beloved through every window of his thought in time and in space, as a permanent union of love and adoration. He should feel emancipated to adore, but at the same time, should be merged together while liberated.

There is only one True Lover**:** God**;** and each one of us is His dearest beloved. The thirst for affection can never be quenched by the imperfect love of mortals. When a seeker learns to love all beings in meditation, then and then only is this thirst for love satisfied.

This love is felt within the divine cave of stillness and silence. It passes through the whole brain and spinal cord and is experienced in the heat of meditation. This fire not only transforms you, but renders you the gift of perfect *ananda* or joy. The experience breaks down narrowness, tears down boundaries, eliminates differences, and frees the seeker or *sadhak* from all the dual polarities inherent in all names and forms.

Every man leaves this earth in an embittered state of unrequited love and keeps coming back until he finds this perfect love of God. When he recognizes the Lord in his own secret cave of the brain and spinal cord, Man acknowledges Him as the only Perfect Lover, and his heart seeks no other affection.

In the discovery of the long lost Lover within oneself there is a giving and a taking of each other. The "Me" discovers the "I". The "Me" becomes the "I" and "I" becomes the "Me"! The unenlightened soul or *chitta* becomes the enlightened soul, The adoration and oneness is mutual and interactive to the highest degree. There is certainty in the merging of the two when the pseudo-soul "Me" becomes the soul or "I".

and the Master explained that only need for affection motivates Man for His Love:

". . There once was a *swami* who fell head over heels in love with a very cultured girl. Not able to contain himself, he told the story of his new-found love to his dearest friend who was delighted with the news!

'What did she say when you professed your love for her?' asked the friend.

'Nothing. I haven't talked to her yet', the *swami* replied.

'What kind of love is that?' asked the friend.

'Well, I have done fifty percent of the work. The other fifty percent is expected', responded the *swami* lamely.

'But, both you and she need to hear that they are loved' said the friend.

'Right, but I do not have to tell Her anything - She already knows because She is my Cosmic Beloved' said the *swami.*

The friend was confused.

And the *swami* continued*:*

'Come my friend, even in the *Bhagavad Geeta*, the Lord shamelessly professes love for the seeker'

'Krishna already described and enumerated the qualities of his beloved'

"He who hates no creature, who is friendly and compassionate to all, who is free from attachment and egoism, balanced in pleasure and in pain, and is forgiving..

"Ever-content, steady in meditation, self-controlled, possessed of firm conviction, with mind and intellect dedicated to Me, he, My devotee is very dear to Me. . [Geeta 12: 13-14]

"I need not do anything more than love the Beloved. Not only must the lover love his Beloved, but the Beloved promises to return His Eternal Love, unasked. . . "

Analysis of Love

When Man longs for love he is in fact longing for God. His restlessness does not allow man to be with His love and does not permit him to practice the *yoga of meditation.* This is the greatest suffering man must endure. The restlessness which causes loss of harmony of the body and mind is the root cause of self-ignorance or *avidya.*

Having made this analysis, one must ask the following questions:
- What is love?

Is "companionship":
- being needed?
- being accepted?
- being married?
- having children?
- a form of self-gratification?
- helping someone? or
- loving things or nature?

Should one's companion be able to talk back?
- Am I in love with the idea of love?

When I say "I love you", is it because:
- you accept me?
- you are nice to me?
- you care for me?
- you are entertaining?
- you are rich or good looking?
- you offer me security or a social status?

Eliminate all the *because* and feel the relief of a new found honesty. Unconditional love, without expectations, leads to no disappointments and thus causes no pain. Those who have truly loved can drop their expectations, can forgive, and can set their companion free.

Which of my senses experience "love"?
- Is it the mind or the ego?

Man must match the reality of the Universe with our own present existence which is generated by the Law of *Karma*. Distortions of understanding in our present life arise from a deep sense of separation from the Universe. Our physical body, which refuses to acknowledge the connection, experiences exaggerated non-optimal life experiences.

We sometimes feel *it is my fault* and we respond with physical and mental reactions which ultimately result in breakdowns. Separated and isolated from the Universe, we interpret issues and situations in accordance with our *perceived* values. Our actions are interventions to correct a *perceived wrong*.

Such delusional thinking creates mental and bodily breakdowns. It would be more prudent to accept and understand the disturbing thought process and heed the implications for changes in our awareness. Settling for substitutes leads to resistance and denial of the symptom itself. This awareness itself heals.

Mind Levels

Mind makes perception possible. Depending upon the success of his meditation, the inner personality of the seeker or *sadhak* acquires specific characteristics:

- His mind as *unenlightened chitta* is unconscious and inert, providing a *tamasic* or dark background of awareness. Meditation makes it *sattvic* or pure.
- The mind as *manas* or emotional mind is hyperactive or *rajasic,* and is constantly adjusting to desires, impressions, and attachments.
- When *self-conscious,* his *mind* is impure or *tamasic*, and is seeking constantly to embody itself as *ahamkara* or ego.
- When the mind functions as intellect or *buddhi* in its pure state, there is pure perception: its clarity becomes disturbed only when it is self-opinionated or self-righteous.
- As "I" the *enlightened chitta*, the pure harmonized or *sattvic mind* is an unalloyed *jiva* or soul or Self.

Chitta:

As *enlightened chitta* the mind is pure *ananda* or joy. As *unenlightened chitta*, it is composed of past memories, habits, and likes-and-dislikes. It is completely under the sway of the *gunas* or qualities of Nature. The *gunas* or qualities of matter are: *tamas* or inertia, *rajas* or activity, and *sattva* or the harmony of the two. The polarity of negative and positive must remain harmonized in equilibrium.

Buddhi:

As *enlightened buddhi,* the mind is intelligence; it is an actively alert mind but in its own stillness and silence. As *unenlightened buddhi*, it is intellect or an aware mind or thought-filled mind, in the field of ego.

Manas:

As *enlightened emotional manas,* the mind rests in a nest of unconditional love, exhibiting gentleness with all contacts. As unenlightened mind it manifests as fear, desire, and attraction to sensory indulgences.

The vibratory frequency of the elements in the five spiritual centers or *chakras* of the astral spinal cord manifest as five frequencies or five phases of the mundane mind. In their evolutionary frequency sequence, they can be heard as 'inner sounds'.

These are the inner sounds my own father introduced me to when I was seven years old. These are the sounds we ask our own children and grandchildren to hear in their own stillness and silence. They emanate from the astral spiritual centres of the divine cave [spinal cord].

- Earth (ego) sounds like a 'chini chini chini' and then a 'chini-chini-chini';
- Water (sensory mind) sounds like the sound of an intermittent ringing of a gentle bell;

- Fire (intellect) sounds like a continuous hum of a conch you might pick at the sea-shore;
- Air (feeling or *chitta*) can be heard as a lute interspersed with the crackle of the cymbal; and
- Space (soul) vibrates with the music of a flute sometimes accompanied by the beat of a drum.

The *yogi* or advanced practitioner of meditation hears the astral body in the sixth spiritual centre as the sound of many waters where the rivers merge in double beats. In the final union of the soul with Spirit, the *yogi* hears the thundering of Niagara Falls.

These are the ten sounds or tones of the Holy Spirit: Aum or Amen or Amin or Hum. Some fifteen years ago, I had asked *Swamini Sharadapriyananda,* my dear and beloved *Guru-amma* or Mother Guru to explain to me what it was that I was hearing during my meditations. She reassured my doubting medical mind by allowing me a gift of an intense spiritual experience in the bowels of Niagara Falls.

She too left her physical body in early 2000. At our last meeting in Madras, now called the city of Chennai, she whispered her encouragement. She wanted me to finish this manuscript. She knew that I had a deep interest in the *Chakra System.* I was afraid to openly admit this fact. My own Master had not taught me anything about the *chakra* system.

My twenty-five year affiliation with the *Chinmaya Mission* would not allow me to openly admit that I had veered away slightly, from the *sankhyan* philosophy. *Guru-amma* reassured my doubting mind with this statement:

> '. . This is about YOUR spiritual journey. *Swami Chinmayananda* is your eternal teacher. At this stage of your life you must follow the path that will take you to your destination in the shortest time possible'!

The underlying psychological reasons for earthbound tendencies are:

- *Ignorance and fear* against a background of unconscious awareness *(chitta* or feeling*)*
- *Desire* wanting all objects *for pleasure* (*Manas* or mind)
- *Anger* if desire of things and knowledge are thwarted (*ahamkar* or ego)
- Knowledge as inward quest for awareness (*buddhi* or intellect)
- Conscious Awareness as the *enlightened chitta* or soul.

Patanjali's Yoga Sutra (Continued)

Having dealt with *Yama* or restraints *and Niyama* or adherence to pledges of restraints, in its basic stages, it is time now to advance to the second requirement of *Patanjali's* Yoga Meditation as prescribed in the *Yoga Sutras.*

If the cave in brain and spinal cord is the abode and altar of *Brahman* (God), the body plays a vital role in attaining the four aims-of-life. The sages recognised that the body also serves as a temple of the Lord and is an instrument of self-realisation. They knew it had to be kept in a good, healthy condition. They prescribed *asanas* or postures in *yoga,* are to purify both the body and the mind. These had both curative [through molecular transformation] and preventive effects on the body and mind.

To attain steadiness and stillness, *asanas* or postures are prescribed before rhythmic breathing techniques or *pranayama* are taught.

II. Bodily Training

A seeker who embarks upon the path of *yoga* should hunger for spiritual knowledge and self-control. One must practice constantly and possess great endurance.

Sadhana or spiritual-effort has nothing to do with theoretical study; rather it leads to a new way of life. Just as milk is churned to butter and burned to release *ghee* (oil in butter), so must the pupil be unswerving in practice to release the knowledge which is already latent in him. He must find his own real identity. When the seeker realises he is a spark of the Divine Flame burning throughout the Universe, then all the past burns away and he becomes enlightened.

Many of our earlier and younger friends disapproved of the intensity of my *vedantic* study under the tutelage of the Master. I was grilled at a Study Group by two of them.

"You are too young to take on a spiritual life in your early thirties" said one of them.

"It will cause you to abandon your duties [*dharma*] as wife and mother. You have to walk with your husband to enjoy the pleasures of life and society" said the second one.

"What is this intense need for God? Are you unhappy in your marriage? Has life been a 'bummer'? What do you need God for? You have money, a beautiful home, obedient children, a doting husband, a successful professional life, and an inquisitive mind. What is it that has caused you so much pain and dispassion that you have put your family on the back burner of life"? said the first one.

"I want nothing except God. I am like a fish out of water without Him. I must find Him" was my response twenty five years ago, and still is.

It took many years to realise that I can find Him in the altar of the divine cave in meditation. Living within the divine cave gives every seeker a personal knowledge of this experience. Allow me to share this with you, but in stages.

Let us start with bodily training which consists of:

1. *Asana* (postures); and

2. *Pranayama* (breathing exercises).

For the practice of meditation, *postures* and *exercises* are prescribed. The purpose of *asanas* (postures) is to become unconscious of the body's physical demands while deep in meditation. Stilling awareness of the physical body allows the seeker to silently harmonise his breath, energise all body parts with life-force, become aware of the divine cave and listen to his inner astral sounds. Until all of these factors are harnessed, one cannot succeed in entering the stages of awareness within. Once the stillness of the body reaches basal hibernation-level, the seeker can expect to survive at basal breathing frequency, sufficient only to support a heart rate that has dropped to a basal level also.

In the late eighties, we were literally stuck while visiting the Bombay Chinmaya Monastery. British Airways had misplaced and could not locate our suitcases. My pregnant daughter and I had to get clothes made, which is not very difficult in India. While waiting for them, I walked into the new Administrator's office. He pointed to some old desks piled with mountains of old files. He asked me to clean out some of the dusty drawers.

Imagine my shock and absolute delight. I found ancient looking papers and notes on *Patanjali's* eight-fold path to meditation. The Master had somewhere along his own spiritual journey commented on them too. What follows is borrowed from this document.

> and the Master commented:
>
> ". . . Any *asana* or posture in which our single-pointed mind can remain undisturbed and continuously turned in the direction of the Self within, that is *asana. . . Asana* is not any painful posture of the body. . . "
>
> " To study the body at the physical level and hold it without any movement is prescribed as a beginning to the elementary students in meditation. But the final goal to be gained is for the individualized ego in the meditator to glide into the State-of-Pure-Consciousness. To awaken into that state and get the body and the world rubbed out of our awareness is the real 'holding the body in steady pose or *deha saamya. . .* "

1a. Asana (Posture) in Meditation

Asanas correct the misalignment of the spine and cure diseases of organs governed by nerves. Since good health is founded on the delicate balance of body, mind, and spirit, the asanas allow the practitioner to remove all physical disabilities and mental distractions; thereby opening the gates of the Spirit.

i. *Sit in a lotus position, cross-legged with your foot on top of the opposite thigh and with your back pulled gently straight. Pull in your lower abdomen and pull back your shoulders by pushing the chest forward. Your head should be thrown a little backwards so that the chin is parallel to the floor. Place your upturned hands at the junction of the abdomen and thigh.*

ii. *Those who are unable to assume this posture may sit on a chair (with their feet on the floor) until accustomed to sit stable and stationary for long periods: for the eventual purpose of samadhi.*

iii. *Ensure that the asana is correct.*
The head and neck must be erect and perpendicular to the floor. The spine must be erect, with the crown of head, the bridge of nose, the chin, the inter-clavicular hollow, the sternum, navel and pubic bone in alignment. This is accomplished by pulling the shoulders back and contracting the lower abdominal muscles. Prevent the body tilting forward during meditation by throwing back the head with chin parallel to the ground. Remain constantly alert and adjust the body throughout meditation as necessary. Unless the seat is firm, the spine will sink and will not allow the diaphragm to move for maximum expansion during pranayamaor breathing exercises. Ensure that you are sitting flat on the base of the spine.

Three areas of the spine "give way" or relaxes during the practice. These are:
- The perineum on which the seeker sits;
- The spine between the sacrum and the first lumber which is held tightened against the contracted abdominal muscles;
- The ninth thoracic vertebra where the center of sternum is pulled forward, with the scapula pulled back.

The first lumbar vertebra feels the maximum tension where the two curvatures meet. It acts as a fulcrum for stretching the spine vertically. *At first, it is difficult to master the art of sitting because the body tends to tilt forward and adjustments of correct posture may cause discomfort. Over time and with regular practice, these will disappear and an unconscious ability to secure the correct posture will be achieved. .*

Now gently shut your eyes and direct your gaze inwards into the cave of the brain through the Kutastha between the eyebrows, as if looking at something behind and above but inside the cave. Avoid eye movements: they tend to create mind activity. If the whole body is relaxed there should be no flickering of muscles or thoughts.
- If your eyeballs droop or remain horizontal [level of the mind and the eye], you will be disturbed by wandering thoughts and images.
- If your upper eyelids flicker when your eyes are held shut and your gaze is directed backwards, you should partially shut your eyes until you reach a suitable comfort level.
- If sleep tends to disturb you, tighten the neck and spine backwards even tighter.

1b. Meditation: Awareness in Body and Divine Cave

Close your eyes and 'watch' or witness your thoughts until they stop into silence. Become acutely aware of yourself sitting in the posture of your choice. 'Look' at yourself from outside and see yourself from all angles of the body. Now 'feel' every part of your body by contracting and relaxing each part as if you were 'energizing' each part with your awareness [feet, calves, thighs, buttocks and back, lower abdomen, chest, hands, forearms, upper arms, shoulders, neck, face and head].

- i. *Now enter the hollow brain cave through the medulla at the base of the skull and above the spine. Roll you tongue back [this opens the mouth of God] and allow life force to rise to the crown of the head [where energy is stored in the seventh chakra] and allow it to permeate both the hollow brain and the hollow spinal cord. Next raise the life-force up the divine cave to the base of the skull. Here make a forward path towards the Kutastha or Christ-Krishna Centre of Universal Intelligence between and behind the eyebrows. You are now in the "silence" of God's altar.*
- ii. *Now travel from the inside of your brain cave and down your spine. As you travel down, charge your cave with divine awareness pouring in through the medulla. Continue this up-and down movements in awareness of the divine cave. Tightening the spine during the process allows you to hold the attention within the divine cave for long periods of time.*
- iii. *Now move outwards from the cave of the brain and spinal cord. Move outwards to every part of the body from the "cave" to the surface of the whole body. "Feel" every movement of life-force energy (while you contract and relax each part of the body. Start by contracting every body part and withdraw the life-current back into the divine cave. After a sustained period of contraction, relax all body parts and allow the life-force refill the bodily space. Continue this for as long as possible. This is energising body parts with life force.*
- iv. *Now <u>feel</u> the outside of the body (during sustained willful contraction and relaxation). Again attend to every portion of the body starting at the toes and moving towards the head; and then relax completely and feel. Start with the toes, feet, calves, thighs, buttocks, back in four parts, left and right sides of abdomen, left and right sides of chest, hands, forearms, upper arm, shoulders, sides and front of neck, jaws, face, and head. After sustained contraction, relax and feel the life-force moving back towards the cave of the brain and spinal cord. Now rest here in the silence and stillness of the altar of God. Feel the whole body charged with Aum. What you 'feel', 'look at', and 'watch' is the power and presence of God.*
- v. *While waiting in silence, imagine the life force entering your brain cave in waves, through your medulla, up to your sahasrahara and down the spinal cord. Move your lips without uttering any sound. Chant "Aum" with each wave recharging the brain and cord-cave; listen with your inner hearing. You are "listening" to the "voice" of Cosmic Awareness. Focus your attention at the Kutastha between the eyebrows where you are "seeing" the "Vision of Cosmic Infinity".*
- vi. *Now you have filled your divine cave with Cosmic Life-force. Send down (by contracting and relaxing) the energy to your face and neck; next to the*

shoulders and both the upper limbs; next, send the energy to the organs of the chest and abdomen to as far as the skin that covers the trunk; next send the energy down your hips and your lower limbs. Next contract the different parts of your body from toes to head and increase the strength of your contraction. Use your will power to "feel" the "touch" of the energy in intense contraction.

vii. *In this meditation technique, you have learnt to engage your eyes in* ***seeing the Cosmic Vision of Infinity;*** *your ears are engaged in* ***hearing the Cosmic Vibration.*** *Your astral body is engaged in* ***feeling the energy*** *it is made of: from your head to your toes and from your toes to your head. You* ***have entered and met the silence of God in the Altar of His Cave.*** *Your speech is engaged in the movement of your lips as they utter the Cosmic sound: Aum.*

viii. *You now know how to bring the Cosmic Energy into the cave of your brain and spinal cord,* ***at will;*** *you also now know how to energize the whole body, using the* ***power of will.***

ix. *Finally, you are now relaxed in body (the body is still) and the mind is silent in the Cave. Now are able to* ***watch the breath****; witness the movement and feel of cool air being inspired through your nostrils and into your chest; also watch and feel the warm air being exhaled through your nostrils.* ***Watch the breath in silence and stillness*** *as long as you can. Do not be alarmed if the respiratory rate drops.*

1c. Asana in Yoga Exercises

i. *While seated on the floor, stretch your legs in front and bend forward with your two hands sliding down the thigh and legs to the left big toe first. Bend your toe forwards and backwards three times and sit up into the starting position. Repeat on the right side. This extends and lengthens the divine cave and stretches the bodily channels or nadis*

The ankle joints and toes are important acu-points for healing muscle and joints. Bending and stretching your body permits the smooth flow of energy from the cave of your brain and spinal cord to the intra-abdominal organs and to your four extremities.

Metabolic dysfunction result from stagnation in body fluid channels (nadis). This ***maha-mudra*** *allows the divine cave to stretch at full length for maximal filling of the Cosmic Energy.*

ii. *Lie on your back with your legs straight in front. Raise your left leg to a sixty degree angle; then rotate it clockwise ten times, then anti-clockwise ten times.*
Repeat for the right leg.

This improves circulation in the gastro-intestinal tract.

2. Pranayama or Conscious Breathing Exercises:

Pranayama is a breathing exercise consisting of the conscious equalisation of inspiration or ***puraka,*** *the retention of breath or* ***kumbhaka,*** *and its expiration or* ***rechaka,*** *followed by another kumbhaka. It emphasizes the retention of breath at the end of inspiration and expiration. It is a conscious witnessing from the Kutastha, between the eyebrows. It is an active vigilant watching, looking, and feeling the energy as prana or breath.*

This practice allows the lungs to achieve their maximum capacity for optimum ventilation and helps cleanse the nadis or tubular channels through which energy flows, thereby preventing bodily decay. This, in turn, results in positive changes in the mental attitude of the practitioner.

Pranayama begins at the base of the diaphragm above the pelvic girdle. The thoracic diaphragm and the muscles of the neck and face must be relaxed, in order to loosen the grip on the senses and the brain. The seeker now attains concentration and serenity.

Use the "Hum—saa—soo—hum" technique.

i. *Breathe with a contracted lower abdomen.*
Inspire, mentally lifting a cool breath, while chanting "humm" and then pause;
Then expire "saa" with a downward flow of a warm breath.
Pause in expiration as long as possible.
Pause at the end of inspiration and expiration.

ii *Repeat this exercise allowing "soo" to occupy the duration of your inspiration and "hum" to occupy the duration of your expiration.*
Allow four seconds for inspiration, four seconds for pause in retention, and four seconds for your expiration followed by a pause of four seconds, before embarking upon the next cycle.

Ordinarily, we breathe 16 times per minute. This exercise reduces breathing to four times per minute.

- In *pranayama*, the practitioner imagines he draws *prana* (the life-force or *aum* is drawn in through the medulla) into the navel or lumbar plexus *(manipura chakra)* and then propels it upwards to the throat or cervical plexus *(vishuddha chakra).* Inspiration is slow and deliberate and feels cool at the back of the throat. Expiration is equally deliberate and feels warm and dry.
- *Kumbhaka* are the pauses required at the end of inspiration and expiration. These pauses energise the spiritual centres of the spinal cord with *aum.*

This imaginative process of concentration is the secret of actualizing everything. Through continued practice of this exercise, the energy is generated that enables the practitioner to transcend earthly moorings. Conscious performance of *pranayama* (normally an unconscious process) allows deeper layers of awareness to awaken.

This exercise can be done not only during meditation but also while awake at work, or while driving, or when among crowds: it helps still the mind's chattering. During *meditation yoga*, the *mala* or rosary should be used: longer and longer duration of *pranayama* should be practiced while witnessing the breath.

The chest is seen to rise and fall with *pranayama*. The use of the upper chest and diaphragmatic muscles facilitate circulation of blood through the body while correcting oxygen and carbon-dioxide imbalances. In essence, *pranayama* stimulates all the organ systems, including the autonomic system, and makes them energetic with *aum.*

Pranayama allows the seeker to consciously control the operations of the heart and breathing, thereby permitting him to enter *samadhi* at will (soul-Spirit union) unencumbered by the functioning of these organs.

> and the Master commented:
>
> "... *Prana* is a technical term used in our scriptures to indicate 'all expressions of Life in the physical body'. To control *prana or pranayama* therefore, is not only regulating the inhalation and exhalation, but controlling and ending all wild manifestations of life's dynamism at the outer physical level. To reject and not allow the world of objects to come and intrude upon our attention is *'rechaka'.* To turn the entire mental and intellectual attention to the Self within is *'puraka'* and to steadily hold the mind in that poise is *'kumbaka'.* This is true *pranayama".*

Once the heart is stilled, the mind's consciousness also ceases. The body and mind are filled with vital-life force or energy, thus allowing *prana* to unite with the dormant primordial *shakti* in the spinal cord. Advances made over time allow for progressive physical control.

The Art of Breathing

Inhalation *(puraka)* is the intake of Cosmic Energy from the medulla and nostril as *breath* for growth and progress. It is a path of action. It is the Infinite uniting with the finite. It draws in the breath-of-life carefully and then gently distributes it evenly throughout the body.

In practicing *pranayama,* breath is like an infant demanding special attention from its mother. Just as a mother loves her child and devotes her life to its well-being, so the *awareness* has to foster the breath. The relationship between *awareness (chitta* or mind/intellect/ego or feeling) and *breath (prana)* is like mother (life-force) and child (breath). However, before such a relationship can occur, the diaphragm and intercostal muscles must be trained and disciplined by *asanas* so that the breath moves rhythmically.

When a child goes to school for the first time, the mother submerges her own identity until the child is accustomed to school. So also, in the case of *awareness: chitta* as life-force can transform itself into the same condition as the flow of breath or *prana,* guiding it to rhythmic flow.

Awareness (chitta) as life-force energy must guide the flow of breath through the respiratory passages for absorption into the living cells. When the breath moves, awareness residing in God's cave of the brain and spinal cord *observes* the movements of the breathing, until one day the breath unites awareness and soul. It is the breath that is the umblical cord that connects every living thing and being with the Cosmic Mother.

- *Inhalation or puraka* is inhaling the cosmic energy from the medulla-nostril from Infinity to the body; the life-force *aum* is stored in the divine cave of the brain and the spinal cord. The cave is the altar of God.
- *Kumbhaka or pause at end of inspiration* is the rest in the silence of the divine cave of awareness.
- *Exhalation or rechaka* is the breath that goes out after inhalation. It is the out-flow of the individualized energy-awareness uniting with the Universal Energy-Awareness. It quietens and silences the brain. It is the surrender of the ego (unenlightened *chitta)* and its immersion with Universal Awareness: *aum.*
- *Kumbhaka or pause at the end of exhalation* is the resting in the silence of Universal Awareness.

According to *Yoga,* the mind *(manas),* which is the source of **emotions**, is located between the navel *or manipura chakra* and the heart *or anahata chakra* In keeping the cave of brain and spinal cord (*awareness)* connected with the emotional center or *anahata* or heart center (by stretching the back straight, pulling in the lower abdomen, and pushing chest forward and scapulae together), the seeker breathes without losing contact with his center of awareness or *ajnaa chakra.*

- *During inspiration, begin by expanding the diaphragm and by relaxing the upper abdomen across a band between the navel and the floating ribs behind (but with muscles of the lower abdomen contracted). Fill the lungs from the bottom up: up as far as the collar bones.*

Yogic Experience of Pranayama

Yogis who are deep meditators, claim that the *energy of inhalation* enters through the nose and is received by the causal body. The *chitta ascends* from the *manipura* to the *vishuddha chakra* (navel to throat) There is contact between the subtle astral and causal bodies. Awareness ascends and unifies the contacts between body, breath, and awareness until it reaches the Self. *Expiration* begins at the top of the chest descending to the level of the navel. Here, the *prana* merges with the Self.

Kumbha means the pot is full or empty. ***Kumbhaka*** is of two types: either a pause at the end of inspiration or at the end of expiration. As previously stated, breath is the bridge between the mortal's body equipment and the soul. *Kumbhaka* is the art of retaining the breath or *prana* in a state of suspension and which rests in Cosmic Awareness. During these periods, there is withdrawal of the intellect from the organs of action and those of perception. In *kumbhaka* the senses are stilled and the mind is silent. The seeker is breathless with adoration, completely absorbed in his ideal within the cave of God (brain and spinal cord).

In time, with perseverance and patience, the practitioner is overcome by intuitive and instinctive feelings of peace and joy. He is in tune with the Infinite. The *chitta* (mind-intellect-ego) is free from passion, anger, greed, lust, pride, and envy. *Prana* (life-force) and *chitta* (mind/intellect/ego) become one in *kumbhaka.*

In the *Bhagavad Gita* (Chapter IV : verses 29 and 30) *Krishna* tells *Arjuna* of the different types of sacrifices *(yagnas) and yogis* or seekers. *Krishna* explains that the *kumbhaka pranayama* is one of the *yagnas*, and that *pranayama* falls under three categories: inspiration-retention; expiration-retention; and absolute retention *(kevala pranayama).*

The *yogi's* divine-cave in the brain and the spinal cord is the sacrificial altar; inspiration is the oblation *(puraka);* expiration is the fire *(rechaka). Kumbhaka* is the moment when the oblation of *puraka* is consumed in the fire of *rechaka* and they (self and Self or "Me" and "I") become one in the flame.

Having understood and experienced this *vidya* or knowledge through personal experience, the seeker who is becoming a *yogi* or advanced seeker, makes *pranayama vidya* or knowledge of breath-control, a part of his wisdom. He offers his knowledge, his wisdom, his very life breath and his *chitta* (soul) as oblations to the Cosmic Soul *(Atmahuti).* This is the state of absolute surrender in which the *yogi* or evolved seeker, is absorbed in the adoration of the Lord.

What is Japa?

The repetition of the single thought (usually a *mantra)* is *japa.* Although the evolving *chitta* the soul, assumes the role of a witness and is free from cause and effect, it is caught up in the turbulent activity of the mind *(manas).* The purpose of *japa* is to disengage the mind from idle talk and thought or feeling and to focus the mind upon a single point which is linked to a single thought, a hymn, or a verse. *Japa* transforms the seeker and transmutes the ego, making him humble.

the Master wrote:

> *Japa Yoga* is the training by which the ever-dancing rays of the mind are compelled to behave in some order and rhythm, and bring out of their effort a co-operative effort a single melody of repeated mantra chanting. In this practicing, the mind becomes extremely single pointed.

Aum used in Japa

Pranayama or regulated breathing, turns the *chitta* of the seeker to the Lord who is residing in the cave of the brain and spinal cord. Here is where the seed of omniscience and the source of all beings reside. Personal experience allows me to share with you that using *pranayama [ham. . saa so. . ham]* as a *japa mantra* while working, walking, driving, exercising, or while amongst crowds is the best way to stop the mind's constant chattering. At other times, the use of *AUM mantra* takes you to the core of your own existence.

Aum, whose cosmic sound is the mother of all sounds in all languages, is the conglomerate sound of all creation, the source vibration that sends forth the whole of creation. It is the Word that expresses Him as the mystical syllable AUM or Hum or Amin or Amen *(pranava)*. From this Cosmic Vibration - *Aum* came earth *(bhuh),* atmosphere *(bhuvah)* and the sky *(svaha)*. All speech came from *AUM.*

> "I am Alpha and Omega, the beginning and the ending, saith the Lord, which is, and which was, and which is to come, the Almighty" . . Revelation 1: 8

Aum conveys concepts of omnipotence and universality. It is auspicious and awe-inspiring. It is a symbol of serenity and majestic power. It is the ever-lasting Spirit, the highest aim. When its connotations are known, all longings are fulfilled. It is the immortal sound. Those who enter and take refuge in It or in Awareness, in the "divine cave" of the brain and the spinal cord, become immortal.

The seeker is miles away from meeting with God within the divine cave. He still sees Him and Her outside himself. He still asks the who, what, where, when, and how's of God, not very different from what we did when we were still children. It must be the umpteenth time that the Master repeated this:

> and the Master explained patiently to my very young children, years ago:
>
> "G is for Generator who can do nothing without Knowledge, so He married the Goddess of Knowledge, *Sarasvati;*
>
> "O is for Operator who cannot operate the Universe without money, so He married the Goddess of Wealth, *Lakshmi;*
>
> "D is for Dissolver who must dissolve matter, so He married *Parvati* who is Energy Herself!"

The Power of Cosmic Light generates *Aum* which not only symbolizes fire, wind, and sun but also feeds back into Its own source of Power and Light, as if: **One with It** in the symbol of *Shiva-Shakti or Purusha-Prakriti or* God-the-Father-Mother. In the **form** of Lord, the **symbol** is worshipped as *Brahma (Creator)* or

God-the-Father*, Vishnu (Preserver)* or God-the-Son*, and Shiva (Dissolver)* or God-the-Holy-Spirit, which synthesize the forces of life and matter.

As Time or *kaala, aum* stands for past, present and future, and yet is beyond and before Time. **As Thought**, *aum* represents the mind *(manas)*, intellect *(buddhi)* and ego *(ahamkar)*. **As Quality**, *aum* represents the three *gunas* of illumination *(sattva),* activity *(rajas),* and inertia *(tamas)*. As a *yogi* immersed in *Aum*, the *yogi* is freed of the effects of the qualities of matter or *gunas (gunatita).*

and the Master commented:

> "Time is *Brahman* [God] alone. The entire Universe of names and forms is brought forth, made to play and disappear, all with effortless ease of the twinkling of an eye by *Brahman, in Brahman.* This Supreme State, when it comes to express as 'total desires' in all minds, becomes God and God becomes the Creator, Sustainer, and Annihilator of all plurality. This conjuring-up of the world or *Karana,* as our dream comes to being in our waking mind, and gets merged into our mind, as Time or *kaala.* To seek this Source of 'time-experience' is the seeker's highest path. . "

The three letters of *AUM* are symbols of man's search for truth along the three paths: knowledge, action, and devotion. The *yogi* or evolved seeker, who has attained the state of stability *(sthita prajna), by* meditating on *AUM*, remains steady, pure, faithful, and becomes great. He now is able to live on a minimum of food intake. He survives upon the life-force.

> "Man shall not live by bread alone, but by every word that proceedeth out of the mouth of God. " Mathew 4: 4

What is Invocation of Light in the Divine Cave?

Divine Light is Aum. Invoking Aum as Light of Awareness in the Altar of God is invoking Life-force Energy in the Divine Cave. The cave is a void that has existed before time and space and occupies the brain and spinal cord. The inner gaze is able to invoke the Divine Light of Infinity and the inner hearing can hear the Cosmic Voice of Aum.

In the newborn, the Divine Light and Vibration enters the cave through the openings in the skull. The individual being enters the divine cave through the Kutastha Centre in the medulla. Individuality of this causal being mingles with the life-force behind the eyebrows in the mind center of the brain. Next the chitta (mind-intellect-ego) descends through the brain-stem and spinal cord. This individuality resides in the various spiritual centers of the divine cave, at the same time energising all the spiritual centres with Divine Light and Vibration .

In meditation, this Light of Consciousness and Awareness is experienced as aum. This meditation technique involves the exercising of Will Power (residing between the eye-brows in the Kutastha or Christ-Krishna Center of Universal Intelligence or site where one views the Cosmic Vision) to invoke aum as Divine

Light of Awareness.

1. Before starting meditation, protect yourself with the "caveat" or protective shield as described in the "Introduction to Vedanta" in the first meditation exercise. Next, establish yourself in the asana or posture of your choice. Do pranayama to regulate the breath and then by watching the breath. Invoke the Divine Cave by first imagining a "void" coursing through the brain and the spinal cord: from the base (buttocks) to the crown of the head.
2. Fill the dark void in the "cave" with the Light of Awareness.
3. Now inspire through the "mouth of God" in through the medulla and fill the "cave" or Altar of God with the Vibrating Cosmic Sound of Aum. Pause at the end of inspiration and "feel" the Light permeating the "cave". Expire and pause inside the "cave" and feel the Light permeating the "cave". Continue to bring in the Energy in waves with each breath. Keep the attention focused at the Kutastha throughout the breathing. Keep listening to the Cosmic vibration through the right ear. Maintain this for at least fifteen minutes or more.
4. Now send this Light of Awareness from the "cave" to your head and neck, and down the shoulders to the tips of your fingers, and to your chest and back (back to front), and also down both lower limbs as far down as the toes. With each pause of inspiration and expiration, say:

   "Every cell of my body is penetrated by the Divine Light of Awareness;
   Every level of my awareness is illumined with Divine Consciousness;
   I have in me the altar of God;
   I am One with the Light of Awareness".
5. Allow the whole body to become a mass of Light-Energy and enjoy Its warmth. **This is called: energizing of the physical-astral body.**
6. When finished, direct this Light in Love to heal a problem area of the body or to find guidance in Its intuitive powers of silence, or to resolve a personal problem. Alternatively, direct the Light towards someone you love and wish to help, or return It back with Love and Devotion to the whole Universe.
   After mastering the concepts of Pranayama and Asanas, the practitioner is led to the next stage of Patanjali's training in Yoga Meditation.

III. Spiritual Training:

Spiritual training consists of four elements:
- *Pratyahaara* (withdrawal of senses);
- *Dhaaranaa* (concentration);
- *Dhyaana* (meditation); and
- *Samadhi* (ecstasy in "oneness").

Pratyahara

Pratyahara is a discipline to bring the wandering senses to the mind source, in the divine cave, which is their true home. Through *pratyahara,* the mind separates itself from the sensory windows of the body and looks within itself, in the cave of awareness in the brain and spinal cord.

Pratyahara is the willful observation of energy while the seeker maximally contracts all twelve muscle groups (feet, calves, thighs, buttocks, back, abdomen, chest, hands, forearms, upper arms, shoulders, and neck-head) and then relaxes them. Maximum contraction when sustained for prolonged periods, allows the seeker to become aware of the pure energy being withdrawn from the body parts and into the divine cave - all within his own astral body. A sudden or slow relaxation of all body allows the appreciation of the same energy entering the body parts from the divine cave to the body. Practicing this for long periods allows the seeker to abide within the energy, away from the senses. The energising of the twelve muscle groups is continued until all awareness of the physical-astral bodies becomes a sustained awareness of the energy alone.

Although *Raja Yoga of Patanjali* has been described a an eight-fold path of meditation, in practice it is a merging of the eight as one practice. This practice is a combined 'watching' by Consciousness, 'looking' at the changes and transformations taking place in Awareness, and an inner 'listening-feeling' of the senses, and mind-intellect.

The practitioner is also asked to watch or concentrate *(dharana)* on his normal and then rhythmic breathing at the same time. The seeker must at all times have his tongue rolled back to touch the soft palate, where he remains connected to the source of life-force as it enters the medulla behind the palate. His eyes are rolled up and back to look at the Cosmic Vision in the *Kutashtha* behind the eyebrows. Here the seeker is connected to the Cosmic Mother. The higher the concentration, the easier it is for the seeker to become disconnected from the physical demands of his mortal beingness.

The mind seeks-gratification through the senses, yet, at other times wants to unite with the Self. *Pratyahara* quietens the senses and draws them inwards into the divine cave.

> and the Master commented on *pratyahara* or the withdrawal of the mind:
>
> "... *Pratyahara* consists in recognizing in all sense objects, the Self as their very essence. The sense objects are nothing but the projections of our own Consciousness, through the mind and intellect equipment. If this understanding is coupled with the understanding that even the contact with the sense objects is nothing but the contact with the Self alone, then *'pratyahara'* is achieved. Self-withdrawal is not the deadening of the mind, never allowing it to go out. Let it go out and let it experience only the presence of the divine. ."

Of the five senses, vision or visual perception has the most influence on the cerebral cortex and consequently the greatest influence on the mind. To negate the impact of physical vision, the practice of meditation requires closing one's eyes. During meditation, the **inner gaze** must be fixed at the *Kutastha* in the divine cave looking at the Cosmic Vision at all times.

> and the Master commented:
>
> ". . . we may start with the practice of 'steady gaze' or *drik-sthiti* which will help to quieten the mind a bit for the contemplation of the Self, but the mind must get merged in that state, and the entire world of objects should roll away from the meditator's awareness. When the mind reaches the higher state of Consciousness, the mind ends and all becomes One Brahman [God]. This is the noblest of visions. Merely gazing at the tip of one's own nose will not take us anywhere in the spiritual life of awakening into the Bliss-state. ."

Once the mind has receded into itself, devotion to Light of Awareness and the exercises of *Asana and Pratyahara* have been mastered, the next step is to discuss concentration *(dharana)* which we have already been practicing, anyway.

Dharana

Dharana is the intense and perfect concentration of the mind upon an inner sound or on a single idea, accompanied by complete abstraction or *pratyahara* from everything pertaining to the world of senses and the world of objects.

Listening to the inner sound through the right ear is continued until it makes you deaf to all external sounds. In the beginning, the practitioner hears loud sounds. Over time they are observed to first increase in pitch. Next the sounds become subtle. Concentration will be seen to change from gross to subtle or even subtle to gross.

The secret of this practice is to remain single-pointed. The mind must not be diverted toward thoughts and must remain unruffled. The practice stimulates our inner awareness to investigate the intellect.

Through *dharana* or concentration, the ego's shell is gradually fractured and its individuality destroyed. This process of fracturing occurs in the mind. To achieve *dharana*, the seeker focuses first at the *ajnaa* in the medulla, and then at the *kutastha* or at the Christ-Krishna center, between the eyebrows .

The mind concentrates on the *ajnaa* and guides the *prana-shakti* or *aum,* the life-force energy, from body identification of "Me", into the divine cave. Here the seeker directs the *aum* to the *kutastha* where the real subject of my search resides: the concentration is on "I".

- The object is the ego or "Me", the individuality of my "beingness", and the subject is the "I".
- Like a laser beam, *dharana* gradually fractures the surface of the matter-identified ego.

- The meditator's concentration gradually becomes increasingly focused and synchronized at the *kutastha*.
- Continued effort at *dharana* results in the merging of the "Me" and "I": 1 + 1 = 1

**Neurophysiologically, with *dharana* or intense concentration, the overall activity of the cerebral cortex (neoencephalon) or conscious and subconscious brain is lowered. With this practice, the limbic system, the hypothalamus, and the brainstem (diencephalon) or unconscious brain, and mesoencephalon are stimulated to a very high degree.

**The unconscious energy of deep sleep (causal beingness) within the dienecephelon or brainstem *(ajnaa)* and paleoencephalon (*kutastha)* eventually becomes stronger than the conscious energy of the neoencephalon (as awake and dreaming "beingness" in the conscious and subconscious states).

The contents of the unconscious or causal or *vasana* mind (desires, habits, likes-and- dislikes, past impressions and ingrained deep emotions) enter the domains of pure awareness. This natural process can cause interruptions in *silent and still awareness* (in the divine cave, while the *sadhak or* practitioner is involved in the practice of concentration or *dharana.*

**Of medical interest. May be omitted if not interested.

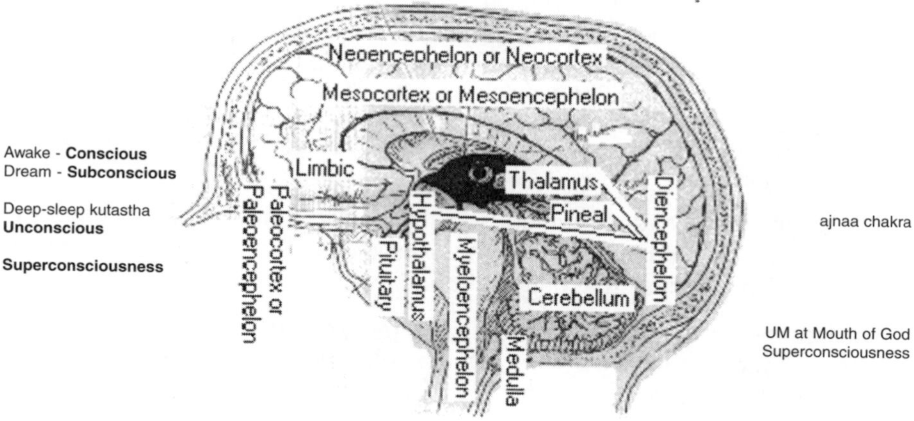

Figure 20. Levels of Awareness-Consciousness in the Brain and Brainstem

Disturbances from unexplained sources may take the form of anger, profound sorrow, or deep emotions. Mental images of the past may also disturb the practitioner, sometimes for months on end.

Persistence in the practice of *dharana,* despite these disturbances, results in the purging of the subconscious and unconscious states of "beingness".

- When wandering-thoughts interrupt *dharana,* the seeker should observe them as a witness until they are purged and the mind is completely cleansed.
- Once this happens, concentration is not disturbed. *Dharana* can then be maintained and sustained for long periods, until the ego shell is completely shattered.
- Initially, the experience of bliss may last a few seconds. There is a new discovery: a bounty of bliss and infinite power which is so precious that one is willing to die for it.
- Once experienced, this soul-Spirit union is realized as a clear, intense, and persistent pleasure which remains for the rest of one's life.

and the Master commented:

". . *Dharana* is concentration. . . Concentration is not tying down the mind to a certain point but allowing the mind to move everywhere and anywhere and trying to see wherever it moves in the presence of the Self. Let the mind go wherever it likes, but, then and there let the seeker experience the presence of *Brahman* [God]. This indeed is concentration. Let the mind appreciate the names and forms it perceived, but along with it, let it also feel the presence of *Brahman. . . .*

"Concentration is not the one people generally go by artificially looking at a picture of a deity and then complaining that when they see the face of the deity the feet are not seen and vice versa.

"Concentration is a technique of feeling in one's own mind a constant and continuous atmosphere of perennial divinity wherever the mind may land. The constant and continuous awareness of the Lord's presence everywhere in and through all the seeker's experience within and without is *dharana* or concentration. . . "

The casting away of ego (our old "security blanket") may cause a temporary instability of bodily and mind functions manifesting as insomnia, hypersensitivity, fear of death, nervous stomach, anxiety, and even palpitations.

The treatment for this is to re-focus the energy by doing a modified *pranayama:*

1. *Focus your inner gaze at the kutastha between the eyebrow and visualize the cave in the brain and the spinal cord which is filled with a void that existed before time and space. Now fill the cave with Awareness through the mouth of God at the medulla. With an inner hearing, hear the aum filling the whole cave from the crown of the head to the base of the spinal cord at the spine's tail.*
2. *Now pant about four to eight times a minute. Slowly, inspire and expire from the base of front of chest (manipura chakra) to the base of the throat*

(vishuddha chakra) for a few breaths, until the body is stilled. The stillness is experienced during the pauses at the end of inspiration and expiration.

3. *Next, visualise the inspiration of Aum through the medulla with each inspiration and allow the inspired air and Aum to merge in the pause of awareness in the cave.*
4. *Repeat the same for expiration and pause in the cave at the end of expiration and rest in the silence of awareness. Now resume dharana.*

Dhyana

Dhyana is a state of mind wherein there is no sensuous thought. It is concentrating upon one thought: that is meditation. It is a continuous flow of perception like a flow of water in a river which is unceasing and absorbed in God-Consciousness. It is the only way known to attain immortality and eternal bliss.

Dhyana is the final destination reached after mastering the art of self-study, reflection, and observation in search of the Self. It involves looking at your most innermost being and culminates in the discovery of the Self. Man is drawn between two paths: one drags him towards desires and sense gratification, bondage, and self-destruction; the other guides him upwards towards purity and realization of the inner Self. To succeed at *dhyana*, the powers of the heart (at the *anhaata chakra)* and the intellect (at the *ajnaa chakra)* must be blended.

Dhyana is like deep sleep with a difference. It brings about a loss of identity and individuality, leading to serenity in the alert and conscious seeker, who becomes a witness to all his inner activities: the seeker or experiencer *(chitta),* of the sought experience *(chit)* and seeking *(dhyana)* merge into one experience of intuitive perception that presents itself as a realization.

Untrained, the mind flies aimlessly. In self-analysis, the seeker integrates the mind and the intellect by will-power. Years of discipline and long, uninterrupted practice of moral injunctions or *yama* and ethical or *niyama* principles, training the body by *asanas* (posture) and *pranayama* (regulated breathing), and restraining the senses by *pratyahara*, ensure the growth of the mind and inner awareness.

> and the Master commented:
>
> "... There is a subtle difference between *dharana* and *dhyana*. ... really speaking, meditation consists in constantly feeling that the seeker himself is *Brahman* [God], not to think that this one before him is *Brahman* or that which he is feeling is *Brahman*. The *sadvritti* or righteous thought, is the divine thought which brings to the seeker the awareness that all this is *Brahman* and he also is *Brahman* which is a condition of the mind, which no more depends upon any of the objects, which no more courts any of these objects. . .
>
> "To lift the mind away from its support stimuli (seeing, hearing, smelling, tasting, touching) is to make it constantly and continuously attentive, alert, watchful, and vigilant, and be aware of the Consciousness alone.

> "That Consciousness in which all objects are removed is *dhyana* or meditation. This condition, when the individual experiences himself as nothing but the awareness-minus the objects or objectless-Awareness is declared as *vikhyatam* or *dhyana*-meditation. Meditation on a chosen 'form' is not *dhyana*: it is *dharana*. As a result of *dharana,* one enters *dhyana. . .*"

Dhyana literally means *meditation.* It is a subjective experience of an objective state. Its purpose is to strengthen and maintain this temporary and infrequent union with Spirit: this happens in the early stages of the practitioner's life. The experience is in one's own psyche. Here, the "being" becomes One with the "Being" by transcending the physical and subtle or astral dimension, and the awareness of oneself and body-awareness disappears.

- The seeker may experience revolving lights at the *kutastha* or the Christ center between eyebrows. He may or may not experience surges of power like the melting of lights flowing into oneself: One may or may not feel warmth or cold at the base of the cord (coccyx) or the lower abdomen (sacral plexus) which falls and rises to the *ajnaa chakra*.
- This experience is associated with a complete loss of consciousness and body awareness.
- It may last thirty minutes or longer.

Breathing is shallow or arrested, especially if the eyes are rolled up to the Cosmic Vision at the *kutastha* between the eyebrows. The heart beats drop to basal level. Some practitioners may even experience a sense of dread.

- This stage is the awakening of the primordial power of life-force that has entered the *brahmanadi* (causal spine) at the coccyx (in the central cave in the spinal cord).
- A warm sensation rises to the *ajnaa* centre and into the *kutastha*. Awareness becomes a 'no thing' awareness.
- There is no operation of mind or body.
- There are no psychic contents (subconscious or dream state) in awareness.
- The ego is partially fractured, and the pseudo-soul (ego) gradually rises towards the higher dimensions of the Self (soul).

There are no experiences of past births (psyche of personality or *karana* disturbing thoughts) in this stage of the seeker's development. Instead, the seeker fears the dissolving of the chastened ego or *enlightened chitta*, the Self or soul with Universal Consciousness or *chit*. He experiences impending death. This is resolved by praying for protection from the *guru* or God or re-invoking the *kavach* or protective shield.

Focus at the kutastha which sits directly in line with the ajnaa chakra (between the eyebrows) and repeat the mantra three times:

***aagama-artham to devaa-naam gama-naartham tu raksha-saam*
kurve ghantaar-vam deva devata hvaana laksha nam
dig-bandha aum bhur bhuvah swaha

iti dig-bandhaha
dhyaanam

Or repeat three times:
"I invoke the Cosmic Forces inside me: give me strength, protection and guidance".

Samadhi or Superconsciousness

Meditation is *samadhi* when it shines as both the subject and the object of meditation: as One. Separate notions of meditator, meditating, and meditation become One. The practitioner is not conscious of either the internal or the external objects. It is a blissful divine experience when both the mind-intellect and ego are dissolved.

Despite intense meditation, the ego: (the "Me - Beingness") continues to stand in opposition to the Self: (the "I - Beingness"). The pseudosoul's power can be temporarily negated in soul-Spirit union, but the ego is almost invincible and continues to disturb this process.

As the bonding of the soul-Spirit becomes stronger (with deeper and longer meditation practices):

- There is no further existence of body and mind (awake or conscious state).
- Similarly, there is no intellect of higher emotions (dream state or subconscious state)
- There is an ideational state of the past births residing as the unconscious state of deep sleep as unenlightened *chitta* or feeling (also called the ideational or causal or *vasana* state of beingness).

Up to this point, the mind (BMI - body, mind, and intellect) was necessary to bring the seeker to this state. Beyond this point, even these are negated for the final experience: a state of superconsciousness of oneness of soul and Spirit.

and the Master commented:

". . . We have to understand that the objects of the world are not merely objects, but objects in a medium of *Brahman* [God], objects playing in the ocean of *Brahman*. Meditation consists of identifying oneself not with the object but with *Brahman* in which the object is playing through the *vritti* [thought]; 'I am *Brahman*'. When I experience this *brahmakara-vritti* [thought that I am God], I totally and completely give up the *brahmakara-vritti* and live only as the *Brahman*.

"This continuous awareness, that 'I am *Brahman*' which admits no otherness in Itself for any length of time is *samadhi*, which is a first-hand experience or *aparokshanubhuti*. This is a subjective experience of the *Brahman* which comes when the seeker ends even the *vritti* or thought that he is *Brahman* and lives as *Brahman* Itself.

"In the one who has become *Brahman* there is no thought that he is *Brahman*, because the subjective state-par-excellence is the state where no thoughts exist,

> when even the thought of that he is *Brahman* does not exist. . .
>
> "The total merger into *Brahman* where there is no entity to say that he has merged is called *samadhi.* Here the seeker experiences what the *Sastras* and the *Vedas* stammer in their inability to express the Infinite".

Conclusion

An existence without awareness of the Cosmic Soul is like living without any bodily communication, emotional interaction, and intellectual connection. Such an existence leads to negative thought forms and emotional reactions, based upon precipitating environmental and situational circumstances. They present themselves as dynamic- generating-symptoms of life and living. The intensity of these symptoms determine the severity and magnitude of a personality disruption.

Entering the pathway of meditation is a means of adjustment which allows the seeker to interpret given situations in terms of known and learned pathways. The outcome of the path is an evolution through the processes of transformation. Through a process of sharing, contact, and support with the Cosmic Soul, there is a profound change in the individual who is able to organize, prioritize, and realize that he is an evolving being.

SECTION TWO

Topics in Section Two

“I Repetition is the Method and also the Path of a Spiritual Journey

This manuscript has gone through eight readings by one person [Carolyn Gray] who did not know the first thing about the Hindus or *Vedanta.* She is a dear friend and her educational background gives her the qualification to judge the document for its language. By the time she was reading her eighth time, she was in tears.

“I have realised that there is nothing that Hindus do that is different from what the Bible asserts. There is just a cultural difference in the way we express it”.

Another manuscript reader found some sections repetitive. Rachna Gilmore felt the book had to be either a manual of instructions on meditation or a description of a personal spiritual journey. I would have to bare my soul. “Show don’t tell”.

The task started as an instructional manual first for my daughters and then for Meditation Groups. My younger daughter reminded me this Knowledge is a Gift from my Master. How true.

The Master was the subtle steering-force of my body, mind, and intellect. The transformation and evolution was the result of repetitive practice. The conclusions were fleshed out and have been presented as facts and information. These are my insights and conclusions but I have no authorship rights to them. They are Universal Truths.

The Master spoke very little and when he did, they were messages to benefit humanity for generations to come. The utterings and writings of the Master, whether through letters to his seeker-families or through his voluminous writings are precious pearls of wisdom. He transformed the lives of many, many thousands around the globe.

Patanjali Yoga Sutras and the *Chakra* System was not his method but he had written commentaries on them. This was the path for me and it is being shared with the reader.

In 1989 I was seated in Mr. Gupta’s car driving from Bangalore to Mysore when the Master said:
“In twenty-five years from now, the world will awaken to a long gone *Swami.* You will not be around and neither will I.

They [the world] will ask: ‘What was that meteoric star that crossed the sky of Time so many years ago’?

Your grand-children will tell the world that their grand-mother knew that *Swami.*”

She was that reluctant student who loved him and used him too. She submitted to him after two decades of close contact!

Svadhisthana Chakra

Second or Pelvic Chakra (sacral plexus)

Preamble

The *svadhistana chakra* or sacral plexus, symbolises the second twin who are the first two *chakras*. Together they represents the art of Restraint (at the root or coccygeal centre) and Adherence (at the second or sacral centre). In the first *chakra*, Man's desires manifest themselves as a list of indulgences desired and promoted by the mind through the five senses. These tendencies are to be restrained.

Most intentions fade into lost promises - unless there is the will to Adhere to the *Yama* and *Niyamas* (do's and don'ts) of any early spiritual journey. Successes here, lead to the third mundane *chakra,* where by constant practice or *abhyas*, the seeker enters the divine cave in a thought-free state of contentment.

Observer-Observation-Observing

Yoga is the negation of thought *(vritti).* Most thoughts have a dualistic value. One value originates as ideas emanating from the ego. The other idea is influenced by emotions. These cause disturbances in awareness. They prevent the perception of the real "I" the soul or Self.

Yogic method demands that, in order for the mind to be open to becoming still and silent, it must be emptied of all its conceptions and assumptions. Once this is done, the mind communicates with and can directly perceive its own real nature. The *observer* (watches), *observation* (looks), *and observed-observing* (feels) the changes. This means that the three: body, mind, and intellect (BMI) become one with the perceiver-feeler-thinker (PFT) from the *vasana* or causal level.

In other words, the old extrovert BMI, through spiritual effort, becomes a changed unit-value *(chhandas)* of a changed-changing body, an introvert and introspective mind *(devata),* and an aligned witnessing intellect *(rishi).* This alignment of the three bodies or *shariras* gives the practitioner his own ultimate Truth, in a single experience. (Please refer to the diagram 'Changes through Meditation' on page 5).

While the early seeker will not really comprehend this experience, its repetitive but improved presence creates a *pattern*, by which the seeker or *sadhak* can measure the value of his own Existence in relation to Universal Existence. Mother Nature now begins to disclose the organic workings of the Life Force or *Prakriti or Aum* in the practitioner. There is a direct perception, and the seeker or *sadhak* sees things as they really are.

This Self-knowledge is the highest form of knowledge. The seeker or *sadhak* begins to understand the realities of the outer world. He understands that the outer world exists as it is, for his own personal experience, and that it is connected intrinsically with his own awareness.

He realises that he is the *rishi* or witnessing **observer** who 'watches' all the shenanigan of the body, mind, and intellect. He is also the metamorphosing person transforming his own inner world as the *devata* who 'looks' and makes this **observation**. The outgoing or efferent impulses and actions are those of a changed person and all actions acquire a *chhandas* or changed quality.

This is because the incoming or afferent impulses or actions of the seeker have a modifying influence on the master organs in the brain. They now release modified neurohormones and neurotransmitters. The whole body now undergoes gradual transformation in the field of perceiver-feeler-thinker (PFT). Now the **observing** of the world is in accordance with the new inputs. He sees the world according to the filters of his own new experiences.

The seeker or *sadhak* now reintegrates all the confusing multiplicity of the world, aligning his senses, organs of action, and sensory mind into a single mental experience of **stillness.** Mother Nature or *Prakriti* or the seeker's physical being is in a state of perfect harmony (*sattvic).* He is not subjected to opposing polarities of his existence. He is aligned with *reality.* He realises that Nature or *prakriti* and Spirit or *purusha* are One. The seeker's mind becomes **silent.**

The seeker or *sadhak* finally understands that if he is to achieve self-unfoldment and self-understanding, he must live in harmony with Nature, both in himself and outside. He must have a healthy body and must master the tools *(pranayama and pratyahara)* prescribed to change the conditions of his physical *(annamaya kosha)* and physiological-psychological *(pranamaya-mannomaya koshas)* sheaths or *koshas.*

The successes in every his efforts can be measured only by acquiring greater self-awareness and self-integrity. Through these visible changes, the seeker becomes a master of his own destiny. This is re-asserted by all Masters of all faiths.

and the Master wrote:

"Success in life [spiritual] lies in one's own bosom, not in the world outside and religion provides the access to it."

Psychology of Raja Yoga

Modern psychology analyses emotions and instructs the patient to right the wrongs of his thoughts causing him psychological problems. *Raja Yoga* insists the seeker or *sadhak* must empty his mind of all thoughts and preoccupation with wrongs and guilt. To accomplish this, he is advised to follow the five disciplines of restraints or *yamas* and five adherence to restraints or *niyamas.*

Restraints are in five *physical disciplines*:
- non-violence in thought, word, and deed,
- truthfulness;
- control of sexual energy;
- non-stealing, and
- non-attachment.

All indulgences through the senses are curbed by making resolutions. It is in the first *chakra* where desire for indulgences take their moorings. Restraints of the five senses are triggered at the first energy level. **Adherence** to restraint of out-going senses underlies the ethical foundation of a dutiful or *dharmic* existence. Five *niyamas* or *adherence* to restraints are observed through *mental disciplines:*
- contentment,
- purity of diet and lifestyle,
- self-study,
- self-discipline and
- surrender to His will.

Yogic **postures** or *asanas* are advised to increase the *sadhak's* vitality and harmonise disturbances in his physical body. *Pranayama* serves to still the breath. Through it, the *sadhak* learns to expand his own life-force energy for both vigour and vitality. Progressive gains made at deepening and extending the various phases of **breathing** still the breath and the act of breathing is at peace. This peace in respiration extends its effect as harmony of life-force flow coursing through the senses, emotions, and mind. The *breath is now visibly silent.*

The seeker or *sadhak* now can silence the senses and mind by **redirecting the life force** back to its own source in the spinal canal. This is *pratyahara.* The life force is now available to focus itself on the **mind in a single search** for the self. This is *dharana.* Some seekers concentrate on the five *chakras* together within the divine cave. Some advise concentrating the mind in the heart area where the element of air is experienced as a void in outer space. This text advises concentrating on the Christ-Krishna Centre between the eyebrows or the *ajnaa chakra* at the base of the brain, in the vicinity of the "mouth of God" in the medulla.

Once the "observer-observation-observing" (*rishi-devata-chhandas or Purusha-Prakriti-Action)* become one, the still and silent mind is able to mirror the Truth as

It really is. The seeker or *sadhak* can dwell at this point and experience himself as the **witnessing awareness.** He is able to observe (witness or *purusha or rishi*) everything that he sees (as awareness of changes taking place as a result of meditation in his causal *prakriti or devata*) with his inner gaze. This is **meditation** or *dhyana. Thought is involved!*

When awareness (object) becomes one with consciousness (subject), there is only oneness. This is **absorption** or *samadhi.* This conscious unification of the seeker's or *sadhak's* life force with the universal life force is the goal of joy and the fulfilment of life. This is how a seeker consciously moves from materialism to his own pure nature of awareness.

Physical expressions of the Subtle Svadhisthana Chakra

Yoga involves awakening the life-force of the subtle energy in the *chakras.* This life- force directs and guides the physical body through the nervous system and into the appendages of the body, also known as the organs of senses and organs of action. It is through these equipment of the central nervous system that man is allowed to make contact with the world of objects and things.

It is through them that all man's desires are satisfied and he is happy. The mind co-ordinates all the needs of the senses. The intellect bases all man's activities in accordance with his past unfulfilled desires, likes-and-dislikes, old habits of millions of past births, and past concepts.

When desires are thwarted, fear and ignorance of the Truth compels the blind neuro-endocrine glands to take control of the physical *chakras* or nerve plexuses in the spinal cord. The Master neuro-endocrine gland in the base of the brain is forced to make physical adjustments in the brain, and the body seeks indulgences for pleasure and temporary happiness. Since desires of the mind require the senses for self-gratification, it is the tongue and the reproductive organs that are most easily seen to respond to the demand for indulgences.

The first or coccygeal plexus or *muladhara chakra* is under the sway of the adrenal glands. All lusts for indulgences are expressed as desire *(kama)* at the first level of understanding. Desire is allowed manifestation through all the five senses. Introspection and restraint of the need for indulgences empowers the seeker.

After overcoming and understanding the base *chakra (muladhara* at the coccyx), the seeker moves upwards into other levels of awareness. When desires and lusts are thwarted at the first base, the second *chakra* (*svadhisthana chakra) or* sacral centre physically expresses itself as *krodha* or anger.

Self-control becomes a habit only through constant practice or *abhyas* of self-effort (*sadhana).* Deciding that he will refrain and restrain from the urges of the senses is just the first step. Adhering to the desire to restrain is the second step. Restraint and adherence to restraints are the twin efforts required to reverse the flow of the out-going senses seeking self-indulgence.

The first two *chakras* in the divine cave are twins. They are symbolically represented by the twins *Nakul and Sahadev* of the *Pandavas* (five brothers for the first five *chakras:* each representing the character depiction of a seeker who has reached that level of self-improvement) in the voluminous epic, The Mahabharata.

The second centre is symbolically represented by *Nakul* the second twin and one of the five *Pandava* brothers, He symbolises adherence to the practices of restraint in *sadhana.* (Please refer to Figure 17)

Awareness involves increasing self-understanding from the point of view of self- knowledge. Many use the word *awareness* interchangeably with *consciousness.* Consciousness, however stands on its own as a substratum. Consciousness is of the characteristic of God or *Purusha* and requires no other knowledge to become aware or conscious. Awareness, in contrast, requires the power of Consciousness for its existence: this is the characteristic of Mother Nature or *Prakriti.*

In the early stages of seeking, the seeker is still very much under the influence of the creative-force manifesting at the second *chakra.* As he evolves and introspects, he notices his faculty of idealistic creativity manifesting. He starts to transform, imagine, forecast, and conceive images, beyond the faculty of his previously out-going senses. He realises, that they were always embedded in his causal beingness. As he stills the body and silences the mind, his inherent idealism seeks validation as the seeker evolves.

The seeker must not be too alarmed when he is forced to acknowledge that even mundane desires begin to hyper-manifest at this creativity level. The seeker instinctively pursues all efforts to extremes, for the experience of self-pleasure. Both extremes are to be acknowledged as existing. With practice of both restraint and adherence to restraints, the seeker makes progress.

Nonetheless, when creativity does not reflect love of the Spirit, Man pursues a dead path. Indulgences, for the sake of pleasure, drain energy and cause fatigue in the second spiritual centre. *Adherence (Nakul)* to *resolve* problems *(Sahadev)* with indulgences must be made through repetitive practice or *abhyas (Arjun).*

The sense connected to this *chakra* is taste. The *tattvaa* or base element for this *chakra* is water, which symbolises imagination. Invariably when intertwined with emotions, *imagination* can work off tangent, and become the birthplace of many personality problems.

On the left side of this physical and astral *chakra* and along the spinal cord, resides the *ida* or the oldest part of the nervous system. In Western terminology, this *nadi* or channel is the parasympathetic nervous system, evolving through millions of years and millions of reincarnations. Here is embedded the true record of all the modifications of the individual as he adapted to changes in environment and world condition. Here is where the self or individualised soul-knowledge of any given individual person resides. This is the inherent quality of this side.

Any interference on this side is an invasion into our own being. The left or the parasympathetic autonomic nervous system which communicates with the right brain translates this invasion by activating the suprarenal glands through the descending right sided sympathetic nervous system. Together, these are the main afferent and efferent channels or *nadis* that influence this *chakra*. When the second channel is irritated through this channel, the person manifests *krodh or* anger.

The channel or *nadi* on the right side of the *svadhisthana* or navel *chakra* is under efferent control from the left brain. Through the sympathetic nervous system, it governs the functions of the liver, pancreas, spleen, and intestine.

All experiences of an individual's action are transmitted to the left brain. The brain in its egoistic nature, demands recognition for all actions by this person. When there are emotional imbalances, the defective effect on this side of the brain is transmitted down the right side to cause diseases in the body organs this *chakra* controls.

The liver is the focus of energy projecting down the right side of the body. While many think the *seat of attention* is the brain, the wise or *rishis* maintain that it lies in the liver. The centre of attention is necessary to project the self or ego into the real-ness of day-to-day living. Over-stimulation of the liver can lead to restlessness of the spirit and a grumbling temperament. It is a recognised fact that both allopathic and *ayurvedic* medicine recognises that both the liver and the eyes can be damaged by the heat [side effects of hepatic metabolic function] caused by alcohol consumption.

Since attention is the ability to project the self or ego into the world, stresses of artificial behaviour dulls the sensitivity of this *chakra*, resulting in depression and lack of enjoyment in life. This is because the person intuitively knows he is dishonest with his own inner being. Sensory indulgences behave as parasites, weakening the experiences of the centre and the organs it controls. There is an ambition to be superior to others or be acclaimed for intellectual superiority, expressing through the right channel. Spontaneity is absent from all ambition. Completed works lack vitality. The results are those of an unbalanced artist.

Through self-development in *yoga*, this channel permits its inherent creativity to flow through the more central channels (from *sushumna to vajra to chitrini and finally brahmanadi*) and for the seeker, a newer dimension is achieved. Through *sadhana* or self-effort, the seeker can become rooted in the soil of divine consciousness. Thus anchored, the seeker becomes an instrument of the all-pervading power of collective evolution by sharing, interacting, integrating and becoming inspired by the Creative Spirit. (Please refer to Figure 15)

The Unmanifest Energy of this centre is that of the *intellect*, which expresses through the mind and senses as *imagination.* Real listening of the mind is only possible when the mind becomes still and attentive. The seeker is asked to hear what is being said without interpreting it.

In dealings with the physical body, perfect attention must be given to body movements especially during exercise. The seeker is encouraged to be attentive to the life-force or *prana* as it energises the muscles being exercised. This is done by *pratyahara* or abstraction of the senses.

The exercise has already been described in the previous section. The practitioner rolls his gaze into the Cosmic Vision and rolls his tongue back towards the soft palate. He watches the movements of his breath while listening to the inner sounds through the right ear.

He observes both sustained contraction and relaxation of every one of the twelve muscle groups of his body. He realises that he has withdrawn from his senses and is one with the life-force energy coursing through his physiological-psychological or astral body. He becomes the energy itself which makes its presence heard through the harp of the water element.

Personality traits or *vasanas* must be subdued and ego analysed. The guiding thought of this centre is purity of mind like the lotus, which radiates purity despite the muddy waters from which it springs. These muddy waters represent reproductive energy, manifesting as desires and imaginations. Thoughts must be refined and controlled.

Daily life translates itself through mental-talk into anything we want to talk ourselves into or out of. The stories of the lives of the *five Pandavas* in the *epic Mahabharata* are examples of the uphill battles encountered in the first five spiritual centres.

Arjuna is advised to address issues that sour a seeker's daily life. *Krishna* discusses these issues in the *Bhagavad Geeta*. The seeker's daily living necessitates a constant vigil in dealing with:

- impulses (*causal trait - ajnaa);*
- false pride (*mada - vishuddha);*
- reactions rather than responses (*karanic habits - ajnaa);*
- self pity (*matsarya in envy - medulla);*
- false modesty and self importance (*matsarya* - medulla);
- selfishness (*moha - anahata);*

All of these characteristics must be replaced with positive traits.

Why practice Yoga of Meditation?

Here, I choose to repeat myself. The goal of meditation is to achieve oneness between the subject of my meditation: **"I",** and the object or the practitioner of meditation, **"Me".** An artist who possesses the innate ability to become one with his art is an example of such oneness.

At this point, despite the efforts made in *dharana* or concentration, the seeker still perceives a distinction between the "Me" and the "I". He cannot seem to overcome this overwhelming sense of difference between the subject "I" and object "Me".

The seeker finds it very difficult to concentrate, as the *ego is activated and becomes stronger during meditation.* The sensing mind is doubtful, and the doubting ego continues to remain separate from the subject. Wandering thoughts continue to plague the concentrator, but through diligent practice of wilfully avoiding *raaga-dvesha* or likes-and-dislikes, all thoughts will eventually disappear.

Concentration or *dharana* is made easier when the practitioner also practices *pranayama* or watching the breath and *pratyahara* or negating the senses through energising the twelve muscle groups of the body, at the same time. When practised for long periods, the mind and senses withdraw into the divine cave and the intellect is in awe of the changes occurring in his physical and astral bodies.

In this final stage of concentration, all thoughts stop and the concentrating ego "Me" is abandoned. Immediately, there is the harmonious union between the subject "I" and the object "Me." The concentrator is filled with a sense of a magnificent vital energy and his consciousness of the body fades away. In this state of awareness he no longer experiences wandering thoughts.

For many, even this objective is difficult to achieve, and if achieved, it is often only of brief duration. If this happens, the seeker is urged to maintain the *sadhana* of *yama* and *niyama.* He is also advised to refrain from all habitual judgements of likes-and-dislikes.

What happens in the Brain during Concentration?

Ordinarily, the brain is in a constant state of excitement from the stimulation of the five senses. For example, the eyes convey stimulation to the visual cortex in the occipital lobe (sensory receptor area) and then to the perceptual area in the psychomotor temporal lobe where the disarrayed sensory stimulation is arranged in *semi-arranged sensory perception.* This stimulus is now relayed to the frontal lobe for determination and actualisation of the perception. (Please refer to Figure 20).

Each of the sensory afferent cortex, depending upon its receptivity, has an inherent rate of excitability as seen on the electroencephalogram - EEG. This makes it difficult to concentrate.

The immobility of *asana* or posture in meditation, reduces physical-mental excitability until the whole brain assumes a single harmonious pattern of synchronised stimulation. For example, in the waking state, the EEG records alternating sequences of alpha and beta waves. The alpha waves frequency is of nine waves per second.

While entering into a combined *dharana* or concentration, *pranayama* or regulation of breathing, *pratyahara* or concentrating on becoming the energy sheath, and during *dhyana* or meditation, the alpha frequency of the EEG drops to around six waves per second. During this same period, alternating alpha waves (which are much slower) and theta waves are also seen to appear and are easily recorded.

Further deeper concentration into the yoga of meditation, results in *localised* synchronised stimulation in the brainstem in the zone of superconsciousness. In this state, the sense of *individuality* of the ego is lost, and one is left with an quiet, alert and vigilant mind**:** a pre-requisite to meditation. At this level of deep concentration, the EEG loses its periodicity and is replaced by continuous alpha waves.

Group meditation has the power of synchronised narrowed or *group focused* consciousness with the innate ability to motivate any positive actions wanted by the group.

What are "Wandering Thoughts"?

Once the meditator has attained synchronised stimulation and the awareness of the body is lowered, he becomes cognisant of wandering thoughts arising from both the subconscious or dream state, and, from the unconscious or deep sleep or causal state of the mind. These thoughts enter awareness only when consciousness is weakened as in the dream state, or during concentration and meditation practices.

The conscious state (awake state) and the subconscious state (dream state) appear as: desires, feelings, emotions, images, and flights of imagination. The unconscious state of *karana* or causal being manifests as clusters of memories of images from past births, first entering the subconscious and then the conscious states of being. Each state of beingness has a competitive adversarial relationship with each other, with each trying to suppress the other.

Seeds of past actions or *karmas* are stored in the memory bank of the *chakras* or spinal cord energy centres and in the causal body. While they normally do not manifest as thoughts, a mixture of impressions do surface as:

- desires in *muladhara* (coccygeal);
- sexuality from *svadhisthana* (sacral);

- gluttony in *manipura* (lumbar);
- aggression in *anahaata* (dorsal);
- human love *(sneha) in vishuddha* (cervical); and
- wisdom in *ajnaa* (forehead).

How Thoughts Disturb Concentration

As the Master so often repeated, the mind is the 'dispatch clerk' of the five senses. Its characteristic is its fabric of emotions. The demands of the senses evoke emotional responses in the mind and it does what it is asked to do, without thinking. The actions triggered are outward-bound contacts with the world of things and beings, for the purposes of self-satisfaction.

Meditation reverses the flow of the senses towards the divine cave. The result is a gradually integrating personality that is both introspective and creative. He has the *rajasic* or creative urges to serve the world, It takes two to three years of daily intense meditation to purge the mind of all its desires, emotions, and mental images. Only then can he serve his community.

In the initial stages, the seeker is disturbed by wandering thoughts involving things and events which surface in the mind from the day-to-day events of living. This occurs for a few months, but gradually, the mind turns to old experiences, made up of desires and past emotions, which lie embedded in the subconsciousness.

Only when past and new memories have been purged, can the subconscious be assumed to be cleared. Consciousness, however, may still be disturbed by *ideas, representations* and *images* of the past, arising from the unconscious state of being. These originate from past memories embedded in his causal being. These also must be exhausted.

How one measures Progress in Meditation

At this stage, the practitioner of meditation feels the lower part of the body charged with vital energy. Softness is replaced by increasing tightness in the lower abdominal muscles. At the same time, the upper part of the body feels empty. This is an indication that one needs to move to a deeper practice *pratyahara in* meditation.

I was recently told an interesting story about why man takes to the path of indulgences:

> "Every part of the body requires acknowledgement. Just as the senses need stimulation. The twelve body parts [feet, calves, thighs, buttocks, back, abdomen, chest, hands, forearms, upper arms, shoulders, neck and arms} require massaging. This is why man seeks body contact for the sense of touch. Instead,

do intense *pratyahara.* Contract and relax every body part to its maximum and infuse the body parts with the loving energy of the life-force"

What about Wandering Thoughts?

There is no need to suppress wandering thoughts. Assuming the stance of a *witness or saakshi*, watch the thoughts until they are finally exhausted. *Pressing the up-turned palms into the thighs* will stop wandering thoughts during all stages of yoga. Once the thoughts stop, the hands should be relaxed.

Revert to pranayama-pratyahara and concentrate on the breath by observing breathing with an **inner gaze, listening** attentively to the movements and sounds of respiration and ***feeling*** *the energy or prana* as a coolness and warmth of physical breathing.

- *Concentrate on the pauses at the end of inspiration and expiration in the silence of the cave, in the altar of God.*
  Now merge with the stillness of the physical and astral bodies and the silence in the cave of Awareness.

This exercise stills the senses of seeing, hearing, feeling, and the mind. Concentrate on the breath rising and falling between the navel and the throat chakras.

Maintaining the gaze upwards and backwards at all times, prevents disturbances from wandering thoughts. Eyes directed below the horizontal line induce thoughts of daily interactions. A gaze that levels the eyeballs in a horizontal position, triggers thoughts of past interactions. Raising the gaze higher may cause disturbances in awareness of memories of previous lives. These too must be *lived* until they are exhausted. *All thoughts must be exhausted.*

Is Meditation a Self-hypnosis?

Self-hypnosis is an autogenic training wherein the practitioner wilfully withdraws from the senses and the mind and from the outside world. Through *pratyahara*, he concentrates on an alert movement of his attention to the energy sheath of his astral body. The astral body is that what you see as a 'blackness' when you shut your eyes.

Through contraction and relaxation, the practitioner contacts *prana* the life-force until his whole being is a mass of energy alone. Having weakened the awake consciousness, the practitioner enters the realms of the subconsciousness-unconsciousness and finally into the blissful superconscious state. The inward journey is a gradual effortless state of merging of soul with Spirit. It is a state of inner realisation that I and the Spirit are one!

This differs from *commercial hypnosis*, where an external source makes the suggestions, and an external energy is required to keep the person's awareness submerged in a shallow state of subconsciousness. The past comes to the level of wakeful state *for manipulation by the hypnotist.*

> and the Master wrote:
>
> "...all hypnotic effects are temporary; whereas once *realised*, it is an experience eternal. God-realisation is a realm from which there is no return. In fact, meditation is a process of de-hypnotization, getting oneself away from one's identifications with one's body, mind and intellect, in order to reach the eternal Consciousness in one's own centre."

What is the Awake or Conscious state?

Consciousness in the awake state is a way to *cope* with the outside world. It allows us to maintain individuality while wearing a mask of *personality.* The subconscious mind governs the conscious mind and accepts things that are unacceptable to the conscious mind. These actions are stored as memories of impressions and images in the subconsciousness: they disturb the practitioner of meditation as wandering thoughts.

When meditation purges the subconscious state, the practitioner of meditation has a changed view of things, beings, and events that occur in his waking state. His world-view is of things as they should be, rather than how he would like it to be changed to suit him.

What is the Subconscious or Dream state?

Dreaming is a state wherein the contents of the subconscious are brought up into the conscious mind to become active and to manifest as thoughts. When the conscious mind ceases to function for prolonged periods of time, the mind becomes less resistant to the external world. It is at this time that extra-sensory perception *or ESP becomes manifest.*

When an individual enters the dream state from the deep sleep, bodily functions become unstable and irregularity in heart and respiratory rates are seen. Rapid Eye Movements (REM) manifest on the EEG as the suppression of alpha waves. REM lasts 15 to 30 minutes and recurs four to eight times a night.

REM is associated with a state of weakened consciousness where the individual is half conscious and half awake - dreaming. The autonomic nervous system is triggered by a destabilised (REM) when the mind exits the from deep sleep (unconscious mind) to the dream state (subconscious mind).

When wandering thoughts occur during concentration in meditation (manifesting in EEG as REM), they are images being released from the subconscious and the unconscious minds. This state continues during persistent efforts in concentration until the mind is completely purged.

What is the Experience of the "Purged-mind"?

Once the mind has been stabilised and freed from invading thoughts, and *pranayama-pratyahara* has been practised for a prolonged period of time, the breathing slows and may almost stop, and the heart rate becomes slow and restful.

The practitioner feels a momentary oneness with some incredible divine power, embraced within the power. There are momentary experiences of oneness of the object and the subject: the "Me" merging with the "I". The practitioner is willing to let go of his own individuality!

If the practitioner's efforts are sincere, the reversal of the flow of life-force towards the divine cave allows him a clear perception of a pure body-mind-intellect. He has the ability to detect the powers of inspirations and intuitions. He becomes acutely aware of the need to move to the next step: from intense concentration to deeper meditation.

Analysis of Thoughts

Water, which is the symbol of this *chakra*, represents the mind. Uncontrolled desires destroy the mind:

- If mind is a flow-of-thoughts, follow each *river and stream* of thought and until it disappears.
- If it persists, then *exhaust it in the action that must be performed* to disempower the power of mind (deeper *dharana-pratyahara* or concentration and disempowerment of the senses).
- Analyse and discard each thought by *dis-allowing emotions to become involved.*
- Keep a diary of the thoughts. This allows one to *exhaust thought and mind in action.*

Analysing thoughts is like making a positive statement and an inward affirmation that our thoughts are in tune with all our present and past images created from many previous lives. Now it is time to enhance the quality of these images. By gazing at these thought-images in your own stillness and silence, you have an opportunity to change the way you think. Travel the path of concentration and open the gateway into a new you as opposed to an imagined *old* you!

How does one purge the "awake state"?

The practitioner must continue to practice restraints or *yamas* and adherence to restraints or *niyamas* and continue to investigate the *urges* of the "Me" in order to modify behaviour in the awake state.

Many a seeker has lamented that they 'slipped' in their efforts after making major advances in their spiritual self-improvement. Old inclinations have a habit of pulling the seeker back to where he started. A burst of anger or a critical judgement has undone me a million times over! The Master called me a 'bull in a China Shop' when all reason and logic flew out through the window! What is interesting is that if I started from the beginning, [with *yamas* and *niyamas*] it was very easy to get back on track.

Yamas are commandments of *physical* conduct. *Niyamas* are *mental* rules of ethics for self-purification. Unless both are embraced, the seeker will repeatedly slip backwards. They are the pillars that must be adhered to if, there is to be success in the seeker's or *sadhak's* efforts at Self-Realisation.

The Master never criticised the offender. He berated the action only. He was forgiving enough to tell me that there would be a day when my sincere efforts would achieve greatness! My rocking boat would surely reach the shores of sanctuary.

and the Master wrote:

"...It is the privilege of man to achieve greatness. Success should have been a habit if only the individual knew the art of diligently using his own abilities and efficiencies. The tomorrow you are waiting for may never come! Introspect, Detect, Negate, Substitute, Grow and Be Happy. Start Today.."

Further Investigation of Speech

Speech is truly the first level of human self-expression. Here, in the second *chakra,* speech must undergo further refinement, especially taking into account the fact that all that is spoken now at this stage, is with a greater awareness.

Pure-Awareness is *enlightened chitta* (mind-intellect-ego complex) - a faculty of *increasing-Consciousness* or *chit* which leads the seeker to better *understanding.* At this stage, language can now be utilised for higher expressions. There is a greater awareness and the introspective being is receptive to his own and the Master's voice (or your guardian angel's) emanating as an inner voice.

Expressions of greater awareness at the mental or *manasic* level consists of *intuitive listening* to the mental speech. When this is developed further, it can lead to *intuitive perception* of both intuitive speaking and listening, for example:

- in the practice of meditation or *dhyana*, mental speech has ceased or is **stilled** and is **silenced;**
- in concentration or *dharana* combined with *pratyahara* or negating of the senses, the mind is silent but alert and the body parts are vibrating with a divine energy of the life-force;
- in the trance of oneness or *samadhi*, the seeker has sunk deeper into the brain-stem level where there are no thoughts possible. There is only awareness that the loved and beloved are one! This is intuitive perception.

The process of listening to the *guru* or intuitive listening is a slow process of perceiving and assimilating all that was ever taught or said to the seeker. Memories of these past communications re-emerge for the development of intuitive awareness in the seeker.

At the time, the seeker is unaware of the messages being instilled into his subconsciousness. Years later, some of these incidents that seemed like enigmas at the time, become clear through life's situations. If the seeker is sincere, he acknowledges that the changes are imperceptible. He must be patient but persistent in his self-effort. Surrender to the preceptor's wisdom is the only way known to man who travels the path of spirituality. He insisted every seeker had to live the extrovert life to the fullest, in accordance with the rules and duties of his life's commitments:

the Master said:

Take time to laugh, it is the music of the soul
Take time to think, it is the source of power
Take time to play, it is the source of perpetual youth
Take time to pray, it is the greatest power on earth
Take time to love and be loved, it is a God-given privilege
Take time to be friendly, it is the road to happiness
Take time to give, it is too short a day to be selfish
Take time to work, it is the price of success.

Man has the habit of giving everything a name, and an intellectual desire to give each object and event a personal meaning. He does that by splitting every experience; he views it through the prisms of his sight, sound, taste, touch, and smell. One experience now acquires five qualities. A seeker on the path of Yoga of Meditation, pulls all these tendencies towards the divine cave in the brain and spinal cord. Merged in the one Life Force - a*um* the *pranava* or Cosmic Sound, he sees all the differences of matter and sense identifications merge into one experience. He realises first hand that all the differences are threaded by the one reality: *Aum*. The seeker begins to see the world of names and forms as the diversity in the single mighty body of the Cosmic Mother. His speech becomes an affirmation of this divine experience.

Speech, at the second level of evolution, is symbolised by the *shanka* or conch of the ocean waters. The sound is that of the waves which one listens to when the mind is silent. Thereafter, even while toiling with the daily activities of living, he hears the hum of the *pranava* in the background of his awareness, and the mind stops chattering *(mauna)* with his mundane wandering thoughts.

and the Master comments:

"...The man of spiritual realisation remains in that inner silence or *mauna,* which is a state beyond the senses and their perceptions, the mind and its emotions, and the intellect and its thoughts. The term 'silence' used here is not the inert silence of sleep or the awesome silence of the grave. This is a 'State-of

Consciousness', which is beyond the realm of the ego, the 'Experiencer' of the pluralistic world of finite things and beings... This "State-of Silence" can be attained by seekers through meditation.."

Meditation Exercises are designed to assist the seeker to listen to *aum* in the background of the mind, during all its activities. This allows the practitioner to delve into his intent, expectations, mental/physical hearings, emotions, body positions, and breathing and to give meaning to words, messages, and ideas.

If speech is words and words are thoughts, then a stream of thoughts is mind. This understanding unravels the mystery of speech. This *understanding* is the primal force directing you to your inner self. Now there is the issue of dealing with your day-to-day life occurrences. For these you invoke your innate powers every time you are challenged by life's happenings. A life force previously used as mere energy for mundane actions is now raised higher and becomes identifiable as a spiritual force carrying you higher and higher towards your final enlightenment.

Analysis on Speech

In self analysis, ask oneself:

- Where does thought come from?
- Is it a desire for self-expression?
- What happens when thought becomes word as sound and then written speech?
- What is the invisible power manifesting through all of this?
- Is it a *power of intelligence*?
- What can this *power of speech* do?
- Can it hurt or protect or love?
- How do I use this *power* in my life?
- Analyse the ripple effect of the *power of spoken words*: what is it that happens?

Does breath or *prana* take part in speech?
What does breath do to the brain?
In the act of speaking, is the tongue involved?

- If so, what "taste" is left on the tongue when something unsavoury is said?
- Is the tongue involved in *my self image?*

One usually ignores the act of speaking. To ignore this action, is to negate symptoms of flawed speech. While interpreting speech and its varied ramifications in action, emotion or thought, it is important to note that the *karanic* or causal-chain-phenomenon exists all around us.

Symptoms of flawed speech appear but they are not the real problem. The seeker must work out the exact point and time when each symptom made its appearance in one's life situations. Thoughts, events, issues, feelings, and fantasies, that are operative at that point, must be analysed. Our language is reflective of our *chitta* or moods and feelings (mind, intellect and ego) and our words in speech embody what is actually happening within our deeper self.

Water and Imagination at Second Chakra

The element Earth, is represented as vibrating energy at the first coccygeal or *muladhara chakra*. Water, is also represented as the same energy or *aum*, where It vibrates at a different frequency in the second sacral or *svadhisthana chakra*. Similarly, the third lumbar or *manipura chakra* manifests the same energy of the element Fire in an even subtler vibration of the Cosmic Sound. The fourth thoracic or *anahata chakra* manifests the same energy of still subtler vibration of the element: Air. The fifth cervical or *vishuddha chakra* manifests this same energy vibrating as the element of Space.

Imagination is born of uncontrolled desires that allow the aspirant to arrange and rearrange images for the purpose of *personal pleasure* and self-image. All wishes start with a thought. Repeated often enough, it gets the momentum of desire. Desire is now given a form and an image. Imagination of this image is now a burning desire to possess. The need to possess is linked with the perennial desire for happiness.

The whole process is like a potter who creates a pot from clay. He uses the water to mould his desired object. His imagination gives it the imagined shape and form. It is hoped that the end product gives him pleasure and happiness.

Pleasures are strong emotions linked with indulgences that translate into, among others, eating habits and therefore involve the sense of taste. There is therefore a need to investigate *taste* which leads to gluttony.

There is an old tradition that had perplexed me for years. When priests go around the temple they mutter away their *sanskrit mantras* and sprinkle water at the same time. The priest was doing the same when he went around and inside the house, in preparation for our older daughter's wedding. I voiced my query and the Master who had already picked my thoughts responded:

> "Ravichandran is blessing the premises with ancient mantras. The water he is sprinkling gives his wish and desire for auspiciousness a definite form of reality. So be it!"

Taste

Svadhisthana Chakra controls the sense of taste. Taste is *developed* in accordance with environment to attain harmony. The objective is survival. Cultivation of taste can be in the field of food, clothes, comforts, manners, speech, and work rules, in fact, the total personality and one's environment.

Heightening a particular taste requires awareness of acute isolation and working on the object of desire. The *desire* is fed by *imagination* which *feeds* the mind until it becomes part of one's personality. Thus, we have coined the saying: 'We are what we eat'. Whether in thought, word, or deed we enter their influence into our personality

What then creates the desires for our tastes? The memory of past experiences of pleasure triggers the need to re-experience the memory of pleasure. Conversely, the experience of harmonious or *sattvic* taste development experiences purity and not pleasure. It is an experience that is felt intuitively and does not influence the need to taste.

Fasting is the best way to see what happens to imagination, desires, and taste. Until the sense of taste is refined to a state of purity, the life-force or *prana* in food cannot influence taste to become *sattvic.*

Dreams should be *watched during fasting* especially since they will indicate the effect of various types of food on the type of imagination. Unrealistic expectations from unrealistic desires must be identified and discrimination used to determine whether the taste is for indulgence or a spontaneous act of refined taste.

The characteristics of an early seeker is a flood of wandering thoughts in the background of wandering imagination which wishes and desires everything and anything!

As a ten year old child, I became interested in the idea of fasting. My best friend in Daressalaam (my future husband's older sister) had started this ritual every Tuesday and as is usual with children, I wanted to be part of this play too!

I began by watching the Arabs in Zanzibar break their fast at sunset. Our family lived in a home attached to a mosque. We were able to see them in the front porch of the mosque from our balcony above. What I did not know was that the Muslims ate before sunrise as well.

I began by fasting all day. I was chubby anyway and could afford to take on the challenge. My parents kept a watchful eye but did not dare to dissuade me. My mother expressed her concerns to my father. She felt that fasting and the stresses of schooling and playing in the heat of the tropics was too much for a growing body. My father reassured her that I would drop the idea once hunger and thirst made its demands on my body!

My twenty four hour fasts became an exhilarating experience every Tuesday. Before 'breaking my fast' my childhood meditation took me into a thoughtless silent mind. Wow, what an incredible experience! I was on an secret adventure every week! I floated on a cloud of an inner sound that carried me through space and an inner peace and quietude which seemed infinite!

Fasting (no food or water for twenty four hours at a time) became a ritual in my life for at least twelve years. This continued until I became pregnant with my first child in Dublin, where my husband and I were studying to acquire 'a piece of paper' that permitted us to make a living for this body, its shelter, and for comfort. We did not know that at the time but now that we have the luxury of looking back on life, we have the wisdom to question all teachings! Colleges and Universities should teach growing youth that there are two aspects of life and living. One materialistic and the other should cater to the secret innate needs of every student! There is a secret of successful earning and then there is the ultimate art of living. It was years later before the Master explained the phenomenon experienced by my habituated mind who enjoyed fasting:

> and the Master said:
>
> "...To withdraw the mind's wandering attention from the world of names and forms, and to redirect its attention steadily to the spring of All Activities in one's own within, is spiritual seeking. To centre our attention on this inner silence and tranquillity and to confront the world of happenings around, is spiritual life. Naturally therefore, fasting becomes important, not necessarily the non-eating of food, but a strict discipline maintained in all our 'intake'...seeing, hearing, smelling, touching...nay, even in feeling and thinking..."

Taste, Greed, and Gluttony

Most people have a blunted sense of taste: the tongue has been desensitised through exposure to stimulants and strong spices.

To experience taste, take food in the mouth and notice the urge to bite, chew, and swallow**:** This urge is greed.

Greed can be controlled. Notice the difference between the experience of eating when the stomach is full, and when one is hungry.

- Notice the same urges with water and other beverages.
- Is it sight or is it taste that stimulates the urge?
- How does the smell or taste of drink and food stimulate greed?
- Which is more important: smell or taste?

Does the taste of food stimulate emotion and vice versa?

Why is food eaten: for celebration, socialising, recognition, reaction to self pity, self-reward?

What compulsions dictate indulgences?

- Is it taste that compels the urge to greed?
- Was I born with a taste for specific foods?
- Is taste a continuous desire?
- Is it a continuous need for self gratification?

Refinement of the sense of taste and the urges of greed is necessary for evolution.

Our urges emerge from the need to impact our lives with the world of objects. Our causal urges, habits, desires, likes-and-dislikes, motivate man who already knows what is of benefit or of harm to him. Yet, we play *shadow dances* with our past and these continue to haunt us from our past and present. One needs to acknowledge, accept, negate, and validate the problem of indulgences for pleasure and apply effort to restrain and adhere to decisions made.

Each psychic centre or *chakra* has important experiences to offer us. Through *sadhana*, the seeker focuses his attention in a special way. It is an opportunity to address the desires that motivate him unconsciously. It is also a means of experiencing a special aspect of his own spiritual unfoldment.

A *swami* or renunciate from Washington who leads our organisational annual walk-a-thons dared us to try an experiment. The 'Friendship Walk' raises funds for alleviation of poor health, poverty, homelessness, illiteracy, and for income generation schemes in women and children in Africa and India. The *swami* asked us to keep a chewing gum in the mouth and wilfully avoid chewing it. We were asked to go about our business walking, if we so desired. 'Watch for the urges to bite and chew' he said!

Indulgences and Keeping a Diary

Indulgences are a function of likes-and-dislikes, aversion and indifference or *raaga-dveshaa,* the delusory power of *maya* which gives an imagined thing an aura of reality.

Maya is the illusion of finitude and limitation. *Brahman* is pure Consciousness which is our real nature. Its characteristic is omniscience and omnipotence. Yet man feels limited! Because of *maya,* we feel ignorant and agitated. We do not have the ability to remain in a sustained state of peace. We experience the outer worlds of plurality. We do not have the tools to experience the oneness in this plurality. Yet the Masters never tire of telling us that this sense of multiplicity and limitations is an illusion. The illusion is created because of non-apprehension of our own divinity.

> and the Master explained:
>
> The Total *Vasanas* of all PFT's (Macrocosmic) is called *Maya.* Therefore, when Aum functions through V it is PFT or *Jiva* functioning as ego; when *Aum* functions as *Maya*, it is the entire Universe *(Jagat)* — it is *Ishvara* of the OET or God. When V is annihilated, *Jiva* (PFT) world (OET) and God merges into one ineffable state of *Aum.*

We live through three states of awareness - the waking, the dream, and the deep sleep states. We experience different states of being in each of these three states. Vedanta declares that all these three states and worlds are unreal when viewed from the perspective of pure Awareness. Each world exhibits a relative reality while we are in that state. When there is movement from one state to the other, the world just abandoned, loses its reality. None of the worlds have a greater claim to reality. The relative reality claimed by the waking world is false superimposition upon the reality.

The Master compares this situation with a famous analogy in *Vedantic* literature. It is like 'superimposing a snake on a rope'! The rope alone is real. Non-apprehension of the rope gives rise to misapprehension of a snake. The snake is an optical illusion -*maya!* The whole world of all our egocentric ideas of a separate existence are superimposition upon the one Truth, *Brahman* or Pure Consciousness.

The seeker is asked to keep a diary of all our delusions and illusions and follow them to their roots. For example, from *raaga-dveshaa* or likes-and-dislikes arise: passion, lust, dullness, laziness, infatuations, possessiveness, arrogance, conceit, aversion, hate, and envy. Recognition of the special characteristics of individualistic likes-and-dislikes should be recorded in a diary and attempts made to develop the opposite positive tendencies. The world becomes vaster and kinder!

> and the Master said
>
> "...If one can give up likes and dislikes then the world becomes double its space for us to move about. Then we do not go about chasing half the things and running away from the other half!"

Cultivation of *positive tastes* can start with appearance, cleanliness, punctuality, handling delicate situations with care, and progressing to good art, books, music, language, discussion, and so on.

From a physical sense, taste must be experienced fully:

- Taste sweet, bitter, and sour foods and then savour the corresponding emotion. Explain why something is distasteful and what is it that one really tastes.
- *Contemplate about thirst and what is it one wants to drink: water, life, ecstasy?*

The Master insisted that the children be discouraged from making judgements on pain and pleasure, comfort and discomfort, happiness and sorrow, or heat and cold. He insisted this tendency would cause them to be pulled by the forces of the polarities of life. Both the negative and the positives were to be accepted with equanimity. Centred in oneself he encouraged them to accept whatever Life gave them as gifts of His Grace!

> My daughter was anticipating an experience of cold nights. The Master insisted children should not be encouraged to dwell on imaginations of pain and pleasure, heat and cold, or happiness and sorrow and he wrote:
>
> "Since you are intuitively feeling it will be cold in the nights, keep a hot water bottle under the blankets and turn your mind to the third eye of the Lord! It is burning hot!.."

The seeker acknowledges that survival is dependent upon basic necessities of life: food, shelter, comfort, and warmth. But, an intellectual analysis of one's self-worth and self-perspective also allows the seeker a tool in personal empowerment. Without *raaga-dvesha,* he begins seeing life from a cosmic perspective. This allows him to become a visionary, free of all conceptual opinions. He develops a personal empowerment capable of friendships under new conditions of unconditional love and service to others.

Investigating Imagination and Desires

The second *chakra or svaadhishaana chakra,* symbolises the element water. Water symbolises imagination - a function of the mind. From this level, man is naturally and imaginatively attracted by emotional kinship, affection, and social compatibility based upon *raaga-dvesha* or ingrained likes-and-dislikes. Personal family ties are the first instincts nurtured by man - these are *tamasic* instincts born of the sense of "Me and Mine".

This tendency can be expanded to a higher or lower level of perfection. One needs to accept *where-I-am-at-this-moment.* The mystery of self-unfoldment is that every experience is a necessity in order to move you along a path to spiritual fulfilment. Community volunteerism is a higher instinct for social compatibility. This instinct is born of *rajasic* or creative tendencies in an evolving mind.

When a seeker sees the multiplicity of names and forms as part and parcel of the Cosmic Mother or the Universe, he accepts all differences and rests in an inner conviction of harmony and oneness with his surroundings. His actions in the world outside are from a different perspective. He is serving the Cosmic Mother. This is a *sattvic* or balanced view of the world. His imagination creates images of harmony. He has no demands. He only wishes to serve his Mother!

When in their undeveloped state, these ***images*** may be pleasant or unpleasant.

- What creates these images?
- Imagination is a product of desire for self gratification and pleasure: a greed for pleasure.

Man when still uncultured, is riddled with desires. These *desires* are pliable at first. When *imagination* gives them a *form or image* based upon one's likes-and-dislikes or *raaga-dvesha*, these desires become *opinions* based upon *beliefs and concepts*, which now, are baked in the kiln of *emotions*:

- These are now hardened concepts with a sense of permanence.
- All the *scheming* is a mental processing mechanism for self-gain.
- The result is the emergence of self-righteousness which we fanatically defend. It now becomes the *birthplace* of our life's problems.
- Rigidity of attitude consumes our lives because it is the only security we know.

- Emotions give our desires *power* to lie quiet but also to re-awaken when the situation permits.

Review all the ***desires*** that one has schemed for in the past but which never came to fruition.

- The Energy from all "scheming" for old forgotten desires, returns into the Universal Energy Source for resurrection in the present or future or in later life.

Insight is required to review all the *hurts, grudges, resentments* that have been left unattended to:

- Discrimination is required to make these *inner hurts* obsolete (by working with the group discussion on pain) in order to dismiss them.
- Once dismissed, there is a sense of *renunciation* which gives one freedom and not self-denial.

Review ***desires that may benefit others***:

- Avoid making new ones.
- Be careful that the mind does not play games of personality and uncultivated imagination and day-dreams of infinite possibilities.
- Instead, directed imagination will lead to creative expressions for the work undertaken.

a parent exhorted:

"Our movies, television series with their pronounced emphasis on sex and sadistic violence are doing the insidious job of desensitising and dehumanising our impressionable youth. How else can we explain instances of youngsters committing murders just 'for the thrill of it'..?"

and the Master said:

"Materialism served by the Pundits of Science can come to only one conclusion that with more food, clothing and shelter, more leisure and entertainment, a little more of general education, happiness can be ensured for everyone, because of the 'sameness' of circumstances provided for everyone..

"Meanwhile the race is on, a desperate race for the acquisition of material goods. To the vast majority they appear to be forever in short supply. To the few who have them in abundance, there never seems to be enough. And so the chimera continues to seduce and confuse us, making our lives a mess of mirages, mistaken goals and wasted journeys"

Fear of slipping into a state of indulgence can breed insecurity:

- Ego will look for a scapegoat and will blame others for its desires;
- Responsibility has to be accepted for self-assessment, effort, work, time, and energy spent on desiring and imagining a work to come to fruition.

Review all the fears and identify the ***source of fears:***

- Look at past mistakes, and into wrong actions, both intentional and non-intentional.

Most fears arise from uncultivated over-stimulated imaginations

- Make a list of your fears and analyse them from their origins to their present state.
- Rebuild the energy to review imaginations and emotions.
- Follow your dreams to problem solve through dream-analysis.
- *Enter the fear (or any problem) by Invocation of the divine cave and enter meditation.*

Watch speech which can be the result of imaginations, fears, and strong emotion. Watch desires and their scheming nature for self-expression in speech.

- Withdraw Energy from speech by problem-solving through meditation, disempowering the imagination that feeds desire.
- Identify if the image is relevant to present life.

Visualise the images created by the imagination of the desire.

- If the image is imperfect, identify a symbol of "unmanifest" perfection.
- Convert mundane desires into a "manifested" vision of ideal action or thing.

Messages or intuitive conclusions are a reflection of underlying dynamics the person is working with. Actions take place in the individual's *moods and feelings* or *chitta* (emotions, thoughts and ego). They start during the early formative and experiential period when a child comes to terms with his past experience (causal essence) and his new exposures in this life. This is the underlying basis of fears, guilt, anger, resentment, shame, and imaginations.

The 'problems' of life and living are imaginations and superimpositions upon the ultimate reality. They may seem real but require man to investigate their source.

> and the Master said:
>
> "...The problem facing us may be great, but the glory of life consists in meeting the problem. Success or achievement is not the final goal. It is the spirit in which you act that puts a seal of beauty upon your life..
>
> "Within the Body there is all perception: the perception of the World. Within the Mind is feelings and emotion for all the World. Within the Intellect there is knowledge, not only of the body and mind, but of the Whole Universe: all of Creation..."

Can old habits be sublimated?

Past encumbrances can be sublimated through the experience of deep concentration or in meditation*:*

- Whenever the practitioner faces stubborn traits, *divination can be practised.* This is done through the Invocation of Awareness in the Divine Cave of the brain and spinal cord. The practitioner is asked to sit in a posture most comfortable for him. Connecting his inner gaze with the Cosmic Mother, he is asked to also connect to the source of the Life-force. He energises every part of his body with the life-force and gathers himself into the divine cave. Here, he allows the Energy of Awareness to acquire a collective sanction to bless everything beyond himself:

Sit in meditative posture and focus your gaze into the space between and behind the eyebrows at the Kutastha or Krishna-Christ Centre, which is opposite the ajnaa centre. Review the brain in Figure 20..

- First visualise the brain and the spinal cord or divine cave as a void, before time and space, and fill the cave with Cosmic Energy through the mouth of the medulla at the base of the brain .

Assume an erect posture or asana:

- Sit flat between and on the buttocks with a straight back, the shoulder-blades pulled together and the chin parallel to the floor. This involves throwing back the head a little.
- Pull in the lower abdomen until the navel is directed towards the spine.
- Pull back the shoulder blades so that the breast-plate or sternum is in line with the chin.
- Rest both palms at the thigh-abdomen junction with the elbows bent, away from the armpits (axillae). Pull in the abdomen in and upwards.
- Roll the tongue back towards the back of the mouth (kechri mudra).
- Concentrate the gaze at the kutastha between the eyebrows and look at the inner vision of the Universe. In deeper meditation, it may depict itself in a kaleidoscope of colours of the rainbow. Penetrate it.
- Concentrate the inner ear on the inner-sound or antardhvani and listen to the Cosmic Sound: Aum. In deeper meditation, follow the sound to its very source.
- Contract and then relax every part of the twelve sections of the body as if massaging it. Squeeze the life-force out of the body parts and return it back into the divine cave; then relax body parts and allow the life-force to infuse back into the 'empty' body parts. Continue doing this until physical body (sthula sharira) awareness becomes an astral (sukshma sharira) awareness of the energy in the physiological-psychological sheaths (pranamaya kosha and mannomaya kosha).
- Watch and feel the movement of air in and out the nostrils during breathing. At first you may start with four seconds each with inspiration: pause: expiration: pause. Ensure at all times that the tongue is rolled back into the soft palate. Remain connected with the Cosmic Mother with your inner gaze. With deeper meditation, the practitioner's awareness watching the breath is accompanied by a realisation that the breath has slowed to an imperceptible level.

During the preliminary stages of stilling the body, practice pranayama by first **breathing through the nose:**

- Inspire by expanding the upper abdominal muscles (above the navel) and the floating ribs on the side of the chest. Fill the chest from its base upwards to the level of the throat, above the collar bones, using the diaphragm to move the chest.

- Expire by slowly relaxing the lower chest (diaphragm) by contracting the upper abdominal muscles.
- Pause at the end of each inspiration and expiration; Repeat ten times until you are comfortable with the pranayama.
- An ideal pranayama consists of starting at the end of expiration: Pause: inspiration: pause: expiration: pause: the ratio in time should be 4 seconds: 4 seconds: 4 seconds: 4 seconds: 4 seconds.

Next, inspire through the mouth and imagine yourself sucking in "cold" air from the base of the chest up towards the throat. A cold sensation will be felt at the back of the throat, while with expiration, one feels a warm sensation leaving the chest. The perception of changes in temperature can be felt more acutely when the head is thrown back a little.

- Inspire and expire while listening to the sound of breathing in the inner ear; or time the breathing with the mental japa of 'Hamm....Saaa....Sooo' Hamm....
- Next, continue the pranayama with mouth closed.

Now practice pratyahara by practising sustained contraction of every part of the body, starting with the toes. Do not make judgements about pain or pleasure. Sustain contraction until the whole body trembles and you experience only the energy of the astral body. Now relax completely and feel the same energy in the stillness of the body.

Next, invoke the Awareness of Aum in the cave of the brain and spinal cord. It should enter through the medulla, rise to the crown of the head and descend to the Kutastha between and behind the eyebrows before descending down the spinal cord to the base of the spine.

- Continue to 'witness' breathing or pranayama to coincide with "Hamm.... Saaa" and "Sooo....Hamm".
- Continue this pranayama until you feel centralised between the manipura (navel plexus) and the vishuddha (throat plexus). You will gradually rest in the centre of the brain-cave as pure thoughtless awareness.

Now widen the Cosmic Vision at the Kutastha in between the eyebrows and into the sky.

- Imagine the earth suspended in the sky and all the stars and planets in the Infinity of the Universe.
- Hold this image and see yourself on earth and inside the Universe. You are a precious divine portion of your Cosmic Mother - the Universe or Mother Nature.
- Expand further and hold the Universe in the Light of your Awareness. By this exercise you have **now harnessed the Light of Awareness in Its ever- expanding sphere** of Perfect Love which encloses your neighbour,

then your loved ones, your home and those of your loved ones. Keep expanding until you hold the whole of Mother Nature or Prakriti in the sphere of Infinity.

- Bless Her or Mother Nature or Devi with your heartfelt devotion and love: Those who know prayers to bless Her may do so, or you may want to chant the Gayatri Mantra; Mrityun-jaya mantra; and Om Namah Shivaya: each, at least three times.
- You may now narrow the sphere and enter your "needs" into the Light of Awareness in your own divine cave of the brain and spinal cord and remain silent in It, all the while listening to the Aum (Hum, Amin or Amen) or the Holy Spirit through the right ear and focusing the gaze at the Kutastha or Krishna-Christ Centre, with the tongue rolled back.
- If wandering thoughts disturb the silence, restart the pranayama until the mind is again clear.
- Before terminating the meditation, feel the devotion, peace and harmony. Now ask for divine intervention to remove stubborn bad habits and urges. This has to be done repeatedly over a long period of time.
- Now narrow the awareness into the divine cave and allow it to dissolve into yourself or direct it towards another who has need of It.

It is to be noted that these techniques of asana, pranayama, pratyahara, dharana and dhyana will be repeatedly described throughout the text. However, at each stage of development, subtle differences are experienced: these should be carefully noted.

> and the Master wrote:
>
> "...The Highest Wisdom has but one Science: the science of explaining the whole of Creation and Man's place in it. There is but one law for all - the Law that governs all laws, the Law of our Creator.."

Mantras of Goodwill

1. *Aum Bhur Bhuvah Svahah*
   Tat Savitur Vareniyam
   Bhargo Devasya Dhi-mahi
   Dhiyo-yo nah Pracho-dayat

We meditate on the Ishvara's (the Sun) glory who has created the Universe; who is fit to be worshipped; who is an embodiment of Knowledge and Light; who is the remover of all sins and Ignorance. May He illuminate (enlighten) our (entire Universe's) intellect.

2. *Trayam-bakam yaja-mahe*
   Sugandhim pushti-vardhanam
   Urva-arukam-iva- vandha-nat
   Mrityo mukshi-ya-ma-amritat.

Aum: We worship the three eyed one (Shiva) who is full of fragrance and who nourishes all beings; May He liberate me from death, for the sake of immortality, just as the ripe cucumber is severed from its bondage (of the creeper).

3. *Om namah Shivaya*
The *panchakshara mantra* is chanted for elemental protection.

Unlike popular *gurus* of the century, Swami Chinmayananda refused to give secret *mantras* to his students of Vedanta. He encouraged them instead to study the spiritual texts and come to their own Truth. For the children, the most popular *mantra* he gave for the purposes of *japa* (turning the beads of the rosary) in meditation was '*om namaha shivaya'.* My daughters use it to this day. Their father has taught it to the grand-children. The grand-children use it to invoke super-human strength when they encounter difficulties in strength and effort. It has become a 'barrier-crossing' of incredible potency!

> On the sanctity of *mantras* the Master wrote:
>
> "...*Mantras* are not mere words. That which uplifts us, when reflected upon is *a mantra.* The 'sound symbol' serve as the train of thought to reach its destination of vivid direct experience. Whatever be the language in which the *mantra* is chanted, the reflections upon them will be done by the individual only in his native language.
>
> "*Sanskrit* is a perfect language and the vibrational effects have a soothing effect on the seeker's mind. Yet this is but a superficial gain compared to the depth-significance of the meaning arrived at through reflection..."

Children of the *Vedic* faith traditionally undergo and observe special milestones in their early years of life and again, as they enter marriage or a life of celibacy. These are again reactivated during death rites. These observances are called *samskaras.* They include, baptisms, entering school for the first time, and connecting them to true teachers, among other rites. Some of these rites were ignored in our parental home because of our distance away from the Cultural Heritage of India. The Master ensured that they were all observed for our children and grandchildren.

> on the revitalisation of *samskaras*, the Master wrote:
>
> *"Samskaras* are rituals of joint celebrations that bring about a sense of social discipline, a pride of belonging, providing a healthy reminder of significant cultural meaning to the rituals prescribed from birth to death..."

Investigating Personality and Self-image (Vasanas)

Self-perception of one's own self-image is usually negative. To possess *self-knowledge*, will remove the sting from the problem. It will not change one's self-image.

- Do not allow anyone to reduce you to the level of low self-image;
- Guard against those doing such harm and invoke the Divine Light of Aum

in the cave of the brain and spinal cord to eradicate such tendencies in oneself;
- Examine your daydreams and identify the images that provoke fear within you.

We all are a collection of multiple personalities veiling the Self in multitudinous layers of *vasana* or causal-personalities (acquired through many previous births) for the purpose of role-playing:
- Each of these personalities should be recognised, acknowledged, and described;
- Each needs to be validated and if appropriate, discarded.

Once this is done, there is a *no special personality* now requiring *survival.*
- What survives once the layers have been discarded?
- What now is my self-image?
- Does the ego compensate the image or does it worsen it?

Through this understanding, one is better able to take responsibility for controlling of these personalities and to complement the changes required for a better self-image. When the seeker feels weak and unable to secure such changes, seek divine help by invoking Aum at the altar of God in the cave of the brain and spinal cord.

Once the concept of self image begins to improve, the energy-spill affects those around, who can see a visible change in the *new Me:*
- Visualise the new self-image and *feel* it in the cave of awareness and down along the senses to every part of the body from your head to the tips of your toes.
- Identify if the image from outside yourself and from inside yourself is valid.
- Determine if changes are occurring and if there are newer goals.
- Am I exercising *My will* (self-will) or has it been aligned to the Collective Divine Will.

Personally motivated will power cannot and will not secure changes in life and personalities; rather, it has to be aligned to the Total Will to secure expansion and energy revitalisation. Expansion into the Grand Consciousness is a learned experience.

There is need to analyse constantly, asking "what role am I playing now"? Am I a mother, sister, lawyer, manipulator, aggressor, victim, aloof etc., until the exercise becomes second nature.

One needs to clarify "Me", the ego to myself who is the real "I"**:** the Self has no personalities.
- *Ego has many personalities, and each is triggered by an emotional stimulus.* Identify these stimuli.
- The *action* in response to the ego is *justification for existence* of this self-image.

- *Grace* is required to change self-image and personality and eradicate the ego.

  Anger was and still can be my biggest personality disorder!

  and the Master reprimanded:

  "You are like a bull in a china shop! How can you undo everything you took so long to build? You are egoistic... Learn to surrender. Learn to smile when you feel insulted. Then anger can never come.."

Liberation from all mind-limitations requires observing one's thoughts, mind, and emotions and learning how the mind functions: Focusing and watching thoughts (*saakshi bhaava)* is the best form of concentration;

- Become aware of the mind's tendency to weave new imaginations and desires;
- Extract all abstract images for they will become conceptualised if not weeded.

This processing involves concentrating on a problem, recalling all past associations and manifestations of the problem, experiencing it through the five senses and the mind, and then emptying the mind during concentration or *dharana*

- Concentrating in the cave, empty the mind until all thoughts have been exhausted. This allows the seeker to receive insights and intuitions.
- The grace of peace, harmony and serenity now becomes a stimulus to continue until a divine image replaces the self-image.

"Will" re-visited

It is easy to be inspired momentarily and forget most of what has been read or heard. Repetition or *abhyas* is the only way to penetrate the hard core of the human personality. Truth must be practised repeatedly until it becomes an established *habit:* this is the difference between *listening* to something and putting it into practice.

Habits are tenacious. Once we perform an action, it leaves an effect or an impression on the consciousness. After several repetitions, the inclination to repeat this action is strengthened. Now, the action becomes a habit in our subconscious and eventually resides in our unconscious being in future incarnations.

> *Habits are nothing but repetitions of our own thoughts;* therefore, they can be changed.
>
> My daughter had to return home to complete her internship after travelling with the Master for an extended period of time. Upon her return she received this letter:
>
> "...How soon one gets addicted..... I just reached here and expect you to be around: a habit of only a couple of months.."

Will Power is the only instrument of man requires to change. To pulverise and eradicate bad habits one needs:

- A *desire to* have a better self-image and *become free from the habit*;
- A *strong will*, born of inner conviction, that there must be a change;
- The ability to determine what it is that needs changing and a plan for action. This requires intuitive guidance and may require introspection and "sleeping over it".

Remoulding awareness requires exercising free will guided by discrimination and energised by will power:

- Discrimination is the key to insight.
- Will power is the power of locomotion.
- Acting on knowledge gets one to the goal.

Will power is easy to develop:

- Watch consciousness all the time and develop the habit of self-examination.
- Examine every thought, action and behaviour for signs of "inclinations" and bad habits. Resist them with will power and discrimination.

With God-given discrimination and will power and with repetitive resistance to temptations for indulgences, the seeker eventually breaks the cycle of acting habitually. He becomes free of old habits by constant vigilance of every action.

The Master insisted that man should be continuously identified with Consciousness. The relationship had to be that of a lover and the beloved. Trust and surrender to His will was the only way known to secure change for the better, in all efforts of self-improvement.

> and the Master said:
>
> "We pray for health, wealth, and prosperity at allotted times of the day. Prayer has become an exercise in beggary! How can you allot special time intervals for loving your spouse, your children, your house, or your parents? Is not 'love' a continuous identification with the beloved? Similarly, 'prayer' is carrying Aum in your hip-pocket at all times and in all actions."
>
> "True 'surrender' is surrender at the altar BEFORE acting! We more usually practice the commoner variety of 'blank-surrender'. We act first and when suffering from the act, then surrender.."

Exercises in Meditation for Children

Ignorance about my very existence as a mortal creates misconceptions about myself and my capabilities. This ignorance is called *maya*. After birth, as soon as the child has the ability to *think* he identifies with his awake but inert *physical or tamasic body,* sleeping *astral or rajasic body,* and deeply sleeping *causal or sattvic* body*: this is maya*, where he identifies with the three *gunas* or qualities of his matter envelopment.

At this stage, he is unaware of his real self. Meditation can reverse this *natural tendency* by teaching. A child can be introduced to *empowerment* through meditation. This can be started by the age of seven years:

- Teach the child (start at age 4-5) to locate awareness within himself and then around himself with the game 'I exist'. Teach the child to press on the tragus or lobe projection in front of the ear canal, with his elbows supported on the surface of the dining table: ask him to concentrate and listen to his inner sound, heard as his own inner hearing.
- Once the child is comfortable listening to his own inner sounds, show him the practice of inner-gazing by focusing at the Kutastha between the eyebrows and show him the Vision of Infinity in front of his gaze as a dark screen with a forward-depth.
- Next teach the child (start at age 6) to become aware of every happening around him; he should be able to visualise his dealings and interactions with every person, name and form in Creation. He must be able to analyse his behaviour with animals, children, parents and friends. He should be able to voice his feelings to a parent or teacher. He should be taught to observe his reactions to situations presenting in life.
- The next step is to show the child to hear the outer or environmental "Vibrating Sounds" entering his inner awareness and inner hearing.
- Now teach the child to observe his thoughts with his eyes closed and focused at the Kutastha: he can now watch his dream-thoughts. This is an exercise in inner awareness of inner thoughts experienced on the screen of awareness.
- *Next, teach the child to stare at the stars and moon in the sky at night or the blue sky, the clouds and sun in the day time.*
- Now ask him to visualise the physical image onto the dark screen in between his eyebrows. Allow the child to repeat the exercise with his eyes open and then closed until he becomes comfortable with this exercise of taraka.
- Finally, make him aware of the entry of Life and Energy entering his divine cave through the medulla: explain that it is the Energy that makes him aware of his body, his thoughts, his feelings, and his actions. He learns the power of empowerment of his body, mind and thoughts.

Children's meditation exercises can be taught one step at a time over a period of years from the age of seven to twelve years.

> The Master said of the Children:
>
> "Deep in the depths of all of us, there is secret longing, a silent impulse, a soaring ambition to do something beautifully great, spectacularly noble. This is a divine summon from the deeper pressure in us, to take us off from the levels of mediocrity into the heights of spontaneity and perfection..
>
> "A child (Man) is essentially perfect, and therefore infinite are the possibilities that lie lurking in him. We as parents, must realise that they have in them all the resources, abilities, energy, and power for building a supremely successful life for themselves and for others in our world..

"Incompetence in life generally springs from false and hasty conclusions that they are impotent, insignificant and ineffective. Spiritual education and practices make them realise that they are part of a whole scheme and are the essential creative essence behind the whole universe which rules the heart in each one of us.."

Conclusion

In the search of Truth in oneself, one must acknowledge that every child brings with him, a Causal personality into a new parenting environment, each with their own personality traits embedded in him. The Laws of *Karma*, Relativity, and Qualities are all operative in each individual child's personal experience.

This is the foundation of the human psyche. His desires, aspirations, and experiences require validation. He now adjusts to his new birth environment by examining situations, routines, events, relationships, motivations, and processes in his new home.

This awareness leads the child to functional precipitation patterns which will now mould the little individual. He is definitely exposed to newer and unfamiliar foundations. The child has to make alternative affirmations. Having dealt with this, the child is ready to enter the field of work. He must follow his innate desires in a new field of activity.

According to the Master it takes the first five years to make initial adjustments. At this stage, he should be helped to go at least to the moon if he wishes to reach the stars!

SECTION THREE

Topics in Section Three

The Soul resides within the Brain

The illusionary power of *Maya* is the mirror through which a wise man views his world of conscious wakefulness. This belief disallows him to take the world of the living, too seriously. Whenever things go wrong he reasons it is a temporary upheaval in his cycle-of-life. He reasons that it is the result of his past actions expressing as reactions in his present life. He does not allow life-circumstances to imprison him. He gains insight and clarity and moves beyond the prison walls of suffering and ignorance.

Where then is his past hidden? Why, right within me. In the brain. All my past secrets are recorded within the causal being of my existence. Its effects are recorded also in the causal being of the Universe. The two interact as one in all Man's happenings. Every action is connected to the Cosmic Mother. Spiritual journeys therefore lead me to this eternal connectedness. I am constantly tied to Her with an umbilical cord of a just and deserving grace and love.

There is nothing fatalistic about the *Vedic* faith. It is rooted into the mains of Infinity. Man must find his own immortality within himself. He must enter the brain cell where all records are imprinted from eternity. Through meditation he is able to recognise himself as Infinite and Immortal. He unravels the Mystery of Life.

He crosses the boundaries of Change. He enters the domain of the Changeless where there is no death. He acknowledges that Change is a wave in the ocean of the Changeless Infinity. He must transform into an angel in the astral dimension and god in the causal dimension.

All he must do is to concentrate on the altar of God in the divine cave. He will find his Oneness with the Creator and Her Creation.

Manipura Chakra

Preamble

The *Manipura chakra* symbolises Man's efforts to better his causal being. In his search for Truth and his own Ultimate Reality, he discovers that he is truly divine. His physical structure is like three tubes, each one filling into the other: the skin and nerves occupy the outermost; bones and cartilage and muscles occupy the middle, and the inner tube is occupied by the physiological functions of respiration and nutrition.

All are co-ordinated by life-force pulsation or *prana* through their contraction, expansion, ascent, descent and in-and-out movements. These *pranic* pulsations are the foundation of living processes. These are the movements a practitioner of meditation is asked to invoke when he is asked to contract and relax every physical part of his body. Through this he withdraws from the senses or *pratyahara* and enters the domains of his energy filled astral body.

Man only notices another's communication and his stance within this gravitational field [awake world of man]. What we 'see' about another is a final resolutions of what is actually occurring on a constant basis within. What we see is the final result of another's physiological-psychological-causal adjustment processes. The external demeanour of Man is the final self-splinting in response to adjustment made for self-validation, self-regulation, and self-affirmation for a foundational security.

A <u>hurtful foundational-state</u> creates pain at all levels of our inner being, manifesting in our thoughts, speech, action, and desires. *Insightful thoughts* lead man through an ascent through the divine cave. He embarks upon a journey of 'Restraints and Adherence' through the processes of *yamas* (physical do's) and *niyamas* (mental don'ts). Repetitive efforts *(abhyas)* allow for new thought-patterns to facilitate the alleviation of underlying emotional and intellectual difficulties embedded in his causal beingness through so many reincarnations.

> "Him that overcometh will I make a pillar in the temple of my God, and he shall go (will reincarnate) no more out." ...Revelation 3:12.

Manipura Chakra
Third or Navel Chakra (Lumbar or Solar Plexus)

Modern thought identifies *chakras* as *physical* entities in the spinal cord and brain. The modern-day spiritualists also assign *functions* to the *chakras.* For example, they link sex to the sacral or *svadhisthana chakra* and emotionalism to the thoracic or *anahata chakra*.

Traditionally, ancient scriptural literature considers them as *astral chakras.* They are centres of concentrated life-force energy. These are energy-dynamos and are sources of energy used for the day-to-day functioning of the physiological-psychological sheaths of the body.

They open or blossom only when they are energised through the *upward flow* of life-force or *udanaya,* coursing through the *sushumna* of the astral spinal cord. Upward flowing life-force energy carries with It *udanaya-pranic* energy or life-force, in conjunction with enlightened mental energy from the senses or *manas.*

This occurs when self-effort or *sadhana* reverses the flow of life from the periphery of the body, to the actualised central nervous system. Intense meditation, (that is, when the mind merges in awareness and *chitta* becomes *chit* in union or *samadhi*), is the key to revealing the *chakras* for what they really are.

When *chakras* are spiritually *open*, there is an awakening of awareness, which is felt subjectively in the *chitta* as a *feeling* of a *presence*. The *awakening* changes your intuitive perception about the relationship of *this presence* as an *omnipotence* in every atom of our physical, astral, and causal bodies. The practice of meditation in self-effort or *sadhana* also purifies the physical body first and then the astral. With this new-found inner perceptual transformation, the physical being's personality acquires a magnetic aura of peace and contentment.

The *new* person innately understands his own true nature and his relationship with Nature. He *knows* that the *chakras* are opened through the *yoga* of self-effort or *sadhana*. He perceives the path he must enter to merge his astral body with his mind-intellect body in the divine cave. He must take the path of transcending all embodiments and enter into his causal beingness or *chitta,* manifesting as *feeling*.

Materialistic individuals utilise the *first three chakras* and their mundane egoistic energy for their own pleasures through indulgences. Through intense *yogic* practice, the lumbar plexus or *manipura chakra,* can be mastered and utilised (without spiritual awakening) by individualised egoistic energised beings for superhuman powers or *siddhis:* these include the ability to manipulate people, to amass immense personal powers and wealth, and charismatic control of things and beings.

An incomplete understanding of spiritual self-effort or *sadhana* can lead seekers or *sadhaks* to flawed experiences. The sectarian doctrines of warring creeds are the result of such imperfect understanding and unbalanced experiences. One requires the leadership of a true and selfless teacher or true *guru* to enter the domains of expanded awareness.

> and the Master explained:
>
> "I asked John if he had tasted a *'laddoo'*. Of course he had not. He was not acquainted with Indian desserts! So I explained in minute detail how it was made, but John just could not visualise the delicious *laddoo.* John wanted to taste it, so I sent the secretary to bring some from the store. John tasted it and experienced the delight for himself.."
>
> "A Teacher must therefore not only be an educated being but he should have experienced the knowledge, so he can share this with his congregation..."

Prana

Five *pranas* or *functional classification* of life-force energy or *prana,* govern the **working** energies and processes of the *astral chakras.* They work at and function from different levels. All these *pranas* converge or exit from the solar plexus or *manipura chakra.* Each of the five *pranas* can indistinctly be related to each of the *chakras,* but these are not rigid relationships:

> ***Udana*** rises from the navel to the head and it acts mostly on the throat through speech. The *vishuddha or throat chakra* and the sense of taste are related here.
>
> ***Prana*** descends from the head to the navel. It is associated with water, food, and air and its main function is to bring impressions of emotion to the heart. *Prana* dominates in the sense of sight.
>
> ***Samana*** works from the navel to the periphery and governs the fire of digestion, the sense of touch and also general metabolism.
>
> ***Vyana*** works from the periphery to the navel and governs circulation and the sense of smell. Through the heart and navel *chakras*, the hands and feet are mobilised.
>
> ***Apana*** works downwards from the navel to the organs of excretion through the coccygeal and sacral *chakras.* It governs the sense of hearing.

These **five *pranas,*** literally meaning five 'breaths', exist in the astral and causal levels as subtle *energy* and their *essence,* respectively; They move through the *nadis* or bodily channels and are connected to the five *Cosmic Pranas* of the universe through the medulla, at the mouth of God. In *sadhana,* their natural flow and direction are utilised for the attainment of higher spiritual knowledge.

- *Udana* is used for ascending upwards along the *sushumna* towards higher spiritual centres.

- *Samana* is mobilised through correct eating habits for the purpose of stilling the body and mind for peace.
- *Vyana* is mobilised for energising all body parts for the purpose of spreading pervasive infinity in every atom of the body.
- *Apana* is harnessed to reverse the tendency for extroversion and ward off negativity.
- *Prana* is *aum*, which enters the body through the medulla. It courses forward to the *Kutastha* and ascends to descend and energise all the seven *chakras* of the cave of brain and the spinal cord. It can be harnessed from the solar plexus in the *manipura chakra.*

The five types of "breaths" or *prana* are therefore only functional classifications of one and the same energy of the *prana* - Aum or Amen or Amin or Hum or the Holy Spirit. It is an all-pervasive awareness, omnipotent, and omniscient.

Swami Yogi Satyam, a teacher of *Raja or Kriya Yoga* (combination of the four types of yoga), advises seekers on the path of meditation to live a *natura*l life for the purpose of creating purity in body and mind.

"Natural living depends upon correct selection of food, dwelling, and company". He admonishes: "No animal eats like man. Every animal has its own chosen food. Man alone goes on eating everything because of his power of digestion. This power has been tapped from the Infinite Reservoir of God's Power, but God's power is being misused for the purpose of sense enjoyments, which lead to physical and mental illness."

"You must become masters of your desires and appetites. When one meditates and cultivates the taste of peace and contentment, man forsakes indulgences and enjoys real happiness."

His advice to seekers include:

- Speak less and listen more;
- Analyse and assimilate what is being spoken;
- Remember wise sayings of good company;
- Practice recharging of the divine cave of the brain and spinal cord;
- Keep genuine fasts and rest the internal organs of the body at least once a week;
- Listen to the Cosmic Vibration entering through the medulla and focus your attention always for a Cosmic Vision at the *Kutastha*; and
- Learn and practice calm deep breathing.

Chakras in Sadhana

Chakras are NOT open to the ordinary person who is preoccupied with his own world and desires and whose predominant aura or magnetic field reflects the functions of active *or rajasic* and inert or *tamasic* activities. However, when harmony or *sattva* predominates, these *chakras* do open to blossom spiritually because of an awakening. The degree and extent of their natural and spontaneous opening depends upon the degree and intensity of Man's self-effort or *sadhana*. Nonetheless nobody does *sadhana* with the objective of opening his or her *chakras*: the aim is only to still and silence the mind.

In *sadhana*, spiritual knowledge is gained at the heart or *anahata chakra*. Energies harnessed at this level *for the ego* exhibit false imaginations of the emotional mind. If *spiritual knowledge and ego* are developed *together* up to this level, the mortal can mislead people with his super-ego.

The aim of *sadhana* should be to still and silence the mind; the awakened mind can now enter the central astral channel of the spinal cord or *sushumna* and lodge through the *ajnaa centre* near the medulla, and into the *Kutastha Chaitanya* between and behind the eyebrows. In this balanced state of beingness, the ego shell is ruptured though the grace of the Lord and *guru.*

Prosperity and Success

Success comes from obeying the laws of Nature. It manifests itself in material successes and acquisition of the necessities of life. The ambition to make money should therefore be coupled with an *intense desire to help others*. This subconscious imperative should underlie all success. Those who ignore or disbelieve in this precept, *fail to utilise the resources of divine supply* and undermine the immortal heritage of mankind.

In the mid-eighties, *Swami Dayananda,* now of *Arsha Vidya* visited and stayed with the family for the first time in Ontario. It was the first time he had come to us after Newfoundland. As soon as he sat in the living-room, he went into himself. When he opened his eyes, he said: "Your material successes will allow you to share it"! My husband protested that his wife "shared too much of it"! *Swami Dayananda* responded with this wise statement: "The art of giving is not born in the genes. It is learnt from elders by example. The children must have living proof that giving of oneself is a privilege".

> "Take no thought for your life, what ye shall eat; neither for the body, what ye shall put on...neither be ye doubtful of mind. For all these things do the nations of the world seek after: and your Father knoweth that ye have need of these things. But rather seel ye the kingdom of God; and all these things shall be added unto you." ..Luke 12:22, 29-31.

Under the influence of ego, the *manipura chakra* physically and psychologically manifests as *lobha* or greed. During *sadhana* or self-effort for betterment, it is invoked with the intensity of Arjuna's single-pointedness. This third centre is also called the *nabhi chakra* and is the *centre of welfare.*

It is the duty of man to be successful so that he may share this Grace of the

Cosmic Mother. The Westerner has accused the people of the Eastern culture of being fatalistic. He reasons that that is why they are so poor and accepting of it, but the Master disagrees:

> the Master said:
>
> "Hindus are accused by both Easterners and Westerners of being averse to wealth, prosperity, and acquisition of material comforts. This is incorrect. We are the only people in the world who perform *'Lakshmi-pujas'* to the Goddess of Wealth, but ***in strict accordance with the ethical laws of Narayana***, Her betrothed companion. We are not averse to wealth and materialism: we adore them!"

Evolution

Prosperity is necessary as a tool in evolution. If man does not have the means to satiate desire, then he makes it a priority to over-seek through intense imagination and becomes lost in materialism and possessions.

There is nothing wrong with wealth and prosperity. The problem is when one becomes obsessed with them. This expresses itself in a selfish primitive mind. However, those who earn more, can give more to reduce disparity and imbalance, thereby helping to reconstruct the collective outlook. Giving in charity is a privilege. The opportunity of physically serving mankind is a rare gift given to the very few. Only they have the mental means to devote their time and share their tangible possessions in the service of others.

> the Master wrote to critical leaders of an organization about volunteers in service:
>
> "Great programs and mighty projects when undertaken, we must have the mental charity and large-hearted love to see the goodness in our workers more than the slips [mistakes] they make. Why look on the dark side only. There is no need to look out for weaknesses and defects. This tilt we must consciously strive to remove from our hearts. Then progress in meditation will be spectacular and with no struggle. Flood the world with Love.."

The quality of *self-satisfaction* that governs the *realm of materialism* is in the stability of the left side of the *manipura chakra*. It brings calmness, satisfaction, inner contentment, and harmony permitting balanced personal growth and spiritual ascent. It enables planning the present and the future and allows clear thinking and logic, lucidity, and an organised lifestyle.

On the other hand, an agitated left channel *(ida or* parasympathetic nervous system) and overstimulated *chakra* (through indulgences) at this level throws the practitioner into a *panic state*. He is prone to commit blunders. Inner poise and self-control are replaced with chronic anxiety, worry, a galloping imagination, and the belief that problems are everywhere.

Patience, not only with others but with yourself, is the balm of the left channel. Frustrated, we find ourselves not meeting our own expectations. *Our temperament and qualities are gifts of our own nature, evolved through many previous births*. In all daily activities, *Nature will take its own course.* Although we make conscious efforts to change, manipulate, and work out our ambitions, work should not be done to obtain a specific reward. *Rewards* come with different faces, depending upon the amount of will exerted and the grace of the Lord.

Calmness at this centre has the ability and power to stabilise others. *Peace* is the essential pre-requisite to prosperity at all levels. It is also intertwined with the blessings of this *chakra* of *ashtalakshmi* of the Mother of Eight Wealths:

- prosperity,
- trust as non-suspiciousness,
- dignity,
- spiritual ascent,
- pure knowledge,
- domestic and collective joy,
- wealth, and
- success.

On a physical level, *attitudes towards food and eating habits*, (like peacefully eating wholesome foods) are an art. Dysfunctional attitudes at this level result in malfunction of the stomach. Diseases result from the dysfunctional breakdown of absorbed foods in the liver.

Indiscriminate fasting as well as *overindulgence in food* disturbs this centre. Fasting has long been used to control thoughts for the *purpose of thoughtless meditation.* For many, fasting is a *habitual rite* without purpose. However, if fasting continues for more than forty days, it progresses to the digestion of the vital organs of the body. Why fast if the mind keeps thinking of food all day? The objects of the world are for our controlled enjoyment and not indulgences. Enjoy the pleasure of Her gifts! *Pranayama* (breath control) with *pratyahara* (withdrawal from the senses) is a better way to control one's thoughts, if that is the objective of the seeker.

The first two *chakras* have a tendency to be drawn into uninhibited, uncontrollable, passionate, and irrational responses of an undeveloped brain. With the third centre, however, the mind begins to control and direct the activities the body.

Magnetic Influence of the Planets on the Physical Body

Surrounding the second or *svadhisthana* and the third or *manipura* centres is a vacuum or void (in the *sushumna)* which is influenced by planets, external influences environmental, and gravitational forces.

- They influence our personality and behaviour patterns (our *dharma* or duty versus outside influences).
- This is the area of planetary influences on our lives.

When the power of concentration or *dharana* gathers momentum, and withdrawal from the senses or *pratyahara* gathers energy into the divine cave, there is stabilisation of the mind and the divine power or *Shakti* fills this vacuum.

- It is only then that our attention is led into awareness of Reality as brief experiences of oneness of the "Me" and "I", where "Me" is *chitta* and "I" is *chit.*
- *Chitta* is Mind-Intellect-Ego or "Me" and "I" is the Soul or Self.

Guidance from a Guru

At this stage of development, when we are ready for guidance, it comes and the guru principle awakens within oneself. The Primordial Master becomes active and incarnated to lay the stepping stones of human evolution.

In the early seventies, we as a family suffered a terrible tragedy when our first brother after five sisters died unexpectedly. There were no flights to or from the fog-bound Newfoundland's main airport for one week. We had to ask a childhood school friend who now lived in Vancouver, to gather the remains of my brother (after autopsy) for cremation. His ashes were sent to India for the final rites, not available to me in Canada. In the meantime, I was looking for a priest to do funeral purification rites in my home. We could not find a priest in St. John's.

It was within this week when my husband, who was the President of the Indo-Canadian Association, was approached to invite a *Hindu Swami to* lecture at the Memorial University of Newfoundland. We were told that a *lecture series in another American University had been unexpectedly cancelled.* The *swami* had written to *Madhuri Acharya* now married to *Vipin* and living in St. John's. *Madhuri* knew this *swami* well. She had worked as volunteer at the Central Chinmaya Mission Trust in Bombay.

I was looking for a *pujari* or priest to do the rites and I urged my husband to invite the *swami.* I attended his lecture series of ten days which were conducted in perfect English. I had never before met anyone, let alone a *swami* who was able to lift me from the depths of my despair. The long lost closeness with my own late father was resurrected after nearly ten years. The Master helped me with the funeral rites but also set me on the path of a spiritual journey.

I personally never accepted him as a *guru* for nearly two decades. I took his teachings very seriously but refused the official 'bonding'. During these years, we the parents of our daughters made every effort that the *guru-shishya* or teacher-student relationship between the Master and our two girls was nurtured in accordance with his commands and wishes.

the Master defined this sacred relationship:

"..*'GU'* stands for philosophical darkness or ignorance, and *'RU'* stands for redemption of ignorance. Therefore *guru* is one who redeems the seeker or *shishya* from the ignorance of the Reality. The hallmark of a *guru* is one who is well versed in the scriptures, sinless, un-afflicted by desires, a full experiencer of the Supreme and who is an intimate friend of those who have surrendered to him.."

".. A disciple is one who submits to a 'discipline', is devoted to a guru, who obeys a *guru's* precepts, and stays engaged in his service for the sole purpose of enlightenment"

For many *complicated* seekers, a true master is difficult to recognise; we tend to seek a *guru* who appeals to our own egos, one with a "personality" already conceptualised.

"No man can come to me (guru), except the Father which hath sent me draw him: and I will raise him up at the last day." John 6:44

I personally never accepted him as my *guru* until eighteen months before he left his physical body. *Madhuri* lived long enough only to introduce me to the Master. She died very soon after this introduction. I returned to Newfoundland many years later with *Swamini Sharadapriyananda.* Ten years later, the old faces were still there. The lecture series and the BMI Chart had to be re-introduced to the same audience, for the umpteenth time!

A Master comes for a single seeker. The inner cry has to be a life and death call for a desperate need for spiritual guidance. Many will hear him but very few will listen. Nobody could see or remember the extraordinary visionary they had met so many years ago. The Master had come to Newfoundland after hearing our inner cries for guidance. He entered our lives to continue where he had left off in our previous lives. We called and he came! The relationship is eternal. The seeker intuitively recognises the awakening of the *guru* personality within his own psyche.

This *guru* personality performs through interaction of the *ida* or parasympathetic, *pingala* or sympathetic and the *sushumna* or central nervous systems, also known as the divine cave of brain and spinal cord. They connect both sides of the physical brain and perform new actions by altering old habits and concepts. This is possible when a practitioner of meditation makes an inward journey into his divine cave.

All incorrect efforts made at this stage of evolution, whether in the name of religion or through the mishandling of the divine-power or *Shakti,* will activate only the parasympathetic left channel or *ida*. When this occurs, the benefits of self-effort towards spirituality or *sadhana,* will not progress from the physical to the astral channels, that is to say: progress into the central astral-spiritual spinal channels of the divine cave of brain and spinal cord *(sushumna, vajra, chitrini and finally brahmanadi)* is arrested.

The Master spent years to break my indomitable pride and I spent years rejecting him and his control. On speech level, we fought like a strict father with a spoilt child, but we also communicated mentally. My revolting heart bled as I pleaded inwardly that I knew he was right! He knew that too because he kept hammering away and chiselling my arrogance bit by bit. Sometimes there was pin-drop silence when my children watched the spectacle. I resented the 'public' reprimands in front of my husband and teen-aged children. "You could have done this privately", I would mentally plead. I wonder what his purpose was!

The left parasympathetic or *Ida* now becomes a storehouse of what is dead in us. It connects with the subconscious (astral being) at the apex of this channel in the right cortex: as the super-ego he is tormented by his tensions, indulgences/ fasts and suffers personality fragmentation.

Siddhic Powers or Miracles

If self-improvement is genuine, spontaneous gains will occur as *siddhic* powers (ESP, psychic abilities etc.). However, it is advisable to ignore these *gains* because they divert the seeker to the direction of desires and libidos.

Practitioners of meditation who become adept at withdrawing from their physical body and entering their energy-filled astral body have *siddhic* powers. The mental or emotional *siddhis* are the common variety encountered as psychics. The intellectual *siddhis* are less frequently seen. Miracles are possible and were always possible. They are poorly understood.

> "Now in the morning as he returned into the city, he hungered.
>
> "And when he saw a fig tree in the way, he came to it, and found nothing thereon, but leaves only, and said unto it, Let no fruit grow on thee henceforth for ever. And presently the fig tree withered away.
>
> "And when the disciples saw it, they marvelled, saying, How soon is the fig tree withered away!
>
> "Jesus answered and said unto them, Verily I say unto you, If ye have faith, and doubt not, ye shall not only do this which is done to the fig tree, but also if ye shall say unto the mountain, Be thou removed, and be thou cast into the sea; it shall be done" Mathew 21 18-21.

The practitioner's spirit is vulnerable to becoming possessed, when allowing the *mind's attention* or *chitta* to indulge in powers of miracles or *siddhis*. At this level, when experiencing the void of awareness during meditation, the practitioner can become filled with a dead-personality or *pishas* from the astral dimension. Their activity is erroneously believed to be manifestations of *siddhis*.

The Master insisted that *siddhis* do not take the seeker to his spiritual destination. The only direct way to the *brahmanadi* or the central spiritual channel of the spinal cord is to follow the strict path of ascent, with the help of a true Master.

When still in my twenties, my spiritual journey took me to the books of *Ramana Maharishi*, brought to me by a Dutch South African friend of my late brother who died in his twenties. Both had just returned after scaling *Mt Kilimanjaro* in *Tanzania*. I studied the books over a period of two years. Perhaps I was too young to understand serious philosophy at that age and was therefore frustrated. I wanted answers to my very serious questions about life. Why am I here in this harsh and unforgiving world? Why does God have no mercy on the drought stricken Africans? Why did the colonialists fill the wells or bore-holes as they were called, with rocks so that the African would have no water, after they left? Why does man hurt man? Why is there so much sickness? Where is this God of mercy? There were no answers. Frustrated, I left the books on my shelf where they still sit.

Many years later, while on my first visit to India, my journey there led me to a renowned saint who had died in the early part of the twentieth century. His burial site in *Shirdhi* has a perennial burning flame. Experts claim there is natural gas source nourishing the flame through a crack in the earth. I was barely thirty years old, then. I began hearing many stories about the *Sai Baba of Shirdhi*. I secretly started a journey of *bhakti* or devotion for this miracle-man. Looking back on this part of my life, I must have scored some successes through my devotion to *Shirdhi Baba*.

I remained on this path for six years. While on the path of *Bhakti Yoga* or the Yoga of Devotion, I made a second attempt to read the two books by the sage *Ramana Maharishi*. My immature mind attempted once more to ask for my own identify, "Who am I"?

We had now moved to another country. We were now in Canada The family met *Swami Chinmayananda*. The meeting was exhilarating and rejuvenated my very soul. Nonetheless, my devotion to Baba forced me refuse him as my *guru!* Instead, he became the spiritual mentor to our two daughters. We, the parents nurtured the relationship as is expected of us. His wish for the children was always a command to be obeyed implicitly. We loved him dearly!

Within two weeks of our meeting with the Master, he asked me to bring the two girls to him in Montreal. I was recovering from a surgery and was able to take time off from my research commitments. At a *satsang* or meeting with the wise, I told him about a recurring dream. I saw a man in long orange clothes with an 'afro-haircut' in my Newfoundland living room. There was also a very large *banyan* tree connected to this recurring dream-image.

"Don't you know who that is? That is *Satya Sai Baba"*, said the Master. Since I was not from India, I was not familiar with any of the Indian saints. I had not heard of this *Satya Sai Baba*.

"He is supposed to be the second *avatar* [re-manifestation] of the *Shirdhi Sai Baba*. He is calling for you in your dreams," he continued.

I was then warned *Satya Sai Baba* was difficult to meet!

After pondering on this new development, I asked the Master if he would take me to this saint who was so difficult to meet. Months later, the Master took me to Ooti a hill-station in Southern India. The Master was 'miraculously' invited to open the Sai Youth Conference.

While flying from Aurangabad and towards Bangalore, the Master prepared me with a warning. He did not want me to get upset with what I was about to see in Ooti. I was alarmed. I was not sure if I really wanted to meet *Satya Sai Baba*. My anxiety would not allow me to accompany the Master on the first day of the Sai Youth Conference. The Master made an appointment for a scheduled meeting with *Satya Sai Baba* on the second and final day of the Conference.

The meeting was an utter disaster! He arrived one hour late and kept the Master waiting in the living room. I was ashamed to have put the Master through this irreverance. I sat at the feet of *Satya Sai Baba*, in the presence of the Master. He spoke no English or Hindi and I understood very little of what he said. He did not recognise me and I could not connect with him!

We now moved to the Conference Hall. Here, I saw *Satya Sai Baba* invoke his *siddhic* [miracle] powers. I was deeply hurt and disappointed. This *Baba* did not know me!

"So many years of devotion and he does not even know me," I thought.

Then I saw a fragrant *vibbhuti* or ash gurgling from both palms of his hands. It felt warm and was perhaps wet. The gray liquid fell with a thud on the cement floor of the Conference Hall,

I had read about miracles or *siddhis* but I never wanted to see them! I was horrified and felt ashamed of the spectacle! I met the Master later that evening in Coimbatore and could not meet his eyes. My own reactions confused me. I could not fathom why I felt so ashamed. I felt responsible for *Satya Sai Baba's* actions! My immature mind would not forgive myself. I had put the regal Master-of-Logic through an unexpected Magic Show!

Later that evening I informed the Master that I had an intense need to retrace my steps to where I had started, before I met with *Satya Sai Baba*. I had to visit the Centres of this new *Baba.*

The Master gave me a chaperone in Bangalore. I first visited the *ashram* or hermitage in Whitefield, near Bangalore. The place was closed except for a skeleton staff of caretakers. They opened the doors and I was able to see the place with the help of the resident priest.

We then took a taxi to Puttaparthi, where the fabled *ashram* or hermitage was still being built. This place also was closed except for a care-taker staff and the construction workers. You must recall I had just met with *Satya Sai Baba* with the Master in Ooti.

At the hermitage we were given unfurnished empty rooms. We now had to buy bedding. That night, there was war within and outside of me! I was attacked by swarms of mosquitoes all night. My heart felt heavy and my confusion and desperation knew no bounds! I was not accustomed to 'roughing it' could not sleep on the hard floor. My mind was in a turmoil. Fortunately, the mosquitoes kept me busy and preoccupied all night.

At dawn, the pesky critters had finally left me alone. I was just dosing off to sleep when I heard someone singing *bhajans* or songs praising the Lord, in the adjoining room. I quickly bathed and readied myself to meet the singer. We met on the balcony outside our adjoining rooms. After the usual polite introductions, she told me she was a renunciate and was now living in Puttaparthi. She was a retired Pathologist from the All India Institute of Medical Sciences in New Delhi, where her husband was still the Dean.

We chatted for hours over a period of two days. We analysed my reactions with the Master after meeting with *Satya Sai Baba.* We both came to the conclusion that my days of *bhakti* or devotion had come to an end. It was time for me to move ahead on this spiritual journey. I was to ask *Swami Chinmayananda* to train me through the Path of Knowledge of the Scriptures *or gyana yoga.*

My recent experiences with *Satya Sai Baba* had left me disbelieving everything and everyone! I was even sceptical of the decision I had made. Never one for backing down when challenged, I reached the feet of my 'future-Master-to-be' and dared him to take me down the spiritual path of knowledge through logic! He accepted the challenge! Looking back at what happened at that time, I must have been a perfect picture of arrogance. The Master was too much of a lover to make any harsh judgements.

It took us seven years to finish the prescribed texts. He gave me my 'homework' and I would meet him every summer to discuss the problems I had. Or, we would write to each other and the Master would write back in terse single statements! They serve me well even to this day!

At the end of the road, the books were read and I was no happier now than I was before. We were alone in the living room and he was watching the trees swaying with the wind from the lake. He was silent. He was a man of few words. I interrupted his thoughts or silence with:

"Now what? What did I gain from this exercise?"
"Use your heart and read the texts all over again"!
I refused, but did exactly what he asked me to do, anyway!

There was a pregnant silence.
"When you find your connection with the Cosmic Mother, you will have arrived" he said.

Thirty years later, I met the orange robed monk and the banyan tree of my dreams of the seventies. Last year I met *Swami Yogi Satyam* in his hermitage lecturing near the banyan tree in *Allahabad, India*! He has been teaching me the higher meditation techniques since.

Intelligence and Sight

Like its predecessors, the third *chakra* also possesses a specific *differentiating faculty*. It relates to the element: Fire and controls the sense of *sight. Sight evokes strong emotions*; strong emotions block clear sight. *Intelligence* (the differentiating faculty), represented at this level, needs expression. The "fire of emotions" must become manifest in Her power or *Shakti* of insight.

Self-transformation through *sadhana* or self-effort occurs in stages. The experience of this graded transformation is a an evolutionary self-realisation. The changes are permanently recorded in the causal beingness. These are gains made on the spiritual journey.

> and the Master wrote
>
> "Self-improvement and conquest over your lower nature, is to be accomplished by the spiritual strength in yourself. Nobody can help you from outside. It is a subjective accomplishment. The knowledge that we have given you, should help you endlessly. Learn to practice it. 'They are in Me, I am not in them'. Always look to a brighter future when you have control over your own emotions. Do not sit and worry over past pitfalls.."

When the aspirant has studied and practised sufficiently to meditate, he gains power over both imagination and emotions. The *best way to control powerful emotions* is by devotion and dedication to the *ishtadevata* (personal ideal) or a *guru* (a realised teacher).

Intelligence at this level is represented by *Lakshmi* (the goddess of wealth) whose Energy has the power to permit insight **or clairvoyance.** The seeker must be clear whether he desires for materialistic success, fame, name or does he aspire for the Self, because, an indiscriminate exertion of this Energy has the power to self-destruct, as well as to bless.

Eyeless Sight

Cosmic Energy manifests as Life Force through the Total Mind: the emotional/thinking-principle or *manas* of Man. The life-force *[prana]* manifests within the divine cave or altar of God (brain and spinal cord) as the astral body *[sukshma sharira]*. Both, the physiological body *[pranamaya kpsha]* and the psychological bodies *[manamaya kosha]* are intimately connected with the astral intellect *[gyanamaya kosha]*. Each of these bodies become more expressive in the three states of consciousness [waking, dream, deep-sleep] and beyond.

and the Master comments:

> "....Just as on awakening from a dream, in the waking-state there is no dream-world at all and the waker realises that the entire dream was pervaded by the waking-mind, so too on awakening to the self, the wise realises that the phenomenal world was all pervaded by the self. The world was a disturbance in the Consciousness Divine. This state is *desa,* the place to be sought..."

When Cosmic Consciousness-Awareness descends into the developing foetus, its first manifestation is in the *eye of universal intelligence and intuition* or *kutastha.* This is where the sixth *chakra* in the medulla reflects as the *kutastha.* The causal phase of the individual will now descend into the brain's cave in the *ajnaa chakra* or sixth centre within the divine cave, directly opposite to the *kutastha.* It must be noted that .before moving towards the *ajnaa chakra,* the soul or *jiva* has perfect recall of his innate divinity.

As the *causal body descends* into the *astral phase of the spiritual eye* in the roof of the divine cave, it acquires an astral embodiment of the mind (emotions) and intellect (thoughts); through the instrumentality of the astral mind-intellect-ego, this individualised being now courses down the brain and spinal cord. This *chitta* personality (mind-intellect-ego complex) makes its first connections with the five senses in the upper divine cave. Next it connects with the five energy centres or *chakras.* Finally, it makes connections with the five organs of action.

As an *astral embodiment* (the physiological-psychological sheaths), the soul or unenlightened *chitta* identifies with the intuitive state of ego perception or *ahankar.* The ego has its own intuitive perception, also called the sixth sense. From here, the astral soul or *jiva* descends to all the five sense perceptive states.

The descent of Man through the five senses or 'instruments of intellection' is of a 'dual' characteristic: one is through the current of the mind-intellect and ego (intuitive intellect or *buddhi*); the other is through the *intermingling* with the current of the life-force or *prana.* This is now the *astral being* with the *power of intuition* as well as that *of the ego.*

The *astral power is of pure life force energy or prana.* The astral being can experience any of the sensations through any of the sensory instruments of intellection. All wisdom must enter through these sense channels to reach the intellect and intelligence.

When Man withdraws his awareness (through *pratyahara* or sense-withdrawal*)* away from materialistic attachments through meditative self-effort or *sadhana*, the e*yeless sight* or the *eye-of-the-eye* regains its divine memory of his divinity and experiences the Light of Consciousness.

Power of Speech at the Third Chakra - Lakshmi

The power of speech evolves gradually through the first two energy centres or *chakras*. In the third *chakra*, speech takes on a the faculty of urgency. There is an uncontrollable need to speak, for self-expression. In its negative form, compulsive talking can take the form of constant criticism, in order to gratify a *need to self-express.*

The *source of language* is unconscious and, therefore, originates from causal beingness. The *drive to express* is also unconscious. Behind spoken speech is a well-spring of past ideas written on a slate of specific previous communications, remembered and not remembered, over space and time.

Man exhausts this pent-up Energy or *prana* in useless chatter and small talk, which is often considered a necessary social convention. Energy spent in this way is no different from physical energy or *ojas,* exhausted in sex acts. Conservation of even this Energy is imperative if the seeker is to evolve. Awareness of the preciousness of this Energy leads the seeker to examine what is going to be said and why.

Attention must be given to both the words and the language being used. With practice, there is an expanding awareness of the power-of-speech. The aspirant acquires a magnetic personality emanating from the astral body, which can speak not only through speech itself, but also through the seeker's mannerisms.

Chanting *mantras* or sacred syllables and *srutis* or chanting *revealed* scriptures like the *Vedas*, can create magnetic fields wherein the words or *vak* create sound or *nada brahma* which is physically expressed as *Aum* vibrations. These are not just limited to the *letters*, but also produce an awareness of *hearing*. There is a gradual transformation in the practitioner of meditation

> and the Master wrote:
>
> "The scriptures, no doubt show us the path to a healthier and more intelligent living, but our determination and concerted efforts alone can help us to achieve it.."

Benefits of Speech Control

Awareness is active in all the three qualities of Nature or *gunas***:** as *rajas* in creation, as *sattva* in preservation, and as *tamas* in dissolution. *Sattva* has the motherly qualities of balance between *tamas* or inertia and *rajas* or activity. *Rajas and sattva* undergo constant change as a result of *tamas.*

Therefore, Awareness constantly changes the states of both subjective and objective creation in the seeker and transfers the changes in the seeker's or *sadhak's* physical-astral-causal body. Man has this creative power or the *rajasic* activating quality in Nature. With this quality, the seeker or *sadhak* actively works at progressive self-improvement, through an inward and ascending journey.

The harmonious or *sattvic* quality of Man preserves (in his causal body) the gains made in spiritual self-effort or *sadhana*. Man has the ability to negate or enhance these *gains* as beneficial effects in his own life, as well as in Nature. If the causal beingness records all the gains and changes made in the seeker's life through *sadhana* or self-effort, then his actions gain a *chhandas* or changed quality. His interactions with the world of objects is from a perspective of an evolved being. He starts to see the Cosmic Mother as his own being.

This evolving seeker now acquires the seven feminine qualities of *Lakshmi* or Mother Nature manifesting as different qualities of Prosperity, in speech, thought, and action:

1. **Speech** *(vach)*, which has been derived from the Cosmic Sound: *aum*, finds vibratory expression in the *hum* of his own atoms. He hears Her in the utterances of birds and beasts. He is able to see and hear it in the articulations of Man. Nature starts communicating with the seeker through this subtle speech. Since speech is the instrument of the highest expression, he uses it as an instrument to do good and spread goodness.

   Man is capable of expressing all knowledge already existing in Infinity as the Cosmic Vibrating Intelligence and Knowledge. These have been physically deposited in revelations of the scriptures, such as the most ancient and authentic scriptures of the Hindus or *vedas*.

The seeker has the ability to connect with these revelations. He has the intuitive power of reproducing and reconfirming these repeatedly, through deep meditation. He sources his own realisations by connecting with Cosmic Knowledge, just as has been done for aeons by sages or *rishis* and teachers.

The 'hums' of the pranic energy are transformed during deep meditation, into inner revelations, through the voice of the sages, living in the astral world or heavens. It is these revelations that illumine and gather mankind within the embrace of Mother Nature's Cosmic Love. It is this power of love that reveals and transforms all.

> and the Master admonished a couple:
>
> "Faults become thick when love is thin. When love rises to swirl around us, when we review in the clear light of love, faults become transformed. There is an inherent beauty in them (faults). This is the magic-touch of love - the miracle played by love. When hearts are full of love, life is a valley smiling with beauty, joy, and romance divine"!

2. The seeker acquires in himself, the Mother's quality of **glory** *(kirti).* He is gifted with the subtle power of expression in speech. His actions have the ability to make it known that his intent is for the glorious achievements.
3. There is a natural ability to be **successful and prosper** *(sri).* There is in the seeker an auspicious power in speech and in action. He is now capable of promoting all forms of success and well-being.
4. His **memory** *(smriti)* is powerful. He has the faculty of continuity of awareness which connects the past with the present. She bestows upon a

successful practitioner of meditation, this legacy which allows Man to draw upon the vast storehouse of universal knowledge and achievements.

5. His **intelligence** *(medha)* manifests as pure discrimination or wisdom. His intellect or thought has the mental power to maintain order and harmony in himself and in Nature.
6. Mother Nature gives the seeker Her power of **intuition** *(dhriti).* His soul-perception is an experience and realisation of Truth. His discrimination (intellect) awakens to the innate faculty of intuition. This is not a new development. It underlies all mental powers.
7. She allows the seeker a gift of **forbearance** *(kshama).* With this the seeker acquires a calm power of stability, which resists all fluctuations and thoughts of duality. He sees himself in connection with Nature.

The *yogi* or evolved seeker, understands that these attributes of Mother Nature can be tapped in deep meditation as one or many of Her thousand names or as "She" alone. As his life and awareness ascends the subtle cerebrospinal centres, he unlocks their mysteries. The effulgence of these attributes illumines him. Nature bestows on the sincere seeker these treasures of spiritual self-effort or *sadhana.*

Further Analysis of Speech and Thought and Sight

The power of speech is similar to the power of thought.
What then is speech and how does one speak?

Why do I verbally articulate what I think?
Do I wish to be heard?
Is there clarity in my thinking?

How is thought reflected in the way I speak?

- In the tone I take?
- In the clarity of my words?

The power of thought can also reflect in the power of sight. In the eyes is the soul of how the mind thinks.

Observe a mantra or short sentence of "affirmation":

- It has the power of sound;
- The power of vibration;
- The power of emotion for expression;
- The power to express the power of thought.

The emotions being expressed may be of:

- hope;
- determination; or
- the longing or desire to become single-pointed.

The best way to know that the emotion is single-pointed is to hear the *mantra* on awakening from sleep. The eventual goal of a *mantra* is to manifest in sleep, in dream, and in awake states.

Observe the breath while chanting the mantra or statements of affirmation:
- Note the voice's link with emotion and the restlessness of the person;
- Have an imaginary discussion with yourself.
- Is the voice strong (does it need to be heard) or soft (does it have a poor self image)?
- Is the meaning clear (clarity of mind and emotions).

The external structure of our bodies is a resolution and re-integration of our experiences of our present existence, sitting on top of our causal personality. We push, pull, turn and twist, move and speak our thoughts, in complete affirmation with our inner re-adjustments.

These compensatory activities, allow us rigidity or effortless grace, depending upon the new thought processes created in our inner being. We think, speak and see what we want to, in accordance with whatever requires validation and re-affirmation, in order to feel secure on this <u>newly created foundation</u>.

Maladjustment manifest as pain, resentment, anger, urge to criticise, have guilt, shame, and show fear and grief. The body reacts with a *trigger reaction* operating as <u>filtered</u> thoughts, speech, and sight.

Analysis of Sight

The inherent elemental characteristic of this *chakra (manipura* or lumbar) is *agni* or Fire. The differentiating intellect or *manas,* expressing through the sense of sight, has all the three *gunas* or physical quality manifestations of *sattva* (harmony), *rajas* (activity) *and tamas* (lethargy). Even with the faculty of sight, we manifest these qualities.

Do I take the faculty of sight for granted? How would it be if one had no sight?
- When I look, what do I see? Is awareness involved and where?
- Can I see without eyes?
- Does the mind interpret what I look at?
- What is the basis of this interpretation?
- Is emotion involved?
- Is the mind coloured by emotions? And, if so, is there real clarity in what I see?
- Watch several people view the same thing and ask them to explain what they see.

Make a note of the **"personal" filters** of my personality when using the faculty of sight. These include:
- Past experiences;
- Emotions;

- Likes and dislikes (raaga-dvesha);
- Previous thoughts of a prior event; and
- Quality of guna for clarity of perception.

Ask what exactly is the "awaring" principle of sight?

- *How is sight involved with food and appetite?*
- *How do surroundings influence the food and the sight?*

Raising the Awareness or *chitta* (as a Power or *Shakti, or* as a feeling of Life-Force and Energy) to the third energy centre or *chakra,* requires the same intensity of analysis through each of the senses, the mind, and its emotion.

- In contemplation, concentration and meditation, control of this *chakra* (sight), endows the practitioner with "insight". It is an achievement acquired after **years** of practice.
- Seeing things as they really are builds self-confidence and makes the seeker stronger.
- The seeker must analyse everything he sees by assessing the involvement of emotions, the ego, sight, insight, the mind's eye, and intuition.

Analyse how I see myself, and answer the following questions:

- How do I see others?
- Do I identify with my family, my co-workers?
- Do I see myself in others?

When I see myself, what do I focus on?

- How do I avoid seeing things I do not like about myself and why?
- In what ways am I intentionally blind?
- What creates these screens of intentional blindness?
- Is emotion involved?
- Am I one who cannot recall what was seen, spoken or heard?

Check the way I habitually look at things:

- Analyse why I am not recording what I have "seen" with both the physical and inner eye?

All issues of maladjustment start in early childhood. When a "new" Causal Being or soul enters the lives of a family that he chooses for validation of his past personality and desires, the environment may or may not be in symmetry with his "agenda-in-hand". He (child) must therefore, make new adjustments.

Over the first five years of life, the child's adjustments are in the region of his old habits, concepts, and likes-and-dislikes. All of these must undergo change to match his new home environment. During this time, a moral environment with insightful parents is the most critical issue during this period, for the development of the future adult.

This fact has also been acknowledged by the wise. Learning to develop new thought patterns is a generic strategy parents must learn. The child who is to become a future adult must be taught techniques of self-worth and self-affirmation. Parents must know how to make positive non-judgmental analysis of the child's wants, without the interference of their own past habitual filters.

Despair and Will Power

Limitations imposed by man's physical body, the vagaries of his mind, and his circumstances, have the ability to thwart desires for success in life. Invocation of will power is usually half-hearted and man eventually resorts to despair, which has the ability to annul the God-given will power.

Man's will power is connected to "mains" of divine will power. If Man had the knowledge on the "what, where, and how" to connect with the Infinite Energy of divine will power, he would have the ability to connect with omnipotence, success, and power. Despair would find it difficult to touch his life!

The "what, where, and how" is done through the practice of meditation. He learns to become balanced with the harmonious workings of Mother Nature. In all of Man's activities, he must remain focused at the mouth of God, or the medulla, through which all Cosmic Energy enters his physical being. He must learn to draw Cosmic Energy from the Cosmic Life-force Source.

Connecting with Love and Cosmic Will Power

Whenever you are caught in despairing emotions, sit in an asana or posture of your choice and assume an erect spine as previously described.

- Shut your eyes and focus your gaze at the Kutastha between the eyebrows and visualise the divine cave in the brain and spinal cord.
- Tense the whole spine for six to ten times from your seat to up the neck, at the base of the skull.
- Open the Mouth of God at the medulla by rolling the tongue backwards in the kechri mudra, previously described.
- Massage the medulla (at the base of the skull near the hair-line) with the fingers of your hand, clockwise and then anti-clockwise.
- Will the entry of the Cosmic Energy through the medulla, directing it first to the Kutastha between the eyebrows and allow It to energise all the energy centres or chakras down the brain and spinal cord.
- Focus at the centre of will power in the Kutastha and focus you gaze there at the Cosmic Vision; at the same time, make sure to roll your tongue back towards the posterior pharynx, and into the source of the life-force.
- Energise the twelve body parts by contracting and relaxing each part repeatedly until you lose all body awareness and have entered the sukshma sharira or the subtle astral body of pure energy. You have entered the domains of Her Awareness through pratyahara or withdrawal of awareness

from the senses and the organs of action. Do this for fifteen or twenty minutes.

- Now rest in this awareness. Watch and feel your breath passing in and out through the nostrils. Make sure your gaze is fixed backwards and upwards at the Kutastha between the eyebrows. Your tongue should be rolled back into the roof of the mouth towards the soft palate. Remain in this for ten to twenty minutes.
- Visualise the image characteristic of your guru [as patience, silence, power] or deity or prophet; allow the image to enter your cave through the Kutastha and allow the image to rest transiently at the Kutastha; now carry the image with deep devotion to your heart centre. Let this image live in your "heart" to receive your deep devotion and love at all times, whether working, sleeping, or dreaming . Allow these characteristic[s] permeate your whole being until it radiates its inherent magnetism.
- Repeat the same, this time bringing the Cosmic Will Power to your own centre of will power in the Kutastha. You are now empowered by Cosmic Will Power and will be able to do anything you put your mind to.
- Pray for upliftment in action, thought and intent; ask for patience, even-mindedness, and wisdom while witnessing the breath.

Watch the Interplay of Sight and Emotions

The next few exercises are divided under two headings. The first half deals with man as he deals with the world of objects, emotions [senses], and thoughts [OET] and incorpotrates their images into his own person. His interactions with the world are directed in front of himself. It is the anterior and inferior interaction of the self.

The second half of the discussion deals with incorporating Infinity into oneself. His interaction is with the posterior and upper half of his physical being, within the divine cave of the brain and the spinal cord. Here the movement is northwards.

I. Look at an inanimate object like a picture or flower for three minutes guarding against thoughts that intrude and dislodge the single-pointedness of sight.

Next, look at a picture of someone dear and compare the ability to concentrate.

Then, look into another's eye without speaking, moving, or blinking:

- Consider and watch the mind and emotions being aroused and record your observations.

Create a picture in the mind's eye at the Kutastha between the eyebrows and hold the image without thought or emotional interference:

- Watch the mental screen and observe the mind;
- See what appears on your mental screen and record it;
- Analyse your thought association.

Images of disturbing thoughts or emotions may be about hurts and insults given and received recently or in the past. You may be feeling regrets that you did not retaliate at that time. This is the time to "deal with it":

- Create an image of the person or incident of your emotional disturbance in your Kutastha.
- Allow the image to descend into your centre of emotions in your heart and allow the incident or person receive your love and forgiveness. Repeat this many times until: You are able to erase it from your memory, where it caused you disturbances.

Remain vigilant and observe if similar problems re-occur. If they do:

- Analyse them and forgive them because they are disturbances, which can become obstacles in meditation.
- Begin with meditation for ten minutes and progress from there using the mind as witness of the activity on the mental screen.

> and the Master wrote:
>
> "Forgiveness is the fragrance, which crushed tulasi (holy basil) leaves on the fingers that crushed them, in a thoughtless act!
>
> "Sandalwood (emits) perfumes, even when the axe that hews it down! The more we rub the sandalwood against the stone, the more its fragrance spreads. Burn it and it wafts its glory in the entire neighbourhood. Such is the enchanting beauty of forgiveness in life.."

Record observations while doing the following exercises on your "sensory mind" or senses or manas and your "feelings" as unenlightened chitta or the mind-intellect-ego complex:

i Look at earth taking the form of an inert stone.

- Express a "feeling" by involving sight, sound, taste, touch, and feel . This is <u>sense-analysis.</u>

ii. Look next at colours, fire as flame and use the technique of sense analysis. Involve the five senses and the emotions of "feelings" triggered by sight.

iii. Visualise AUM, the Holy Spirit as an "image". This technique allows the seeker to convert subtle issues into intellectually acceptable "concepts" in your mind; over time, with the advent of wisdom, your intelligence will "feel" Aum intuitively:

- Look first at the alphabets of Aum.
- Next "see" and "hear" Aum entering your divine cave of the brain and spinal cord through the medulla with your inner intuitive gaze focused at the Kutastha between the eyebrows.
- Take in a breath through the mouth, with your tongue rolled back and "feel" Aum, the Holy Spirit, first fill the divine cave. Next hold the breath in inspiration for a few seconds. Now let Aum energise all the chakras down the spine, and allow the Holy Spirit radiate from the energy-centres or

chakras to the various parts of body they control, down as far as the peripheral skin.

- Next, expire and observe the emotions evoked.

iv. Look at a dot on a white background and stare at it without blinking for as long as you can until your eyes water (trataka). This technique sharpens your ability to recall images from memory or sight into your inner gaze.

- Watch their effects on your "feelings" as you breathe and again as you stop breathing.
- Compare the differences or similarities staring into an eye or a dot.

v. Think of the navel (the location of the third chakra) and imagine a silver disc looking like the moon located here. This technique allows you to draw from the imagery of concepts in your mind's eye:

- Now focus at the brow between the eyes and bring the silver disc to that spot.
- Imagine the disc as the silvery moon emanating a cool feeling.
- If the mind becomes active beyond the sight, mind and coolness, add to it love, peace, and light.

vi. Visualise the most perfect Master in your mind's eye while seated at meditation (some may require to stare at a picture of such an ideal), until the eyes water: Using the trataka technique.

- Seat the ideal in a meditative posture and place him/her inside your divine cave behind your inner gaze.
- Observe and record your emotions and feelings.

vii. Look into the sky and visualise Divine Light Aum Shakti, both seeing and feeling It, first with your eyes open and then with your eyes closed.

- Hold the vision in the inner eye as long as you can.
- Some may need to practice trataka by watching a lit lamp or actual images.

viii. Look and see everything; then analyse and understand what is being seen. What do I actually see inside of me? What do I feel and what is its effect?

- Place a coloured dot, quarter inch radius on a plain background.
- Stare at the dot without blinking until your eyes water.
- Continue by lengthening the time spent staring.

Breathe in, a cold breath and expire hot air while staring. The varying temperatures are sensed more acutely when the head is thrown back slightly at the neck and the tongue is rolled back:

- Relax your hands and the lower abdominal muscles during expiration;
- Then tense your hands and the lower abdominal muscles during inspiration and observe for a few seconds before expiring.
- Write down your observations.

Now, compare looking at a dot with staring into someone's eyes.

ix. Look at your own face in the mirror or stare at a portrait of yourself.
- What do you see?
- Resentment? Pain? One who can be trusted?
- Does your face look deceitful, or is there divine Light shining through?
- What kind of face is it? Is it kind or what?

Close your eyes and visualise what you saw physically with your eyes. Make notes on: what, where, when, why, and how you see the images in your inner gaze.

Prolong the times of trataka or staring pauses, and then make notes, until the power of sight is made acute and images are clarified to be what they are meant to be.

- *Now project the image in the sky.*

II. Now look at the vast infinite sky. Every star, sun, and moon remain securely suspended in the vastness of Infinity. Look at the earth. It too remains securely fastened within this void without any harnessing or mooring. Imagine the earth walking and talking with all the cosmic persons in this Cosmic Creation.

- Look, listen, and feel the earth enjoying the total presence born of joy. Note that you are using the same senses you used in the previous exercises to visualise vastness, infinity, purity, friendship, and omnipresence,
  The earth is happy to see the plants, birds, beasts, and humans safe in Mother Nature's warm embrace. They are all growing and evolving.
  Keep looking at this Cosmic Vision.
  Watch the infinite space, the sky, and the ocean.
  Feel the infinite warmth of Her embrace as Mother Nature nurtures the stars and the planets. They are firmly secure in space and fear no tumbles or falls.
- Now enter your own silence and watch the breath coursing in and out through the nostrils. Watch the breath for a few minutes. Listen to the Cosmic Sound of Infinity within the divine cave. Keep looking at the Cosmic Vision and incorporate it within the divine cave until it merges and sees its own immortality and infinity. Feel the immortality. That You Are - tat twam asi.

Dual Existence

As soon as a being descends from his causal state of combined consciousness and life force into a foetus, he establishes his astral existence. The individualised soul enters the energy centres or *chakras* in the cave of the brain and spinal cord. Consciousness resides in the crown or *sahasrahara chakra.* The individualised being directs the soul into the medulla or *ajnaa* centre, as the *chitta,* or the combined mind-intellect-ego complex.

The sensory mind or *manas,* enters the future body as the five senses of intellection, locomotion, and astral functions of physiology-psychology. He now descends into the domains of a physical-mental-physiological mortal. Playing the mortal in a world of objects, emotions, and thoughts (OET), he loses the memory of his own divine state.

This memory loss is not permanent. As soon as he embarks on the Yoga of Meditation, Man retraces his journey back to his own divine source. Through the practice of the eight-fold path *[Patanjali's ashtanga yoga* of universal commandments: *yama and niyama or* rules of self-purification, correct posture or *asana,* breathing techniques *pranayama,* sensory withdrawal or *pratyahara,* and concentration or *dharana],* he gradually stills the mind and recalls the silence of his intuitive ego - the sixth sense. This stillness and silence is progressive, depending upon the frequency and duration of his meditative efforts or *sadhana.*

At this stage of the practitioner's development, *dharana* or the practice of concentration in the seat of meditation, takes him to partial-union with the object of concentration - the subject "I":

- The seeker or *sadhak* first focuses on the body as he gradually retracts towards the subject of identification**:** the *stillness* of the body and mind.
- Next, he experiences ("Me" experiences of *chitta* as feeling) an "entry" into the subject "I" *(chit)* which has the characteristics of divine purity**:** the *silence* of the mind.
- Finally, "I", the enlightening soul, experiences momentary partial unions with an all-encompassing power of Universal Intelligence in the *kutastha chaitanya*, which embraces all things including the practitioner**;** the experience is that of a *still and silent* Awareness of Consciousness.

Purpose of Dual Existence

Man is not only an isolated individual as a "soul", but he is also a "social being"; extending his being outwards, through the senses. In doing this, he develops the rules by which society is governed. *Man's greatness is that he embodies society.* The purpose of a dual existence is that this *individualised being* possesses an inner-force which directs him to *serve society* as a *social being.*

> Swami Bharathi Krishna Tirtha wrote:
>
> ".. From the standpoint of science, we need not be apprehensive that our study of religion and the practice of the principles inculcated in us, will stand in the way of our material prosperity. The two go together. There is no difference and there can be very little conflict between the two.. And if at any time we find that there seems to be a conflict, we may be perfectly certain that we have misread our scriptures, or misunderstood the laws of nature around us. It is not possible that we have understood both correctly when we find an irreconcilable antagonism between the two.."

Through self-analysis, man realises that God exists and the universe as he perceives it, coincides with His or Her making of the Universe. He recognises that *this inner-force is the same that animates all of Mother Nature or Prakriti.*

After enjoying the play-acting of my present existence as "Me" the materialistically satisfied ego becomes restless again and begins his search for his origin as "I". In this search for his origin, his feelings of "duality" lead him to the discovery of himself as the "I" everywhere. The combined force of consciousness and cosmic energy, as *Shiva-Shakti*, is like the sun and the sun-rays. (Please refer to Figure 1)

In *pratyahara* or withdrawal from the senses and in *dharana* or concentration, this experience of partial union is the first stage of entering meditation or *dhyana.* This is the stage when the practitioner exits from his physical being and enters into his astral being. Here, an experience of expansion occurs and, occasionally, he senses an integration with all of creation. He leaves his gross physical sensations and becomes subtle energy!

Experiencing Partial Union

The burden of the subconscious (astral being) and the unconscious mind (causal being), must surface into the realms of consciousness as "wandering thoughts and images", and dreams. These all must be dissipated to allow the mind to become transparent.

At this stage of the practitioner's development, the mind will enter the astral dimension and expand beyond the bodily shell of the practitioner. The mind's ability to expand has no limits. It is able to extend spatially and temporally. This includes making contact with the subject "I" - the Self.

When the practitioner opens his eyes, he is aware that the body "Me" (object) and the "I" (subject) are separate. This dual perception or double vision is a perception at two levels of being:

- Perception through the senses as a physical being; and
- An inner perception as an astral being, as energy.

Over time, the practitioner can look at physical objects with his physical eyes, as being separate from himself. At the same time, he has the ability to become one with the energy of the subject, in the astral dimension. Here, everything - both animate and inanimate, sentient and insentient, possess energy. This energy now becomes available to the practitioner as progress is made into meditation.

> and the Master wrote:
>
> "...When M and I are transcended, (when V is exhausted), PFT-awake gets 'enlightenment' of its Pure State, the Aum-state, the God-state of Consciousness."

Defining Energy and Partial Union

Oneness or *samadhi* occurs when the energy of the physical being merges into the energy or *prana* of the astral being. Next, the combined "physical-astral being" merges with his own causal beingness and experiences first a *stillness,* then a *silence,* and finally both *stillness-silence.*

This is not a state of hypnotic trance or a hallucination. *Hypnosis is* a mental impression that one is being drawn into past experiences stored in the subconscious and unconscious. The recipient experiences issues of which he is already aware.

Conversely, in *partial union,* the awaking mind undergoes a new experience, previously never experienced in his awake state. When the practitioner persists in meditation, the mind expands beyond the limits of the physical body and enters the astral dimension. The seeker then realises that the life-force he experiences is the same energy in all things.

Defining the Astral and World of Matter

The physiological and psychological life force manifests in the psychic or astral dimension of energy or "lifetrons", which is an extension of the physical being, matter. This, too, is the energy of physical atoms.

When the practitioner enters the astral dimension in meditation, he transcends his own psychological-physiological connections of individual beingness and expands into the astral dimension of energy beingness.

Astral energy channels through the five astral senses. It is its physical counterpart that makes contact with the outer world. The practitioner can retract into his astral brain and also into the causal astral centre of his intuitive mind. Here he remembers his divine right!

Psychics

Individuals who are able to recognise that they are able to move from the physical to the astral world (psychic world) may die before making any further progress in their spiritual lives. They may be reborn in another lifetime, with memories of this experience. In this new manifestation, they experience psychic phenomenon termed psychic-gifts.

Psychics are individuals who have reached a partial stage of enlightenment in previous incarnations. This is comparable to partial union in meditation, which is the result of the incomplete shattering of the ego shell ("Me") in the astral dimension.

Practitioners with psychic abilities are encouraged by *yogis* to pursue the path of inquiry instead, especially focusing into the functioning of the Ego. Preoccupation with this faculty (psychic phenomenon) will cause one to lose sight of the ultimate goal of man: for ultimate happiness and oneness in *samadhi.*

There are psychics who interact with the astral mind on an emotional level. More evolved psychics interact at the astral intellect level. *Yogis* living in the astral heavens enter and leave the different astral heavens at will. They guide spiritual seekers in their different stages of development.

Analysis of Energy, Mind, Imagination, and Dreams

Energy has no form and is therefore shapeless. During self-effort in *sadhana,* life-force or Energy or *Aum Shakti,* which normally descends from the cave of brain down the spinal cord, is made to ascend to the brain-cave towards consciousness.

Progressive self-effort in *sadhana,* involving the practice of the moral restraints of *yama* and adherence to the rules of *niyama,* gradually raises awareness. The practitioner's awareness now becomes progressively chastened. Intense practice by repetition *(abhyas)* of postures (*or asana),* withdrawal from the five senses (or *pratyahara*), and breath-control (or *pranayama),* takes the practitioner towards the *Manipura* or navel *chakra.* Here, "She", the energy, gathers potency and subtlety but also tangles with strong forces such as, desires and imagination, emotions, and sight.

Concepts and images at this stage are soft and clay-like and can be moulded, before they are hardened in the kiln of emotions and self-will to become passion. One can be passionate about names and forms, as well as ideas and *concepts.*

Once we adopt concepts, they become prominent memories in our lives. Over time, they acquire the *"power" to modulate all future actions.* Our actions are now dictated by such powers; for example, emotions *cause intentional blindness.* These concepts now become appendages to our personality revealed as *habits* of procrastination or self-pity, and the desire to compensate or be vengeful.

Through the repeated practice of *pratyahara* or wilful withdrawal from the senses, the seeker experiences this awesome energy, free of all body awareness. He experiences this both in contraction and relaxation of his energising exercises. This recognition, affirmation, and validation of the existence of the energy, now becomes a *habit.*

Instinctive habits are established patterns of thinking, feeling, defensive reaction, and compulsions. Habits colour what we do and do not wish to see, smell, taste, hear, touch, or feel. They manifest as our likes-and-dislikes or *raaga-dveshas!* All aspects of our existence are under the influence of these past habits.

The best defence against this *raaga-dvesha* of personal opinions is the power of positive thinking. Replace negative thinking which force us to react under the influence of our emotions and ego with positive thinking. Cultivate the **visualisation of ideals** within the mind's eye. Ideal responses must be projected and observed in the mind. The *meeting with energy* during *pratyahara* makes it easier for seekers to reach their ideal.

As the **mind interprets everything** from every sense, emotion, and experience we become increasingly aware and more sensitive to the objects of contact and the processing of the information in the mind.

Networking and co-operation occurs between senses, objects and the Cosmic Body. Self-importance now takes a back seat, and the sense of isolation from the Self is dissolved.

Because **images** of past lives appear as **dreams**, they must be observed. Their power of control on the unaware "sleeping" mind is remarkable. The mind transfers these images of causal beingness and messages into consciousness translating them into actions as habitual actions. It takes courage, prayer, and humility to clarify the dreams, which determine our "unconscious" actions.

When in the depth of meditation, when body awareness has dissolved into the astral body and there are no more thoughts to disturb awareness, there is here a divine stillness and silence of an immense expanse of Infinity. Here a recurring image of yellow blooms [which I have never seen before] touch my face, as if I have walked into them. This is an example of an image from my causal unconscious state, making an entry into my astral subconscious state. These may surface as dreams or during meditation.

Analysis on Imagination, Mind and Energy

Let us investigate, next, "My world". Do I like it, and if not, can I destroy it for a new one?

"My world" is the result of "blind" habitual thinking patterns:

- It arises out of my own experience of sight, smell, sound, taste, things, people, illusions, and beliefs.

What are these beliefs? What is their foundation?

What would happen if each of my beliefs were appraised in the opposite?
Does that disturb me?
What are facts?

Review where, when, why, and how your beliefs became crystallised. Observe if there are any emotional upheavals within myself if someone opposes my 'facts and beliefs'.

Notice how focused "Me" becomes when each fact and belief is analysed.

"Me" is becoming more central (as "I") to the hub of the revolving wheel-of-life.

- Functioning closer to the centre brings newer insights.

What are my habits and routine tasks?

- Review where, when, why, and how these habits and "facts" became part of "Me".
- Observe any emotional upheavals within myself when someone acts differently from my way of doing things.

Review your own actions-and-reactions as a "mechanical habitual behaviour":

- How do I react?
- Am I defensive to criticism?
- How do I act when I feel hostile?
- How do I react to the aggression of others?
- Does the aggressor's appearance affect me?
- What emotions do I experience when witnessing a conflict?

Behaviour patterns function first through thought patterns. Relationships with the world of objects, emotions and thoughts (OET), are the dynamics of how an individual patterns his needs to care for himself in a better, efficient, and more destructive manner.

He ensures his needs are met without further disruptions in his foundational causal being. Man then uses his imaginative thought processes to energise the new adjustments he must make for his present existence. Some of these adjustments are self-destructive and even counter-productive.

De-coding self-destructive tendencies in a particular individual must be analysed. A Spiritual teacher has the intuitive power to rebuild his social life-history in terms of his physical, emotional, intellectual, and behavioural dynamics.

Information gathered from such analysis, leads to crystallisation of new insights that are helpful in transforming the individual seeker the *guru* is working with. He is taught to avoid *raaga-dvesha* or likes-dislikes through meditation. This speeds his evolution through repeated prescribed practice and meditation.

Behaviour Modifications and the First Three Chakras

All our shortcomings are "imagined" and can be overcome by intense examination of the three senses: sight, smell, and taste. The meditation practices and group discussions in the first three sections have all the tools for *yamas* or "Don'ts" and *niyamas* "Do's" of human conduct.

- With imagination and emotion under control, I gain mastery over myself
- Every small step counts because it is disaster to hold on to imagined conditions, circumstances, desires, and hopes.
- All my dreams are but illusions and awakening from them may be cruel but necessary.

- To see things as they are helps build self-confidence and inner strength.

Straight thinking implies meeting situations as they are instead of:
- imagining their meanings; or
- foggy thinking; or
- doing nothing about problems; or
- being overwhelmed by problems and worries.

Insight is connected to concentrated thinking.
- Intense concentration can be developed by cultivating straight thinking and utilising physical, mental, and emotional tools to review the depth of all actions and reactions.

Review how long it takes to analyse a problem through concentration.
- While concentrating, analyse how I analyse problems: are the images real or abstract?
- If there is no image to hold on to, can I see myself as a Mass of Light or am I a body without destiny?
- Notice new thought trends and new dreams and record changes because these are connections to the inner Self.

Study the changes in thoughts and dreams and you will enter the innermost being which now becomes the guiding force of all your activities:
- The guiding-force motivating the seeker now gathers Energy from which can be drawn the required drive and enthusiasm to face any mundane problem, including obstacles in self- development.

What are my problems, my "dark clouds"?
- How did they form?
- Can I see them developing at their earliest stage; how does one prevent their formation?

In what areas of my personality do I act under compulsion of emotions?
- Are my emotions more valuable than reason?
- How can I trigger the thought processes that stimulate reason - "First think and then act"?

What is "brainstorming"?
- Do I use others as sounding boards in order to clear my own thinking processes and permit effective action?
- How do I obstruct an act through emotions and "mind tactics"?
- How do I obstruct by criticising or making judgements?

Watch my actions and delay-tactics of:
- Not doing work. Blaming the past and procrastinating into the future.
- Remaining "emotionally blind" to justify inaction.
- In what areas of living do I use delay tactics: work, study, and personal relationships?

Through mental exercise, watch the mind's awareness:

- Concentrate on objects and pay attention to them;
- Record observations and dreams;
- Do energising exercises by beaming out "awareness" from the cave to the periphery of every part of the body
- Reflect on daily events, meanings of words or ideas.

It is through self-analysis and self-healing that one realises that old habits, concepts, and opinions are embedded in the Causal Being through millions of previous rebirths. The thought-form and emotional content, resides embedded in this awareness. The right to survive, self-thrive, self-love, self-accept, self-commit, and have self-confidence, are all defensive mechanisms to self-serve.

Self-healing begins with the same knowledge while engaging oneself in *karma yoga, gyana yoga, bhakti yoga* or *hatta yoga. (*Please refer to Types of Yoga). Aside from these paths, *raja yoga* (combination of the four yoga paths) restores integration with the Cosmic Being in Awareness and Consciousness. *Raja Yoga* is the only process known that systematically leads Man to his own Reality.

Emotions or Mind and Energy

Emotions are the biggest stumbling block in the aspirant's life, clouding it with pride, false modesty, vanity, drive, and competition due to false illusions. In the practitioner's life there must be no competition. One grows slowly out of these habits through reflection, or the ability to mirror an event, and to assess the level of performance at all levels. One's own attitudes must be investigated to prevent actions from being hurtful to others.

Pain, however, must be treated as a great teacher for self-improvement. There must be an inner understanding that pain of previous lives lead to problems in the present and in future births to come.

Development of latent potential is Divine Law. If you do not develop your potential you will lack purpose in life.

Helplessness, due to lack of self-mastery, is against the law of *karma.*

Emotions exert a powerful influence on the practitioner. The *Manipura Chakra*, located at the level of the navel (lumbar or solar plexus), is the seat of both lower and higher emotions .

Spontaneous reactive emotions to minor stresses in life, have a hypnotic effect on the aspirant. Through positive thinking, base emotions can be given concrete images of higher idealism. Reactions to situations can manifest in the higher emotions of devotion, service, and concern, which have the power to move both fire (third *chakra)* and water (second *chakra).* The intellectual power of reasoning has the ability to balance chastened emotion.

Analysis of Emotion

An emotion is like a drop of water which is so small as compared to the ocean, that it can be wiped away very easily. If left unattended, many drops take on a form, a flow, and an erratic direction.

- Think of a lake. It has depth and appears murky. It prevents clear sight to the bottom.
- Water takes on a shape and form of its own unless it is given boundaries: this is the story of emotion, uncontrolled and unregulated.
- Can I see things as they really are when overcome by a torrent of emotions?
- To overcome this "blindness", I must remove the clouds of emotions [which distort the intellect], through reasoning.

Review all issues and emotions of jealousy, attachments, self-pity, procrastination and self-justifications

Disorders of underlying causal beingness, negative thought forms, emotional outbursts, individual life-stories since childhood, are all predisposing factors capable of precipitating dynamic situations [emotional] of all descriptions and magnitude. Only Man is able to make adjustments and give himself a re-interpretation of what is really happening.

The Master repeatedly accused me of being too emotional. I clearly did not understand what he meant because I reasoned that there was nothing wrong with being emotional. It took me years to understand that there are two levels of emotionalism. One is reflexive and reactive to life situations [which I was being accused of] and the other is reflective.

Refining Emotions

The "image" of the divine cave or a *guru* or any deity or an ideal gives one focus for prolonged concentration or *dharana* and worship.

- Worship is an expression of empathy, gratitude, love, and loyalty.
- Once one is elevated to the ideal, the monotony of concentrating-meditating in a predetermined period of time disappears. The aspirant now is fired with enthusiasm to reach greater heights of refined emotion.

  and the Master said:

  "...'Idol' is 'Ideal' symbolised..."

Create an Ideal Altar - a Place of Worship

- *Sit in meditation in the asana of your choice. Rearrange the posture and straighten the back with shoulders together. Throw the head backwards so that the chin is parallel to the ground.*
- *Roll the tongue back, turn the gaze towards the Cosmic Vision, and watch*

the breath coursing in and out through the nostrils. Look inside the divine cave and find the ideal image of righteousness of God or the ideal inner sound in your divine cave. Here, righteousness signifies the infinite nature of omnipresent God. Rest here in your own stillness.

- *Next, attempt to feel love for God in the divine cave.* ***Next feel the divine cave filled with Light. Light here signifies the wisdom of existing in singularity. [non-dual or advaita]. You and the Light are One.***
- *This exercise is difficult and demands great awareness, discrimination, and gratitude. The exercise will also help in the invocation of Aum as Light: a physical-astral reality. Start by concentrating on any sound you hear. Gradually hear your inner sound. They change as you go deeper into yourself.*
- *Concentrate the gaze at the kutastha between the eyebrows. You will* see lights or an eye. Enter the centre of the eye. There is Light here. Enter it and become one with the Light within the divine cave.
- *You are now on the platform of the Light of Wisdom and are listening to the sound of Oneness: AUM, Amen, Amin, ar Hum.*

Here in the Light there is no pain, nor is there pleasure. There is no good nor is there evil. There is only harmony. There is nothing to "think" about. There is only the seer, and seeing what needs to be seen as Light.

Make sure that you are looking at the divine cave with your inner gaze (seen) focused between your eyebrows at the Cosmic Vision:

- *Roll your tongue back towards the pharynx;*
- *Watch the breathing at all times - (seer);*
- *Feel and become aware of the whole energy filled astral being - (seeing);*
- *Listen to the Aum through the inner ear;*
- *Listen to the inner silence until you [seer-seen-seeing] become One with the sound. This Light of Awareness filling the divine cave is personal wisdom or vigyana..*

Thoughts have a way of disturbing this peace. Most emanate from the conscious and subconscious levels of existence. Think of ways to replace a negative emotion with its opposite, (in day-to-day living) such as:

- *gloom for cheerfulness;*
- *anger with love and mercy;*
- *criticism with acceptance.*

Those unfamiliar with the use of images or Light as ideals in meditation may find the exercises described above as idolatry. To them, I will render what the Master said:

> at a *satsang* [meeting with the wise] the Master was challenged about 'idolatry'. To illustrate the logic of 'personal preference for each seek' he told us the following:
>
> "A leader from a small province in India was elected President and was asked to

move to New Delhi with his ailing wife. On arrival, they were shown their 450-room palatial new home and were asked to choose and occupy whatever rooms they desired for their permanent Aresidence.

"The ailing wife became hysterical with the prospect of caring for a 450-room residence. She had to be pacified there was enough staff to care for the palace. Hearing this she became even more distressed that she would have to manage a hundreds of staff members. The Administrative District Commissioner soothed Her Excellency and assured her that he would serve her without outside interference from the staff or involvement with other rooms.."

This allegory was used to illustrate his point:

"Truth is One without a second. His attributes are like a thousand rooms. The seeker is asked to choose the room [God's attribute] most suited to his personality. The rest of the attributes take care of themselves..."

Identifying "I" and "Me"

Notice how "Me", the ego depends on "I" for its existence in hearing, touching seeing, tasting, smelling, feeling, and thinking:

- *Where is this consciousness felt in my personality?*
- *Where is the awareness of this consciousness?*

Become aware of "my centre" in the divine cave and "see from the mind's eye" all that happens to me:

- *Observe rising emotions in others and see if they are directed towards me?*
- *Observe the harmful emotions that can manifest against others. Create a more ideal situation and become a giver of "positivity".*

Balancing Different Emotions

Both benevolent and destructive emotions must be balanced through reasoning. This is done by recording daily events without imposing an emotional overlay:

- The seeker must take full responsibility to develop and cultivate balanced emotion, addressing both the creative and destructive facets of his emotional traits. The polarities muse be harmonised.
- With correct effort there will be co-operation from the Higher Self.
- Results create a sense of gratitude, which translates itself into "worship" of the ideal.

Gratitude Solidifies Worship

Make a list of things for which you are grateful for in your life and in the lives of others with whom you have been emotionally involved:

- *Now identify your needs. Identify the controlling pressures of your needs.*

- *Ask, if these "needs" are wants of my little will?*
- *Are these "needs" met?*
- *Must I have all these needs fulfilled?*
- *Do I have the capacity to leave "my needs" at the mercy of "Your Will"?*

Do not waste time criticising others and yourself. The secret is to replace the negative habits with positive affirmations. This will lead to an acute awareness of a newer dimension in you. The chastened emotions become more available for gratitude and worship.

> and the Master said:
>
> "..There are some 'lame' individuals who are activated to function in the world outside by their inner worry: so addicted are they to their worries that if their worries are removed, they seem to collapse without their crutches.
>
> "..You deposit your worldly possessions in the Bank for safekeeping. Why don't you deposit your actions in Nature's Bank for safe-keeping and stop worrying about the Future.."

Recording Dreams

Through dreams we can contact the Higher Self, the beloved Master, the *Guru.* By writing down the dreams immediately upon awakening from sleep, the trends of messages being given can be discerned.

Even as a child, I had a terrible fear of darkness. We lived in Zanzibar where I spent my early school years. The children of the school whispered among themselves that the 'big house' we lived in was haunted. I would 'see' things that others could not and wake up screaming. My father would allow me to crawl into his bed, until the next time.

I was now twenty-two years old and already a doctor. My father realised that I had not out-grown my fear of 'seeing things'. He was always concerned about this.

I was now tweny-five years old. My father was being taken to the crematorium. As I wished his physical body farewell, I unwittingly promised to wake up every morning at 0400 hours to light a lamp for forty days [continuously].

The prayer room was in the next room of our three bed-roomed home in Dodoma, Tanzania. Every time I got up, the fear of darkness and what 'I might see' filled me with terror. I would fly into the next room and fly back to bed. It took me one hundred and thirty days to do a forty day vigil. I was rid of the terror but I have never been able to completely remove the fear of 'seeing things'.

When the Master left his body, I feared seeing his astral body. My daughters 'see' him and talk to him but I do not wish to see him. I have asked him to come to me in my dreams.

1991 Ottawa: When he was so frail, I worried that he would leave the body right in my arms. As usual he picked my thoughts:

"You wanted to mother me in your last life. You have your wish now" and I shuddered with alarm. Then he said kindly,

"I am not going very far...close your eyes and I will always be there."

When he did physically leave us, I feared seeing his astral presence. I begged him never to frighten me.

"Come to me 'physically' as the face of the Sun, whenever I call upon you, come hail or storm. Talk to me when I need you. Show me your face when I feel troubled or wish to 'see' you with my physical eyes...and when you wish to speak with me, come to me in my dreams or in my intuition during meditation..." My Master has never failed me yet! I also know that his promise

"I will be there with you" will come true when I finally exit from my mortal moorings!

- *If you do not dream, or do not remember dreams, write the first thought that comes to mind immediately upon arising.*
- *Leave space for interpretation.*
- *Leave space to record events and mental preoccupation which occurred before the dream.*

Note how the mind attends to perception of time and space in the context of events in your dream:

- *Compare this with how the mind shifts with events irrespective of time and space.*
- *Become aware of the "reality of time and space" in life while awake and in sleep. In dreams, there is no time or space. There are only images on a screen of awareness.*

Record symbols seen in dreams and create your own "dictionary" of their meaning.

- *Discover how the mind expresses ideas repeatedly when they are meant to be "personal" messages.*
- *These are messages from the "inner guru".*

Worship

Worship is the transmutation of raw emotion into a channel of spiritual energy which manifests as a high quality feeling of reverence for the object of our love, desire, and devotion. To keep worship alive, it is critical that the prayer and ritual not become mechanical. Regimentation for the sake of stabilisation creates boredom and the personal experience of elation and the fire of enthusiasm eventually dies.

To keep the spirit of worship alive in yourself:

- *Stare at the image of the guru or deity with the eye and connect the emotions by aligning yourself with His Supreme Intelligence.*
- *Now close the eyes and create the image in the mind's eye.*
- *Transform this emotion of love into channelled spiritual energy of intense feeling for oneness with the object of your love.*

An alternative to eyes aligning with emotions is aligning sound and voice with emotions to give vent to admiration, gratitude, and humility of the soul residing in the divine cave as the Universal Intelligence *(Kutastha Chaitanya).*

> and the Master said:
>
> "...To serve the Almighty, who is manifested in all living creatures, with whatever faculty each one of us has, is the greatest worship, the highest spiritual living..."

Another Analysis of Sex

It is time to look at sex again.

Analyse the compulsions that manifest as lust versus the spontaneous feelings refined by strong emotions. Make note of *compulsive action* versus *compulsive emotion*, which is spontaneous and arises from feelings of goodness and selflessness. Compulsive action benefits me. Compulsive emotion is a giving of love to the other.

Now let us review **sex without affection:**

- Is it an impulse generated by an idea of what was seen or heard through another?
- Is it a game of seduction or conquest?

Are **sex and spirituality** different?

- Are they the same energy manifesting in spirituality and sex?

By yielding to spontaneity, is the door to Higher Awareness left open?

Man comes with many conflicts and confusions about identity, worth, vulnerability, and procreativity. He either de-values himself on issues of intimacy, or he raises his awareness through trust, consideration, respectfulness, and peace between himself and his partner.

Past traumatic experiences embedded in his causal foundation can lead to difficulty in showing love in committed relationships. The personal pain of fear, insecurity, guilt and resentment, lead to faulty thought patterns. Conflicts lead to issues around self-worth, right to exist, right to love and also, faulty opinions of sexuality.

Readjustment through meditation and moral living allows a seeker to enter his own inner being. There is a transformation in his understanding and the power of intuition allows him to make adjustments. This leads him to correct thinking about the purpose and spirituality of Man's sexuality.

Awareness as Divine Energy

Many tell us that God is a fabrication of the mind. If the mind is a string of thoughts, is there an awareness that links it with consciousness? The third *chakra (manipura)* is important in that the seeker is now becoming increasingly self-aware as a result of *sadhana* (self-effort in the inquiry into *yama and niyama).*

Awareness is a progressive knowing illumined by the Light of Consciousness, where Consciousness stands alone and mighty.

The Master used an instinctive act of a single individual to explain that all awareness is connected to a greater Cosmic Awareness. It did not make any sense at the time. Nearly three decades later, we marvel when we meet the children we taught at *Bal Vihars* or Junior Childrens' Sunday Schools and *Yuva Kendras* or Youth Clubs. These young adults are not only successful but have the right values towards children, parents, elders, communities, Nation, and the world! A self-sustaining act of worship.

> In the early 1970's *Swami Chinmayananda* writes from Los Angeles about a single "instinctive philanthropic act" of an inspired Muslim girl [Malek Sultan Hussein Walji] who met him for the first time:
>
> "..good and bad actions of each of us set the entire Universe into action: in fact you cannot pluck a blade of grass without making the stars shudder. The entire Universe is an organic whole....God!!! He is *Jagadishvara"* (Lord of the Universe).

Malek had instinctively given away her worldly savings in a rental investment in Mt. Pearl, for the purpose of cultural meetings for the Indians. Three decades later, it has transformed itself into a million dollar place of cultural interaction in St. John's, Newfoundland. The people of St. John's have forgotten the initial act [Energy] but that one instinctive act remains connected to the mains [Consciousness] of the Cosmic Mother!

Scientists would reject the above emotional statements. How then does one convince the doubting-Thomas that Consciousness and Energy are interchangeable? Scientists say that Energy and its manifestations or Matter are inseparable. Einstein also said that Matter is Energy multiplied by the square of Light, which remains constant. If we assume that manifestation of Consciousness is Light, then:

- Consciousness is the Energy (both *Purusha and Prakriti*) of Light; and
- Its expression is manifestation, first of all as the *pranava*: Aum or Hum or Amen or Amin or the "Word" of the Bible.

The *physical* expression of this Energy is Creation:

- She *(Prakriti* or Mother Nature or *Shakti*) is the womb and cause of Creation, both as Microcosm (me) and as Macrocosm (universe).

- Both are manifested forms of this Light Energy - *Aum.*

Everything, which is manifested, is a variation of this vibrating Energy *Aum*, holding and gelling all atoms, molecules, names, and forms together.

Self-analysis or Sadhana

Are all our attempts to analyse, codify, organise, and record efforts at self-gratification for self-importance?

- Can we now use this habit to analyse, codify, organise, and record to clarify our preconceived concepts and ideas, by tuning into the finer forces within, during meditation? Yes, we can.
- The seeker will arrive at personal conclusions guided by the *inner guru.* This innate Divinity in each one of us lies hibernating and semi-asleep within us. Awareness of the *guru's* existence within depends upon our awareness of Its presence.
- Arousing this innate Energy of Divinity is what *yogis* mean by raising the *Devi Shakti* [Powerful Mother as Energy] in the divine cave.

There is a misunderstanding in scriptural commentaries about raising-the-*kundalini!* Withdrawal of the life-force through *pratyahara* helps concentrate the energy into the divine cave of the brain and spinal cord.

In the cord, the energy of the first *chakra* or earth is transformed to water, and then to fire, and to air, and finally to space. This is an astral transformation which increases the subtlety of the *tattvas* or elements at the spiritual centres. The transformation is towards a subtler astral beingness. The gradual elevation of the subtle nature of the practitioner eventually allows him to enter his own causal dimension.

There is no rising of a serpent or *kundalini!* There is only an evolution and therefore a 'rising' and spiritualising of the physical-astral *chakras.* The "Me" becomes more of an "I" over time and constant practice. His final fight is the acknowledgement and dissolution of the ego!

Power of Spiritual Knowledge and Tantra

Just as the learned exert power over the illiterate and the rich over the poor, those who experience Divine Energy can exert games of "power" over those who do not understand spiritualism. These temptations must be avoided as they are detrimental to the practitioner's inner growth.

Some individuals have the misconception that *tantra* is a hypnotic therapy to cure self-created problems through the use of potions and drugs. *Tantric* philosophy is a strict science demanding control of all body parts. The seeker first gains complete control of his central nervous system by training and rehabilitating his five out-going senses. This training in meditation eventually transforms every cell in the divine cave as well as in the body.

The interplay of undeveloped senses and our own need for inner-growing in consciousness, can play havoc in the lives of uninitiated seekers. If such seekers of *tantra* serve new initiates, they have the ability to lead them astray. When this knowledge of *tantra* is incomplete, invoking their powers through teaching and *tantric worship* is unwarranted and dangerous.

Experts in the practice of *tantra* regard it as an esoteric and secret spiritual practice. The secret is based upon a novel outlook to life. The teachers of *tantra* require the seeker to look at life differently from the way they are accustomed to. They must outgrow social and human outlooks and develop superhuman divine view to beings and things. It is a secret science and must be taught by a qualified teacher.

The *tantric* philosophy is based on the concept that Man must accept the dual nature of manifestation inherent in everything. Nothing is single [black-or-white, good-or-bad, pain-or-pleasure] because everything is bi-polar and everything in-between is also part of that polarity . They believe that sorrow is caused by a uni-polar existence, an unnatural way of living.

To the *tantric,* the things of the world are not obstacles and desiring cannot be overcome by rejecting the desire itself. Everything is a subject-object relationship. Desire can be overcome only by another but higher desire! *Tantra* also holds the dictum 'that by which one falls is also that by which one rises.'

The practice is not only difficult to master but also very dangerous. When instructions of *tantric rituals* are not followed accurately, there will be problems in achieving the spiritual path.

Tantra has become very popular in the West. A Macleans article in recent years was a clear example of the misunderstanding of the dictum that 'the impure, and the ugly things of life are things which have been wrongly seen out of context'. This statement has to be understood from the platform of untuitive understanding.

Teachers of *tantra* teach a seven-fold path. Each path is a graduated movement through different stages of involvement with the object of desire. By rising to a particular condition, the seeker transcends his relationship with the desired object. In the first three stages, the seeker engages his animal instincts *(pasu bhava).* The next two stages engage normal human instincts *(vira bhava).* The last two stages engage spiritual inclinations *(divya bhava).*

The first four stages are linear movements naturally outwards and along the natural currents of the senses. The secret training involves first the outward indulgence followed by the assimilation of the outward instincts into his own being.

During this phase, he gains perfection through acquisition of wealth, power, and sex. It is these tendencies that *tantra* intends to harness first and then overcome. An untrained mind and a teacher who is an impostor can lead practitioners of *tantra* towards a fall! The remaining phases of training are secret practices that are never discussed.

> My daughter wanted the Master to comment on: the Age of Evil - the present 'Iron Age', and on *tantra*.
>
> "..*Kalyuga* [the Iron Age]: That is only a measurement in Time. Seek the Timeless and ignore the *tantra:* [esoteric ritualistic practices]"

Sai Baba and Siddhis

Psychic or knowledge of the power of miracles *or siddhis* does not imply having inter-personal mastery. Those who display these powers have not transcended ego identification. Instead, true seekers look for the Power behind the knowledge. In fact, seeking the Truth rather than being satisfied with the power to control is the duty of every aspirant.

Recently, J.C. Sorcar, a Bengali magician made the Taj Mahal disappear to hundreds on on-lookers for a period of two to three minutes. He claims it is not mass-hypnosis. He has the psychic power to dissolve physically visible atoms into invisible astral energy. This is *siddhi* and can be performed by masters of psychic energy. They are invoked by advanced masters only for encouraging spiritual seekers along the difficult path of spirituality. Even mediocre seekers have these abilities. Serious seekers acknowledge their presence and ignore them. *Yogis,* on the other hand continue to serve even after terminating their physical manifestation.

> *Shirdhi Sai Baba* appeared on the scene in the mid nineteenth century and left his mortal remains in 1916. He 'came from nowhere and was above all religions'. He trod both the Islamic and Hindu way and guided disciples on both sides, compelling each to recognise the validity of the other. He did however perform 'miracles' and left no 'guidance for devotees'. His continuous protection in time of trouble, is invoked even to this day. When he was alive he made some definite and pregnant statements:
>
> 'I shall remain active and vigorous even after leaving the body'
>
> 'My shrine will bless devotees and fulfil their needs'
>
> 'I am ever living to help those who come to me and surrender and seek refuge in me'
>
> 'If you caste your burden on me, I will bear it'.
>
> 'If you seek my help and guidance I will immediately give you it".
>
> 'There shall be no want in the house of my devotee'.
>
> '*I give to my people what they want in the hope that they will want what I want to give to them'*, **and this is the most potent of his statements.**

My Master once told me a story about *Sai Baba*. It seems while *Shirdhi Sai Baba* came to introduce himself, the present *Satya Sai Baba* is here to give his devotees what they want, even if this is through the medium of *siddhic* powers. His *siddhic* powers are making vast numbers of devotees that seek succour in the shrines in Aurangabad, Bangalore and Puttaparthi. The third *avatar* [reincarnation] will demand that these devotees take from him what he wishes to give to them - the *karma phala* or fruits-of-action, of spiritualism.

Paranormal Ability in the World of Meditation

In the early stages of meditation [deep concentration or *dharana*], there occurs a partial union of the physical realm [energy in the physical atoms of the meditator] with the astral realm [energy in the physiological-psychological life-force of the meditator]. This is what is meant by the gradual transformation and transmutation of the grosser to the subtler starting from the first *chakra* to the fifth. This transformation is associated with an awakening and rising or ascension of the dormant power or *shakti* of the Divine Mother in man. The characteristics of this transformation include the development of the sixth-sense:

- This permits access into the astral dimension which allows the practitioner to develop paranormal abilities *(siddhis)*.
- The practitioner can then perceive phenomena in the material or physical world without the assistance of the physical senses.

Astral World and Beings

The beings of the astral world are spiritually similar to living physical people. Apart from the fact that they do not have a physical body, they resemble humans in their capacity to experience strong emotions and desires; indeed, the intensity of desires and emotions is much higher through the sensing mind than through the physical senses.

Many who enter this dimension after physical death with strong physical attachments have difficulty overcoming the mind-level astral dimension. In our world, most people have strong attachments to material things. In the astral dimension, the being exalts in the emotional and mental aspects of being. As long as the being (spirit) is focused on the mental/emotional aspects of being, he is confined to the lower dimensions of the astral world.

Siddhas or Psychics

Efforts in *Yoga* (meditation) in the physical manifestation allow the disembodied being to ascend into the higher realms of the (psychological/physiological) astral world.

Rebirths of emotional/mental people may result in physical births. Born with entrapments of the lower astral dimension (mental-psychics), those preoccupied beings may possess supernatural powers *(siddhas* or psychics). Individuals would do well to avoid or ignore such powers, which leave them confined to the lower dimensions of being.

Slightly more evolved are psychics with intellectual astral tendencies who have been around [angels] to help physically bound mortals in their time of need. Highly evolved *yogis* remain in their higher astral world for world-level visionary work for the sake of man-kind. All are psychics but each is more evolved than the previous one.

Foundation of Spiritual Unfoldment

Disciplines of the body, mind, and speech are the foundation of spiritual unfoldment; perseverance in these threefold austerities makes the *yogi sattvic* or calm. His whole being is harmonised with his true Self. He is overcome by devotion for Nature and serves Her without any desire for the fruits of his actions.

Through intense and frequent meditation the *yogi* works *at his own behaviour* from within. He acquires virtues of body, mind, and speech: he is worshipful towards all Nature's manifestations; he pays homage to the Spirit and to Its creative power of Nature; he communicates with Her in meditation; and, his actions are pure, honest, sincere, desireless, and wish no intentional harm to anyone.

The seeker's *speech* is disciplined and supported by an inner perception of the truth which penetrates his conscious, subconscious and unconscious states of beingness. Here, in his causal state of superconsciousness, the seeker experiences the Truth. Through continued practice of deep meditation, he increasingly becomes one with this Truth. His speech now becomes kind, forceful and truthful *(satyam)*, wise and pleasant *(priya)*, and beneficial *(hitam)*. It engenders peace, understanding, and well being and is free of harsh connotations.

Ecstatic meditation renders the mind tranquil, placid and content. The ego is retrained and there is quietude in the heart. This gradual inner purification makes the seeker desirous of the same well being in all his outer actions. There is now a divine purity in all his actions.

He understands the law of *karma* knowing that any attachment to his attainments binds the soul in the sphere of manifestations. He frees himself from the longings of the fruits of his actions.

He meditates deeply with intense love and desire to become One with his Eternal Lover, God. Even if he fails to find Him, the seeker never stops seeking Him. With each thought wave, and with faith and perseverance, the seeker sinks deeper and deeper into the ocean of himself, until all obstructions of past lives are eradicated. Eventually, he will become one with the Cosmic Ocean.

and the Master wrote:

"...Blessed as he is with an Intellect, Man is self-conscious. The self that he is conscious of is not a happy one and therefore he wants to be happier. According to the Knowledge of values, he goes about struggling to get various things...but he finds himself wanting in spite of various achievements through the struggles.....He is knocking at the wrong doors.

"...There is no object in the world that can be called 'happiness'...If happiness is not an object, much less a quality of object, it cannot be in the external world....But Man does experience happiness now and then. Perhaps, Happiness is within Man..."

Conclusion

Considerable adjustments have been made by now, through Restraints-Adherence-Constant Practice. Re-interpretation of situations have by now, lead to major re-evaluation of personal behavioural, emotional, and intellectual patterns of life style.

Circumstantial and cultural influences of isolated nuclear families must be evaluated, especially as it affects a growing child in the first five years of life. Parenting in accordance with moral and ethical values, must be the provided, until the age of eighteen, so that the child can face his "youth-hood" with the confidence. Only then will his foundational structure be innately self-guiding, self-supporting, and self-validating.

SECTION FOUR

Topics in Section Four

Brain and Spinal Cord are Bodily Field of Dharmakshetra - Kurukshetra

Raja Yoga brings the polarities of outgoing negative *tamasic* forces [one hundred *Kauravas*] and positive *rajasic* forces [first five spiritual centres or *Pandavas*] together within the field of *Kurukshetra* [war zone in the spinal cord, in a spiritual sense]. Once there is harmony between them, the *sattvic* force has the ability to rise towards the higher brain centres

Control of the senses is ensured through withdrawal of the life current into the altar of God. There is no suppression of any sensory demands. There is a transformation in thought and therefore also in the direction of the flow of the life-current. The ascending journey is towards *Dharmakshetra.*

The physical location of *Dharmakshetra* in the brain is indicated in the ancient *Purusha Suktam* with the following verse:

Om sahas-sra-shiir-shaa purusha saha-sraakshah saha-sra-paat
sa bhumin vishvato vrit-va-atyata-tishta dash-aangulam

Oh Infinite Lord who is endowed with a thousand heads, eyes, and feet and fills the Universe; who is in every atom of manifestation from here to Eternity. You can be found in me [my brain] between the *kutastha* to ten finger-breaths above it [crown of the head].

Anahaata Chakra

Preamble

The *anahaata chakra* is symbolic of the Real underlying soul intuition of every Man. It has the ability of giving or receiving Unconditional Love for his Cosmic Mother. Man can serve by gradually identifying with Her through meditation. Successful efforts through the first three stages of *growth* have created new habits and concepts that justify such happy changes becoming embedded in the foundation of the causal being.

Healing oneself is a power gained through correct interaction with Creation. There is this voice from within telling you that you have all the knowledge of all your past experiences in your many past lives. In early life, this manifests as *ojas* or physical energy compelling you to do what you want and desire.

Once Man desires God, he aligns these desires with what is best for him. He becomes a channel of *prana* or creative life-force, patterning his outer world exactly as the images being impregnated into his transforming causal being. He uses his body, mind, intellect, and the unenlightened soul or *chitta* to live his life correctly. His life becomes a journey of responsibility.

The central nervous system is the final common pathway through which all knowledge of life is received by the *rishi* or experiencer who 'watches', and integrated by the *devata* as experience as it 'looks' at the changes being made. The new transformed brain cell now triggers the master glands of the body to release transformed neurohormones and neurotransmitters to change every old cell of the body. All subsequent experiencing is a transformed experience with a specific or *chhandas* quality.

The central nervous system of man is designed for evolution through the power of his own will which resides in the *kutastha* or the Krishna-Christ Centre of Universal Intelligence. Once Man desires immortality, meditation ensures that his thoughts are transformed. He learns the Science of Concentration and discovers this Infinity through regular and intense practice of *raja yoga*.

There is a gradual self-evaluation over the years of such practice. The seeker discovers and realises that he the mortal and the Cosmic Mother are one. He diverts all his outgoing currents inwards and up the divine cave.

There is now a synthesis of his emotions and his thoughts. His thoughts align with the upward and inward flow of the life-force. There is a re-arrangement of all his body structures starting at the DNA molecule. Every cell of every system in the body is transformed. The distance between the outgoing life-force or *apana* and the in-coming life-force or *prana* gradually shortens until there is complete synthesis within the astral being.

Anahaata Chakra
Fourth or Heart Chakra (cardiac plexus)

The heart or *anahaata chakra* is located in the chest. In its untamed form, it manifests as aggression in the life of an undisciplined mortal. Yet, it is this same *chakra* that is intimately connected to the mesolimbic pathways of the midbrain system. It is the area which projects to areas of the brain that deal with emotions, moods, psyche, as well as psychotic behaviours. Addictive alcohol and drug behaviours that are seen in some people originate from these centres, especially in cases where and when the personality has gone awry. (Please refer to Figure 20)

The mesolimbic pathway is also connected to the hypothalamus-pituitary master glands and thus to the neuro-endocrine functions of the body. Another effect of this control is that it dictates how the blood will flow to the gut and the kidneys. There is therefore, a direct control on digestion, renal functions, and the blood pressure.

A strong "heart chakra" is the basis of a healthy personality. Nourished with love, it emanates warmth and happiness. It is Nature's way to suck nourishment from the soil of *Prakriti* or Cosmic Mother. When the *anahaata chakra* evolves, it has the ability to merge into the vast compassionate Collective Spirit.

> and the Master wrote:
>
> "Expand! Unfold your within and discover therein an accommodation even for the cruel, for the desperate, for the wily. They need your love and help more than others. Run to them always with love, extreme humility, full devotion, and complete sincerity. They are delirious; they may kick you back. With more love nurse them: they need all your tender and patient love.."

The capacity of the brain can be limited when the heart centre remains stunted. Excessive right-sided autonomic activity (through the *pingala* or the sympathetic nervous system) results in feverish efforts to win, out-smart, run, and race. These tendencies burden the physical heart into succumbing to *heart attacks* at a young age.

This hyperactivity of the right side shifts the attention or *chitta* (mind/intellect/ego complex) to the mental or emotional plane, and the practitioner loses all ability to appreciate the joys of the heart. If this attention or *chitta* is allowed to swing far to the left *(ida* or parasympathetic nervous system where old habits of past lives are embedded), there arises a split personality, which suffers extreme opposites in behaviour patterns, for example, the psychosis of schizophrenia.

Movement towards the central channel (the *sushumna* of the central nervous system), can release the seeker, permitting him to rise. He now *enters his own centre* through the heart *chakra,* and moves into the limbic cortex of the brain. Here, the seeker resides as thoughtless awareness, until he is enlightened by *Aum Shakti* [power of the Holy Spirit] for the purpose of joy and fulfilment.

The *mind does not love; it only desires*. Because the mind is *conditioned* to desire over many births, the feeling of love is confused with sex, selfishness, and possession of the object of desire. The desire of the mind is satiated only, when the novelty wears off and excitement dies.

The heart centre is the *chakra* that experiences bliss, ecstasy, and pure love. Here, there is no domination or possessiveness, which both stifle relationships, and is also responsible for fracturing relationships between friends and marriage partners.

When unconditional love or *prema* is misidentified with conditional love or *sneha,* it suffers disappointments because it is restricted to male-female relationships or inter-family relationships: this misunderstanding in Man results in loneliness. Creation is the best testimony of the pervading power of divine acts of love. We magnetically attract what we quantitatively and qualitatively give out.

> and the Master admonished a couple:
>
> "..It takes two to quarrel. It also takes two to make up! Without invoking love this cannot be accomplished. Flood your mind with love; look into the eyes of the other and embrace the one with whom you have tangled. Words are not necessary! Both will be moved to tears of joy which wash away all quarrels for the time being. Try this! You will find this true every time. This is the power and strength of love.."

Meditation to Activate the Chakras

The will to heal your inner being is the strongest force ruling your life. It has the power to look at past experiences and transcend them as lessons learnt from your past. You let go of the memory and re-evaluate how you must live and progress forward. Your past becomes a benefactor of all future mental processes.

Efforts made to move towards the third *chakra,* have allowed the seeker's mind to come to grips with the primal urges of the undeveloped brain. Sincere efforts of *Yama - Niyama* (Universal Moral Values and Rules of Self-Purification) at various levels of ascent bring about the *control of desire*.

By leading you into situations, you are forced to experience the inequities of life and those living around you. Your refined being is drawn to change them. Your spiritual heart makes a spiritual decision. You see others suffer. You have learnt that it is possible to open your own heart and transform your energy into an act of love which manifests as service for the purpose of a common good.

"Me", is now beginning to make its presence felt as "I", the ***aum***. "Me", the *chitta* (mind-intelligence-ego), must continue to gain perfect control, by moulding itself into the ascent process, through the fourth *chakra*. Progress in spiritual life is not an instinct. He must be introduced to the Holy Spirit, *aum*: a Master who has experienced the Holy Spirit is the only person authorised to introduce *aum* to a sincere and ardent seeker.

Meditation in Divine Cave

1. Sit in the asana [posture] of your choice. Position yourself so that the spine is erect, head slightly thrown back, chin parallel to the ground, and the hands lying upwards at the thigh abdominal junction.

2. Roll both the eyes back as if looking at the kutastha [Krishna-Christ Centre of Universal Intelligence] above and between the eyebrows. Now look at the cosmic vision beyond the body and then withdrawn within the brain cavity. Roll the tongue back.

3. Stabilise the breathing by doing the Ham'saa..So'ham technique: 4 seconds or more of inspiration:pause:expiration:pause.

4. Stabilise the autonomic nervous system by inspiring through the left nostril and expiring through the right nostril and vice versa.

5. Now watch the breath coursing in and out through the nostrils for another few minutes.

6. Place your gently clasped hands on the medulla at the base of the skull. Contract and relax the perineal muscles of the excretory organs of the body at the base of the spine until you enter the astral centre.

   This exercise physically massages the muladhara or first coccygeal centre. Entrench your will into the awakened astral centre while you rest your hands back on your thighs and watch the breath coursing in and out through the nostril.

   Exercising this centre gives the seeker power to control his five out-going senses. This centre is traditionally known to have the tamasic qualities of lust or desire [Duryodhana].

   Next replace your clasped hands at the back of the head. Reposition the spine, the tongue, and the eyes towards the divine cave. Watch the breath.

   Now contract and relax the svadhisthana or second sacral centre by contracting the two buttocks. Continue until you enter the astral domains of this centre. Now relax the hands back on the thighs and watch the breath.

Maintain stillness of the body with eyes and tongue rolled back.

This exercise gives the practitioner control over the mind. The practitioner gains flexibility of personality. He is able to live under every circumstance. Like the element water, his personality moulds with the shape of the vessel undergoing transformation. The practitioner achieves all his ideals in this life.

The first two astral centres of the divine cave are ruled by the two planetary angels [ashvini kumars], otherwise represented as Sahadev [dam] and Nakul [sham]. Obedience to the teacher is their innate characteristic.

7. Return your clasped hands to the base of the head. Roll the tongue and eyes back. Reposition the spine with an arch backwards.

   Physically locate the manipura chakra or third lumbar plexus. Contract and relax the para-umblical and the lumbar muscles until you have entered the astral level of this centre. Now drop the arms and watch the breath while looking at this centre. Watch the breath wile still focused in this astral centre.

   This astral centre has the power of Indra [lord of mind and senses]. The practitioner gradually gains even-mindedness. He is able to live under happy and unhappy circumstances. His inner vision clears [danda] to give him a uniform outer vision. There is no aversion to differences in taste or smell.

8. Return the clasped hands back at the base of the head. Roll your tongue and eyes roll back and re-align the spine. Regulate the breathing and watch the breath.

   Physically locate the anahaata chakra or the fourth thoracic centre. Contract and relax the scapular or shoulder muscles until you enter the astral domains of the centre behind the heart and within the divine cave. Now drop your hands and watch the breath while within the fourth astral centre.

   Transformation at this centre renders the seeker even-minded with the perception of touch. The entire skin surface and the tongue has the incredible power of Bheem [one of the five Panadavas]. He is able to withstand luxuries and aversions of the skin and tongue. He has secured even-mindedness under all circumstances. He overcomes tendencies for likes-and-dislikes [bheda].

9. Return clasped hands to the base of the head and roll both tongue and eyes back with the aligned spine securely positioned. Regulate the breathing and watch the breath.

   Locate the physical vishuddha chakra or the fifth cervical centre within the divine cave. Physically contract and relax the back neck muscles until you enter the astral domains of this centre and have become entrenched into it. Drop your hands and watch the breath while witnessing this astral centre.

Ascent to this level gives the seeker the power of righteousness and patience. There is a complete transformation in every atom and molecule of the seeker's body. When the centre awakens, he is able to connect with the Power of Universal Intelligence [Krishna or Christ]. He does not require any astral visions of the heavens. He is able to see heaven with this very physical manifestation [Yudhishtra - the fifth Pandava].

10. Re-position yourself with spine erect, eyes and tongue rolled back, and folded hands behind over the medulla at the base of the head. Watch the breath and locate the ajnaa chakra or the sixth medullary centre.

    Contract and relax the occipito-cervical muscles at the base of the head and neck until you enter the astral centre within the medulla. Entrench *yourself within this astral centre. The Universal Intelligence Centre or Kutastha resides here and reflects in front behind the eyebrows as the spiritual eye. Bring arms down to rest position while you watch the breath and remain absorbed in this astral centre.*

    This is the centre of the internal sun of Awareness. Every planetary awareness revolves around It. The seeker must penetrate the eye of the sun to enter the domains of Consciousness.

11. Reposition yourself with the spine erect, tongue and eyes rolled back, and hands folded over the base of the head. First stabilise and then watch the breath.

    Enter the sixth astral centre as previously shown. Entrench yourself into the spiritual eye and enter the central star. You may require to magnetise the divine cave by rotating the whole head [at the neck] 360* - first clockwise and then anti clockwise [14 times each]. The head clears and the seeker is able to 'see' the cosmic vision through the inner eye.

    Realisation dawns that the seeker has been living a dream-state. Every level of his existence [physical-astral-causal] is a dream of God - he is That God.

    He realises he is AUM in all three states of being. He visualises AUM-Consciousness. He sees his own being held within this One Consciousness.

    He experiences inner peace because he knows that the Light of AUM is also the creativity of God. He suffers no illness. He meets all prophets and saints while in this physical body. He leaves his physical entrapments at will.

    Worship of the seven candles within the Divine Cave in meditation is considered the highest worship of the Prophet of all Righteousness. No Hindu would dare start any work or ritual without first invoking Ganesh, the elephant-headed lord who removes all obstacles. His head and trunk symbolise the divine cave.

This meditation exercise allows the seeker to enter the depths of Kutastha Consciousness. He must reach the singular stream [spiritual river] of his own causal spine to experience the disappearance of the seven astral centres. This is what is meant by baptism by dipping into the spiritual river *[ganga-shnaan]*.

The seeker must have the patience to overcome the powers of the three physical qualities or *gunas [tamas-rajas-sattva]* of the interacting physical, astral, and causal bodies. Longer and more persistent meditation is the path.

Analysis of the Heart Chakra

Man easily feels trapped and limited by limiting circumstances and endless restraints. The journey of a spiritual life is to go beyond these self-imposed limitations. Offering food, shelter, and material means, give immediate satisfaction to the primal urge to serve and love others.

Most volunteers end up suffering 'burnout' and stop all their activities, not knowing why they have lost their enthusiasm. They realise that there is an eternal problem of want in the world and the social worker is not sure if they have made a difference!

What is required is a change in the awareness of both the giver and the receiver! Material wants are necessary but what is required is the giving of the volunteer himself! It is love, generosity, and kindness that helps the world. The act of giving gifts is only a manifestation of what is required at that moment for your own inner growth. What needs to be given is an offering of spiritual qualities which are bigger and of higher value than already existing in your own being. The inner self needs re-evaluation, re-packaging, and re-offering!

What follows are exercises to understand the outgoing senses first. All physical senses must first be analysed and sharpened with an inner understanding. The astral senses can then be overcome by entering the astral divine cave [dealt with in the previous section]. Controlling senses is not a suppression. It is a shedding of the lower for a higher desire. It is a sublimation. It is as automatic as shedding a favourite teddy-bear as the child matures to newer and more valuable life-interests. Every level of this growth must be understood and discarded as the need arises.

Now, imagine the heart centre [for likes-and-dislikes] is a hexagram of triangles, each representing a particular sense faculty (smell, taste, sight, sound, touch, and emotions). Each triangle must be examined and concentrated upon. Each should be analysed in group discussions and conclusions made. The exercise is about keeping my centre free of likes-and-dislikes, past habits, opinions, and concepts. Once the senses and emotions are freed of their encumbrances, each of these senses acquire a heightened 'sixth sense'. This is wisdom.

Smell

Now, the pool of "seeing awareness" (the circle of six triangles) is still. Move to the triangle of smell, and smell the fragrance of perfumes; someone now drops a bag of foul smelling manure and the smell of perfumed fragrance is erased with the stench.

Does the awful smell disengage me from my centre of balance which resides in the heart or *anahaata chakra*?

Allow the smell to fade and smell first vinegar and then the perfume again.

How did these odours affect me?

Could I recall the changing smell acutely?

Could I keep myself balanced within the circle of six triangles?

Continue with the circles, exercising each through taste, sight, sound, touch, and emotion.

- I am now complete.
- I feel balanced.
- I have overcome and understood and controlled my desire for sensual pleasures, or have I?

I am not yet complete:

- I have only understood the logic of all this study.
- I know that some day this mundane body must die and that the spirit will go on its way while the body will disintegrate into a pile of dirt. I need to embrace higher levels of comprehension.

Taste

Smell and Taste are like twins. Both need to be understood together.

Smell is about controlling the senses for self-pleasure and taste is about controlling the emotions of the mind making its incessant demands for pleasure and indulgences.

- Can I obey the commands of *yama* and *niyama* while making efforts to transform these two out-going forces?
- Am I able to invoke these two doctors of angelic of personality to rehabilitate my desires for indulgences?

Sight

Now begin with the triangle of sight.

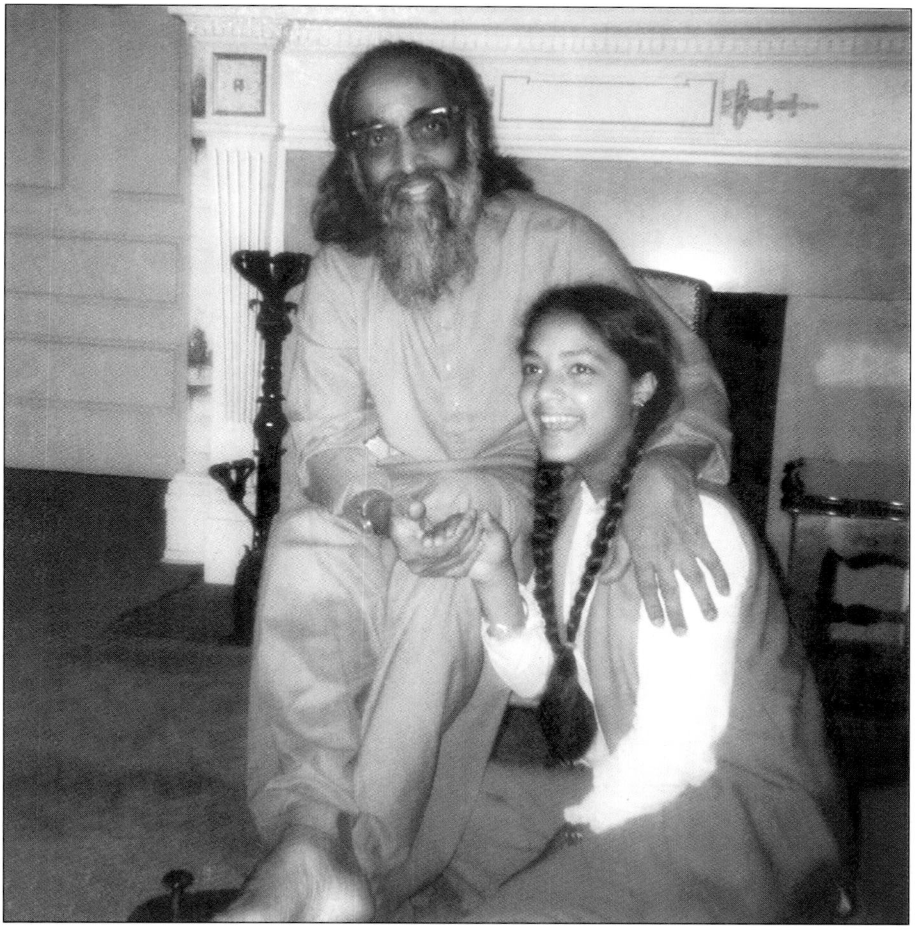

Swamiji & Bina in Montreal

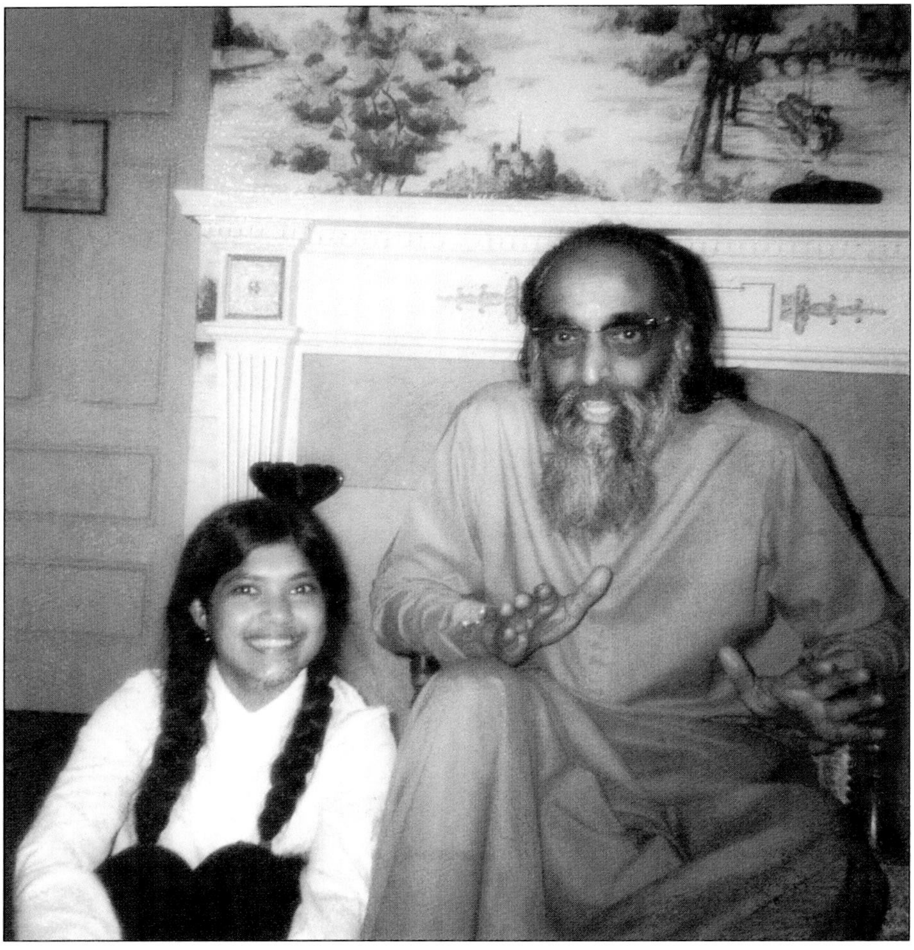

Swamiji & Meena in Montreal

How balanced is my sight?

Imagine "sight of awareness" to be a still limpid pool. Now throw a rock into it.

Can I accept the agitation on the water surface with equanimity?

Does the suddenness of the change pose a threat to me?

Have I the power to remain even-minded in both states of life's ups and downs?

This sudden change may be reminiscent of someone with whom I am dealing: abrupt, unexpected, and outside my control.

- Can I keep the triangle of sight in balance with the other senses?

To attain unified vision under all circumstances, one needs to have conquered smell and taste. There must be no like or aversion.

Now repeat the exercises for the senses of touch, hearing, and the mind. Create exercises of self-evaluation for each of the hexagons of our personality until it is understood that they are all false personality-moorings brought from of past lives. These anchors need to be cut asunder for a higher journey through meditation.

Life can be overwhelming to the uninitiated. Everyone has embedded with them, both unconscious (causal) and subconscious (psychological-physiological) errors of commission and omission. Man [reacts in this life] to these causal past acts.

Analysis of reactions to sense stimulation, gives the seeker the parameters of his nature, personality-patterns, and thought-content. Reactions emanate from his very core-content to become his normal range of structural reactions from all levels of his being: physical, mental, and intellectual (BMI).

All old structures must be dissolved and the seeker on his spiritual journey evolves as he becomes filled with new inspiration. The old structure was there to protect your tender inner being. With the input of new information, the old idea of separation of Self from the Universe is replaced by the Knowledge of the Self and his relation to the whole.

The *sadhak* or seeker realises that there is a Cosmic Will working in his inner being. His subconscious motivations are brought into full view. He learns his lessons from his false expectations. The ego is chiselled down further and the seeker grows with renewed intensity.

Love

When working with the *chakra* of the heart centre, it is important to realise that, in all relationships of friendship and love, the purpose is to deepen the Spirit.

A new-born, who has just suffered the shock of birth, is but pure unadulterated spirit. When it responds to its mother, it is responding to her spirit. There is, as of yet, no physical relationship. Such friendships are also nurtured by spiritual Masters when they meet new students of spirituality.

> The friendship between my children and the Master is interesting. He worked hard to become part of their Sisters' Club. This incident took place in Montreal, within two weeks of our meeting with him in St. John's
>
> The children were very young and I was myself not sure of the "old man" as I privately called the Master! He was busy answering letters from his devotees all over the world. In the front room of the hotel suite many of his visitors, including us, were waiting for *satsang* (meeting with the wise). The children had already started writing and sending him 'love notes' on tiny pieces of paper. The Master stopped writing and called them both in.
>
> There were peels of laughter from within. I had to peep in. The three were seated on the bed, one child on his left and the other on his right and they suddenly sang to him: "Wise men say, only fools rush in...but I cannot help falling in love with you..." The children were dumb enough to sing the whole song and the 'old man' was swaying side to side with his eyes shut.
>
> I began to think: How could they? I was horrified and embarrassed. Everyone outside could hear them! I wished the floor would open up to swallow me. I imagined the visitors thinking! "This young mother [me] has brought them [children] up with no idea of any ethics on how to interact with a spiritual personage".
>
> Then there was this horrific rhythmic thudding and squeals of laughter. I peeped in again. The three were jumping together on the bed and reaching for the ceiling. Loving without expectation: only children are capable of that. Only a *yogi* has the ability to go down to the level of the children. The Master was now a member of their Club!

The <u>Mind does not love: it only desires</u>.

- Conditioning of the environment gives desire false notions of needs that are transformed into a feelings of sex, possession, and selfishness.
- This feeling is confused with unconditional-love which is always detached. The mind views every object and person as its <u>possession</u> and insists on having all its desires satisfied. This is the only way the *mind feels complete*.

Once the mind is satiated, it detaches from the object of desire and loses interest in it. All relationships based upon physical attraction die.

What one person sees in another in a physical union is *self-projection* in the other. Only when the spirit becomes one with the spirit of the loved one can a relationship survive.

Bliss and ecstasy of love can be experienced only in the *heart centre* where there is no domination of the other.

My younger daughter could never bear to share the Master with anybody or anyone, except, perhaps with her older sister. Even as a little girl she would grab him by his hand and take him away from visitors. Much later, they [the Master and the younger daughter] made a solemn promise to each other: he would remain alive as long as she wanted and needed him as a Master.

She was now much older and with him in Sidhbari at the foothills of the Himalayas. One day the Master gradually went into congestive cardiac failure. As was the 'unspoken-law': nobody could treat him unless the Master allowed the physician to touch or treat him! By the time he reached the Army Hospital at the Himalayan foothills, he suffered a cardiac arrest. The team of physicians had started CPR and defibrillated him once. The monitor started to squeal its ominous single monotone of asystole. My daughter looked at the faces of the physicians declaring their worst!

She jumped on the stretcher and lifted the Master by his shoulders and shook him violently: 'No! You are not going anywhere yet! You promised you would not leave until I am ready to let you go!" To everyone's surprise, the Master spoke: AYou were here to bring me back from the jaws of *yama* (Angel of Death), but you will not be there the next time!"

He lived a few years longer, becoming even more physically incapacitated! During this period, two priceless video serials were recorded for posterity: the *Bhagavad Geeta and Vivekachudamani.*

The Master and my daughter met again in Tristate in 1993. As usual, in his room, they both held hands while he taught her his wisdom! She felt embarrassed that she had him imprisoned with herself. She kept reminding him [for the first time in her life] there were people waiting outside for him. The Master said: "I want to be with you. I do not wish to share myself with anyone!" She insisted and they both went to meet with the visitors.

Weeks later, while flying from Washington he developed chest pain which progressed to congestive cardiac failure. He always told my younger daughter "I will die in my own juices"! When my daughter and I reached San Diego in California, the Master was in the Hospital. Never before had I seen such 'helplessness' in this divine giant-of-a-man who had ruled and guided my own and the world-family! Our hearts bled as the vigil began. Devotees from all over the world began to pour in!

He underwent a very successful coronary-by-pass surgery. While still intubated, and with a blood pressure mechanically supported, we were told he had stabilised. We decided to leave for Canada!

My daughter visited him in the ICU and held his hand. They spoke. She scolded him. "You get better! How can you just lie there! Get up and honour your Master. You cannot honour *Tapovanji Maharaj* [the Master's Guru] lying on your back!" And the Master winced!

She then asked for permission to leave California. He squeezed her hand and she bid him farewell, until the next time! By the time we reached home [Canada], the Master had exited from the body! This time she was not there to stop Lord *Yama* [Angel of Death]! She again returned to California with her husband. She wished to touch him for the last time, once again: They [the devotees] would not let her touch the Master or his things she had guarded for years during their travels together! In despair, she asked another girlfriend [Jyoti B.] to write on the crate that took his embalmed body back to India. Red lipstick was used to emblazon on, her anguish: "I Love You like Crazy."

My husband met the devotees and *Swami Tejomayananda* [the present head of the Organization] in London and together they arrived in New Delhi. As befits a Man of such stature, the Master was lowered off the plane first. My husband saw the red scrawl on the crate for the first time from his window and a lump rose in his throat! The witnesses who watched the crate being lowered gasped as tears filled every eye there!

She grieved bitterly for months! Then a realisation dawned on her: for the first time in her life with him, she had been willing to share the Master with the visitors. She did not need the *guru* in his physical form any more!

But for this family, it can never again be the same! Nobody and no one would understand it, anyway!

Mercifully, only recently someone did! Seven years after the Master had physically left us, the family shared their anguish of profound loneliness without the Master. Grief has different faces. The family needed validation that he is still with us and always will be. *Swamini Sharadapriyananda,* who also had the good fortune of being his student, recognised him as her very own beloved Master. We grieved together! Although she too has now become a resident of the astral world, *Swamini Sharadapriyananda,* our beloved *guru-amma,* reassured our older daughter with the following : "The world knew you two sisters as his children and you still are. Continue doing *Swamiji's* work and establish *Gurudev's* vision: **Love all Mankind** through Service."

Love is the flow of sap to all people who care, share, and are aligned with the all-pervading Power of Divine Love:

- The self-confidence which love generates becomes a shield against all negative influences of the environment.
- Personalities do not become crippled with fear, insecurity, and egotism.
- We attract to ourselves what we project to others.

A strong *heart centre* is the basis of a healthy personality. Nourished with innate love, it emanates warmth and happiness to anyone seeking its nourishment.

- Love becomes compassion, *compelling us*, without thinking, to reach out to mankind.
- It is a spontaneous act and not a moral compulsion or a mental decision.

The brain, in this situation, loses its identity and becomes the free Spirit.

- It is important, therefore, not to act by compulsion or egoistic reasoning in the affairs of the heart by functioning from the "mental plane". This level of thinking is blind!

Habitual reactions shift the subtle psychic activity to the left side of the brain, and the seeker loses flexibility to catch waves of joy of the heart. He reacts through the *pingala* or right sided sympathetic response. Allow attention to be mobilised, so that it can swing towards the moderating influences of the left-sided *ida* or the parasympathetic nervous system and the right brain.

- Over time, this balancing act takes the practitioner into the central channels or *sushumna* and prevents extremes in behaviour patterns.

It is difficult to reason everything at the blind mental level:

- Linear thought processes of the emotional mind lead one into the labyrinth of self-related problems like obsessions, concepts, and opinions. It is better for the intellect to analyse thought through sight, smell, taste, sound, touch, and feel so that the door of the heart may open.
- The mind (emotion) is blind. Although it is the dispatch-clerk for desires to be executed through the senses, it can be harnessed to think. Through the intellect, every act must be screened.
- The central channels will suck dry the preoccupation of the right channels (motivated by habits, reasoning, and compulsions) and open the heart centre.
- The seeker's energy as *chitta* (mind-intellect-ego complex) now ascends to the limbic areas of the brain to become "thoughtless awareness." (Please refer to Figure 20).

This is what is known as "turning within" versus turning the beads of the *mala* or rosary. Here, there is no "I" or "Me," only the merging of a deep "human unity" with the One - perfect love.

Symbols of the Fourth Chakra

Symbols have been discussed whenever they are of assistance to the practitioner of meditation. Symbols of the fourth *chakra* take on a new meaning. They are capable of taking the seeker to higher levels of awareness.

The heart *chakra* is the celestial-wishing-tree or *kalpataru,* that emits a mellow flute sound of the element: Air. During meditation, the practitioner can rise up to this spiritual center in the spinal cord. The activation of the astral sound at this center is related to *Vayu* for the element Air. It has the quality of differentiation, molded by feelings of compassion, mercy, and spiritual experience.

The merging of *Shiva-Shakti* is represented here by two triangles. *Shiva* is Consciousness and *Shakti* is Awareness. One cannot be without the other. The interlacing of two triangles is such that they point upwards to symbolise the aspirant's ability to rise to greater heights, with effort. Intelligence is symbolised by *Isa*, an *unmanifest* Energy of *Shiva,* the Lord of Speech, who is worshipped in the heart.

Shakti, the *manifest* Energy of this centre (also symbolising the energy of intelligence), must be pure:

- Spiritual experiences during deep meditation are fleeting but, with expectations eliminated, advances will be made. Mental worship is offered here for *moksha* or liberation.

Awareness in Heart Chakra

Each *chakra* has a subtle level of awareness and represents man's evolutionary processes, as he ascends the spiritual path. *Anahaata* or the heart *chakra* controls:

- Air and touch;
- Breath; and
- The power of speech.

The seeker's breathing pattern determines the character *(guna)* of his speech. He does this by setting up currents in the air to match the character of his speech. The noose *Shakti* (Divine Mother) symbolically holds is a warning not to get caught in the emotion of hearing oneself speak. We are asked to analyse why we need to verbally articulate that what we think.

The **refinement of senses** must be a persistent effort. Speech must be refined to become the *sabda* or sound of the heart rather than of the tongue. Once this is accomplished, speech has the quality of awareness of surrender, stillness, and intuition at its deepest level.

- From this level of growth, the Spirit can enter the domains of the Selves (souls).
- Here, *Devi* of Thought and Speech is empowered by word-power or *mantra* that purifies the universe around where sound travels. The more persistent the *mantra*, the more expansive its reach for purification.

> In the text *Chhandi* or Mother-who-Destroys-Thought:
>
> She is extolled as Existence, Intelligence, Awareness, Time, Change, and the Energy that survives dissolution. She is suspiciousness, goodness, the ultimate doer, a refuge, and Mother of Light and Consciousness.
>
> She is Energy and of the Nature of Qualities, remover of suffering, the Vital-

Breath, Energy-of-Unity and discipline. Pure beauty, vibrating and articulating with determination. She desires union with good and gives courage and fortitude to slay all wandering thoughts. As the 'thousand-eyed-one' She illumines every life-of-confusion and is the slayer of anger.

She spreads true-wealth in the form of humility, knowledge, faith, nourishment, self-sustenance, and displays constancy in removing ignorance, and nurturing an intellect of love and restraint. She removes fear from all difficulties.

Having destroyed all thought, the seeker realises that it is She who supports the manifested world on the substratum of *pranava: Aum*. Illumination of Truth and wisdom dawns and the seeker acquires the Light of Discrimination, free from egotism and attachment.

Sovereign and soul of the Universe, She protects it from afflictions, terminates disturbances and hostility and blesses mankind with whatever they desire for a collective good. When perplexity and impossible behaviour wrecks havoc in the worlds, She will appear in Fearful Forms to annihilate evil as phenomenon of dissolution and destruction.

Sadhana to the Level of Awareness

Concerted efforts at refinement empower the *mantra: Aum*, which finally acquires a self-generating energy manifesting as the *Devi or Shakti or Prakriti* or Mother Nature Herself. She blesses the aspirant with waves of joy, flooding the seeker with an awakening of Her benediction and rousing feelings of surrender and profound devotion.

- Here, Mother Nature gives boons that must be kept secret. Speaking about them unwittingly puts the aspirant on the throne of the *Devi,* which is Hers alone.
- Speaking of the boons ends the Divine love affair. To prevent this, surrender to Her by stilling the mind and receive Her messages through intuitive perception.

The Heart Centre is our own personal temple. The Mind must create the necessary atmosphere for feeling the mood. Here, let us worship the *Ishta* or Ideal. This is also the abode of mercy, feelings of mercy and forgiveness, and understanding coming from the heart: these must translate into words and action.

Just below the Centre lies the wishing-tree or the *kalpataru*, where the seeker can pick words of truth and sweetness. This is the innermost courtyard to the *chakra.* The only way to enter this area, the Most Holy, is in an attitude of awe, gratitude and wonder. In this place one discovers the Divine within and the awesome power of the mind. The experience is that of psychic energy within the Temple of the Most Holy. It is from here, that all spiritual energies manifest.

and *Swamini Sharadapriyananda* asserts:

"Spiritual perfection is described as a motion without movement. Movement implies a shift from place to place but spiritual evolution is a psychic ascent which has no space or dimension.

"Layers of ignorance form concentric circles of varying dimensions surrounding the Supreme and covering It up!

"To the man of ignorance the world is a riddle clothed in mystery. He is tired of living but is scared of dying. He plods on not knowing the why and wherefore of this world..

"To the *sadhak* [seeker], the world is a field where he can work out his salvation. To the *evolved sadhak* with devotion, the whole world is a beautiful manifestation of his beloved Lord and he loves and serves the world.

"To a man of Realisation, there is no world at all but One Truth.

"*Raja Yoga* is the science that directly deals with the mind's functions....when the mind finally has reached the perfection of integration, objects are removed and the mind becomes Awareness...."

Feelings or Moods

The nineteen elements of the astral body are intelligence *(buddhi)*, ego *(ahamhara),* mind or sense consciousness *(manas),* feelings *(chitta),* five senses *(sight, smell, taste, touch, and hearing),* five instruments of action *(procreate, excrete, talk, walk, and manual dexterity),* and the five *pranas (metabolic functions of the body for digestion, assimilation, elimination, circulation and metabolism).* (Please refer to Figure 9)

These nineteen powers of the astral body make the physical body grow as well as sustain and enliven it. The centres of life and consciousness reside in the astral brain and the astral spine in the six astral centres or *chakras (medulla and the five centres below).*

The finer forces of the soul (will, feelings, intelligence, consciousness) are manifested through the *kutastha* between the eyebrows, and *ajnaa chakra* in the base of the brain. The coarser functions of the mind manifest through the senses and their instruments of action. The deluded soul functions through the body as a limited ego.

The enlightened soul or *chitta* (mind-intellect-ego complex) residing in the *ajnaa chakra* functions through the inner chambers of super-consciousness. The centres of super-consciousness include the Centre of Universal Intelligence or *kutastha,* the Centre of Universal Awareness in the *ajnaa chakra* opposite the *kutastha* in the base of the brain, and the Centre for Universal Consciousness in the *sahasrahara chakra.* The life-force or *prana or aum* energises the divine cave through the mouth of God in the medulla.

Feelings or *chitta* is the thinking-principle of the person and includes *pranic* life forces, sense conscious mind, ego, intelligence as intuitive intellect or *buddhi*, and ego. When the *chitta* is disturbed, it manifests as agitated thoughts and emotions or *vritti* in man's awareness.

These must be neutralised through a fervent desire to return to the Self through devotion, restraint in word and action, discrimination, dispassion, and meditation. These qualities can be developed early in childhood. Growing children have a natural tendency for attachment with an object of their identification. Parents must connect their near adolescent children with an ideal peer, god-parents, and or perfect teachers.

We had both become parents in our early twenties. We were forced to become disciplined parents of two children, especially since we had still not finished University. By mutual agreement my husband would be the loving parent and the mother would be the disciplinarian! The father of the children promised never to contradict me in matters of discipline.

By the time our daughters were on the threshold of adolescence, it was obvious that one of my daughters would give me a run for my money! The older one was always obedient but this mother could never be sure if lessons were learnt! The younger one dared this unreasonable mother to the limit with her impeccable logic.

It was at this time that the Master stormed into our lives. I was consumed with concerns. The growing girls were discovering, as all growing children do, that their parents are human. They would soon be looking for their ideal in peers! The Master sensed my concerns and became their ideal parent for the rest of their lives! The Master adhered to the cultural law that the mother is the first *guru* of the children. He softened the blows on this unreasonable mother of two new teenagers, but the Master never contradicted my decisions!

There were many grey zones on moral issues! The children were growing within a home environment of an older time-proven culture, in the midst of a new materialistic culture. Neither were incorrect. We had to make the merging compatible, through mutually acceptable modifications!

By the time our daughters were in University, the Master had become their closest confidant and I had acquired the name of a 'witch' who must be obeyed!

The younger of the two children carried this for years. The Master sent her up to Northern Ontario to do her Internship over two years. Her daily meals were frozen packed and flown to her every week, but I was still the 'witch'! The Master never contradicted her! She was now married five years and the Master physically left our little world.

She was now pregnant with her first child and she had become increasingly introspective. We became 'friends' once more. After two daughters of her own, she reminisces that her younger child is doing to her what she did to me! This is a perfect example of how an identification with a ideal in teen years can transform itself into a enriching personal realisation and experience.

We as parents are grateful that we never had children that hurt us physically, mentally, or intellectually! We delight in seeing how they are nurturing their own nests. Values-with-a-Vision is the hallmark they will inculcate in the grandchildren. All good things have a habit of magnifying themselves. To this Master, we offer our eternal thanks!

> My very young daughters were arguing about who would hold on to which limb of the Master visiting us in our home:
>
> "Never mind about the *Swami*.. You are the younger one, so you hold on to His body and the older one can get His face! He is very just and merciful. Request Him to exchange your positions. In fact it doesn't matter.
>
> "If a devotee can have His feet, it is sufficient. You must feel He is the entire Universe of things and beings! The entire Cosmos is His Dance! He alone IS. In Himself He is ever Motionless, Infinite One Essence.. when we see Him through our mind-in-tension, we see HIM as the World. Quieten the mind in Love, Purity, Joy.. the World disappears into the Divine Vision .. the One God: the Reality.."

Man forgets what it is that he loves and adores most in life. Fortunately, inherent in Man is the memory of his own divine origin. When Man seeks perfect identification with his ideal, he will naturally strive to attain his state of existence-knowledge-bliss once more. As children, they do it through the senses of touch and the Master knew that in his wisdom. He allowed the children to touch and maul him.

As adults, he encouraged the seeker to study the philosophy under a true teacher. He knew that once this *book-knowledge* has been realised as his own experienced wisdom, Man wants to learn about the *path of return* through the yoga of meditation. He wants to be free of the prison of his past actions or *karma.*

Emotion

The potential to produce "Many" *(Prakriti)* from "One" *(Purusha* or Spirit) is Her Creative power or *shakti.* The workings of this potential together constitute *maya* or the cosmic delusion of multiplicity. The individual soul or Man, identifying himself with this *maya* is the deluded soul under the influence of ignorance or *avidya.* He is the body-identified ego, expressing outwardly and subject to the laws of manifestation.

To recapitulate, *Maya* is the power of delusion resulting from the Law of Qualities or *gunas* of inaction, action, and the harmony of the two: or *tamas, rajas,* and *sattva.* Personalised ignorance or *avidya* manifests as individualised delusion or elaborate feelings of what I like-and-dislike or *raaga-dvesha.* Under the influence of the sensory blind mind or *manas,* feelings or *chitta* express as emotions of fear, attachment, desire, and repulsion. These are Man's own creation!

Emotions are personalised thoughts reacting to materialised ideas of His creation. They are Man's own ideas of sense-conditioned feelings. They result from interacting with materialised ideas of God's creation. But ideas are fleeting and move in time and space: they change through their very movement. However, the underlying ever-existing awareness perceiving the operation of the ideas is constant: the only constant in the willing, imagining, and remembering.

When Man is attuned to his divine intelligence or intuitive mind, he becomes pure, noble, and wise. Eventually, the inner magnetism of the Spirit will lead his individualised awareness to seek the path of ascension through the *free choice of right action*. This links Man to the uplifting power inherent in Nature's Laws. Attuned to the Cosmic Mother and Her will, Man's action acquires a divine potency that blesses the doer as well as the Collective Cosmic Spirit.

> and the Master wrote:
>
> "The most intelligent thing is to act as the occasion demands, always truthfully, honestly, without ego, vanity, or boastfulness. Meekly, as the servant of the Great master, act! Act because we are His servants, and our action is only the accomplishment of His plans.
>
> "The greater our surrender to His will, the greater will be our intensity of devotion for Him...the more constant our mental remembrance of Him, and the surer our action in parallel with His will...and His will, ever works itself out to success.."

Freed from the manifestations of Nature, Man awakens to its Natural Laws and becomes One with It. He gradually becomes a perfect reflection of the Spirit. He experiences and realises that he is the One in many and the many in One. He exists in the Eternal and in the relative states of the One. He is the wave of the same Essence.

Refined Touch and Feelings

Air and touch are expressions of the heart centre. Air signifies lightness and cannot be grasped. Breathing is vital for survival. *Life-force grasps on to breath*, yet its *touch is light*, when all self-gratification have been renounced.

Breath connects the physical body to the Spirit. If the grasp is loosened, the *touch of breath* creates a feeling not explicable by words.

Ascent to this level of awareness, through *sadhana*, takes the practitioner to different types of emotions or feelings:

- *Sattvic* feelings convey an awareness of a mystical connection. Touch is that of giving without asking for anything in return.
- *Rajasic* feelings are governed by a *need* to accept and be accepted.
- *Tamasic* feelings also need acceptance, *without* judgmental preoccupation.

Touch and Emotion

As awareness of the power of *Shakti* or the Holy Spirit increases, all the details of the practice of meditation must be given complete attention (the what, where, why, when, and who of each detail that was previously taken for granted).

After examining *touch*, one must analyse *emotion and emotional impulses*. If touch is refined, there is a corresponding refinement in feelings and a growing awareness that the practitioner's understanding has changed.

- This awareness leads to the recognition that previous tendencies caused feelings of hurt.
- By using discrimination (which is also an awareness), the habit of reacting with revenge and anger is controlled.
- Awareness now becomes a tool for a more balanced form of living.

Analysis on Touch

Touching love is both the physical attraction on a human level and the craving for the divine. In it there is a heightened energy of perception of the good within the loved one. As the experience magnifies itself, the lover expands his perception to include the beauty of Nature. He experiences loving everything. He unites with the divinity of Nature.

Investigating 'touch' is like visiting the *lover within*. Finding the *loved one within* is a discovery that you are seeking**:** the opposite of your own self. You are seeking to harmonise the opposites within. The inner search and meeting with the *other half* is the meeting of two lovers!

To investigate "touch", analyse your answers to the following questions:

- Am "touched" by a smile or generosity?
- Where do I express the feeling?
- Do I feel it all over the body like "prana"?
- Can touch be transferred through a healing touch?
- Can it comfort another?
- Can touch be thought of as an irritant when nervous, tired, or angry?
- What does the phrase "keep your distance" signify?
- Does the touch of another soothe?

Can hands - the vehicles of touch - build as well as destroy? And how?

How do I perceive touch?

- Are there prohibitions on what can and cannot be touched?
- Does touch evoke feelings of emotion?
- Do I recall what I have touched - and in what detail?
- Do I really experience touch, and can I recall the experience?

The perception of touch is experienced on the vastest area of the body all over the skin and the tongue. To become even-minded at the skin-level is to have acquired the valour of *Bheem - the pandava!* He has the ability to be not-wanting whether amidst poverty or luxury. He can even suspend the need for the breath!

Is thought involved in the memory *[chitta]*?
- Is experience a memory of a thought evoked by the sense of touch?
- How does touch affect the other senses?

In order to analyse touch, conduct the following exercise:

i. Touch an object for three minutes. Go through objects of different consistency (for example: touch wood, a metal, or a glass object that is sharp, rough, smooth, or soft or touch another person. Observe your thoughts/reactions and note them down.

ii. Rub your hands on a spotlessly clean cloth and wish that your hands were clean. The cloth is now dirty. What does this mean?

iii. Touch the fingertips of a partner with your fingertips:
- What thoughts are generated?
- Are there impressions?
- Are there reactions?
- What do these mean?

Now leave space between the finger tips:
- What do you feel?

iv. Do "akhanda" kirtan (continuous inspirational chanting) for three hours and feel the vibrations from the various parts of your body:

- Feel these at the end of one, two and three hours, noting the differences in the intensity of vibrations over time.

v. Fall asleep with a stone held in your hand:
- Continue to hold it during sleep
- Can you awaken with it still in the hand?
- Recall your dreams and write them down.

Insights arrived from these exercises are more valuable than experiences described by others. The seeker must make personal discoveries about himself and take responsibility for personality tendencies.

An inwardly "wounded" causal-astral being, does not manifest himself overtly. His experiences in his awareness, motivate all his thought patterns, emotions, and feelings. He may exhibit structural distortions of behaviour, tendencies or thoughts. Decoding these aberrations, lead him to his own Reality, through the process of intuition and love for the Cosmic Mother.

The union of the Lovers within must be experienced by taking several remedial steps. Once the seed of desire to know your other-half is sown, use the energy to its best advantage. Give each the opportunity to do your best while on the path of mutual spiritual self-discovery.

Take responsibility for negative as well as positive situations you create in your environment. Appreciate life situations that offer opportunities of self-growth. Change life-situations to make necessary changes to benefit the relationship of the lover and the beloved. There is no need to magnify life-problems! Instead, utilise the energy to concentrate on options and solutions. Finally, take time to meditate daily and drink from the common fountain of love and ecstasy.

Mind Power

The most important work must be done on the first three *chakras*, which lay the foundation to subtle changes based upon experiences and conclusions reached over time. This may happen without awareness or understanding of what is really happening during initial *sadhana.*

The seeker has arrived at this point due to the forces and compulsions of a changed life-style. The seeker must clean the cupboards of the mind that have become filled with concepts and ideas accumulated over the many births, including the present one.

Once this space is cleared, the Void experienced in meditation becomes a place of extraordinary experiences. Some of these experiences can cause discomfort as well as anxiety, such as, when the body or parts of body expand in a mass of Light. Although such a psychic or astral experience is intriguing, it is best not to get caught up in it. The seeker will however, naturally ask why or how did this occur?

Every aspirant functions primarily and predominantly through one of the five senses. The seeker's sense level now becomes dominant trait in his astral experiences. This predominance of sense identification is by choice or through circumstances of *sadhana.* It is through this sense that first psychic manifestations come into being. The experience, however, is not to be dwelt upon.

All efforts from this stage of being should be directed towards channelling the Energy to self-development. The psychic experiences, at this stage of development, are rarely a source of guidance or inspiration. Clairvoyance and clair-audience are also not tools of self-development.

The Fourth Chakra is where one undergoes both spiritual and psychic experiences. There is a difference in the two types of experiences:

- **Spiritual experience** is unforgettable and cannot be repeated at will. It is a source of divine energy for our further development. Mastery of the self becomes a self-sustaining source of energy that flows permanently through the seeker.

- **Psychic experience** is repeatable, leaving one with no after effects, except a sense of having enjoyed something, like an experience of the senses.

The *ability to have perfect-recall* requires practice, time, and effort. Perfect recall is necessary so that the seeker can make written observations of events and dreams. As well, observations of personal changes in feelings, hunches and insight must be made. These observations of increased sensitivity, if pursued will lead to higher degrees of perception.

Success is not a static state. After reaching the peak of success, one needs to descend. Only the wise ones have the ability to foresee what is coming and moving towards you. The battle must continue. Both retreats and successes are advances in *sadhana.* Re-evaluate, re-assess, re-group your thoughts and become re-inspired by the urge to meet the other-half within.

Meditation is a process of self-transformation from the dense to the increasingly subtle. Austerity is a prerequisite. Withdrawal from the senses and their preoccupation must be mastered. Once the practitioner is able to withdraw into his divine cave, he ascends in subtlety from one spiritual centre to the next, until all the first six centres transform to Light Energy. From this level, the merging of Awareness with Consciousness is imminent.

Memory and Mind Control

Your talents, hopes, dreams, fears, concerns, and memories are embedded in the very cells of your causal body. You carry it in a seed form in every one of your life's adventure! Your creative energy or life-force summons you to overcome all fears of the dangers ahead where the Light promises to illumine the path of life.

Travelling the spiritual journey is like venturing into new territories, but a helpful map is embedded in the old memory bank. The pathway may look different, but all roads lead to the same Reality.

The inner *guru* or guide already lives within you. Although seemingly distant, the Master is more than you! The Master brings you loving information for your spiritual growth. He allows you to grow larger than the outer limits of your own psychic energy field. You are being pushed towards outer planetary fields and under beneficial celestial influences, always under the Master's ever-loving protection. Here, you begin to make contact with other guides at a much closer level. With new information and inspiration, they entice you further along the path of your spiritual journey. Your spiritual family now becomes the unconscious environment you live in.

The rejuvenated memory is heightened to the extent that one is interested in the subject. The centre of this guiding force is the heart *chakra.* Its energy field knows the core Self. It is surrounded by a cloud of causal beliefs, desires, wishes, feelings, attitudes, expectations, thoughts and memories. Changing the way you think, behave, and desire opens the windows of the causal cloud.

Memories of the causal state does not disappear with age, but age definitely differentiates what is important to remember. Recollections and observations are products of thought associations that can recall the past. When they are coupled with present observations, one can understand their own reactions to the environment around them, including mannerisms, clothes, situations, and events. These reactions may leave the seeker puzzled, and the "triggering" stimulus, may not be too clear in the memory.

Coincidences of the same thought in two minds or recurring thoughts voiced by many, prove that there is always an interplay of the mental forces all around us. Once one is aware of this ability, sensitivity can be increased. Exercising this awareness consciously, for the sake of a collective good, is encouraged. The seeker's emotions should be directed to the goodwill and good health of Mother Nature.

Keeping the mind single-pointed and focused is an effort at mind-control. The mind becomes receptive to a clearer awareness that, if tuned into the Higher Self, leads to mental powers of clairvoyance and clairaudience, and telepathy between *Guru-shishya,* mother-child and husband-wife.

When mental powers are developed, the merry-go-round of mental conversations ruminations of self-justification, self-glorification, and self-gratification that silence the inner voice of the mind also stop. Insights come in flashes of awareness, in moments of inspiration when the mind is quiet.

Over time, the Inner World of the seeker begins to evolve all by itself! Your Master takes you to his own home where his light shines benevolently. He comforts you when in need and understands the deeper meaning of your upbringing. He becomes your true friend. He will explore your questions, your ideas and your desires, and give you the right answers. In challenges of life, he will be ever at your side as the next story of our life with the Master indicates:

> My three-month old grandson who was reduced to a mere one kilogram was operated on for a congenital heart defect. By midnight, [10 a.m. in India] we were called back to the Toronto Sick Childrens' Hospital. Before leaving for the Hospital, my daughter called the Master but he could not be contacted at that address. She asked the telephone respondent to inform the Master that her child was not doing very well post-operatively. He had already had three cardiac arrests.
>
> We arrived at the Hospital and found the infant's pacemaker non-functional, his liver functions were abnormal, the kidneys had shut down through hypotension, and he would not stop bleeding from every puncture and bodily aperture. The Hospital wanted a consensus to shut off the ventilator if he arrested again.

My children and I normally communicate telepathically. My daughter pleaded for guidance but I felt helpless. My husband said: "Today your role as mother is being tested, but more importantly your role as a *shishya* [student of the Master] has come to the forefront. Control your emotions and remember the Master's teachings.."

My daughter stopped crying and thanked my lifeless grandson for giving her the honor of carrying him for nine months in her womb and allowing her the honor and privilege to serve and love him for a few months. She then mentally placed the child in the Master's lap. "I now give you back my child. Either he comes back to me as a normal child or you must take him. I do not want a vegetable!"

My daughter started to chant the *Devi Mahatmayam* [An Adoration to the Cosmic Mother], which took them four hours to complete. She and her husband had asked Mother Nature also, for Her compassion. They then returned to us in the 'Quiet Room'. She cried on her dad's shoulder while my son-in-law sat at my feet. It was time to instruct the nurse to turn off the ventilator.

We were all very tired and unknowingly fell asleep! It was 6 am and I was awakened by the male nurse who was not only excited but crying: "Doctor, doctor there has been a miracle! The child is alive. All the problems have been reversed."

I knew instantly that the Master had given my grandson a 'gift-of-his-own-life'. I also knew instinctively the Master would have to pay for this act. On August 3, 1993 our Master developed my grandson's post-operative complications after a successful coronary by-pass surgery and shed his body. In 1995 I met Anjali S. a devout admirer and devotee of the Master. We were told that the Master disappeared in his room at around 1000 hours local time in India [midnight in Canada when my daughter called him before leaving for the Toronto Hospital]. He reappeared from his room at 1600 hours Indian time [0600 hours in Canada] and said cryptically: "It is done"! My grandson was suddenly and miraculously alive at 0600 hours!

Group Discussion on Mind Power

Spiritual journeys are inroads into your own life. The talents you acquire, the power you have discovered within, your insight and inspiration should be put to use in your daily outer living. The paradise you have discovered within should become manifest in your outer world. You discover that the outer world changes as you experience the inner changes.

When asking questions, seek the answers from within. If the answers do come, question:

- Where is the awareness coming from?
- Are the body cells independently aware?
- What causes the mind to think of pain or a need?

Is the mind the manager of authority?
- How did it become so?
- Through auto-suggestion, self determination, or self hypnosis?

What gives events in my life details?
- What interplay of forces bring about the ideas and concepts created from these events?

How does the mind invent something?
- Was the idea there in the *Hiranyagabhaya* or the Cosmic Golden Egg (Cosmic Causal Seed of Total Ideas residing in the Cosmic Causal Brain of *Ganesha or Ishwara*)?
- Does the mind have to be focused on a single-point?
- Does the inventor have to surrender all preconceived ideas and opinions?
- Must the mind be "emptied"?

When the mind is emptied, does it relax?
- Can the physical body also be relaxed?
- Does breathing play a role in this mental and physical relaxation?
- If so, is this increased receptivity a necessary prelude to spiritual awareness and inspirations?

Not infrequently, the mind is incapable of processing the psychic experiences of the seeker:
- The mind now is led to make premature assessments of the experience; these are translated into "doubts"!

Begin to record in detail all psychic and spiritual experiences in detail:
- This will help to clear doubts which cause the aspirant to become depressed or lose enthusiasm for the study at hand.
- Faith and persistence of effort leads the seeker to small victories.
- The secret is increased control of both imagination and emotion, until they lose their power. Faith in one's ability to become master of the inner disturbances becomes a self-generating energy dynamo of hope.

It is critical not to expect immediate results. Impatience is a form of arrogance of the ego that destructively undermines faith, hope, and will. Conversely healthy doubts stimulate queries and promote a healthy expansion of awareness. Doubts given strength with the power of imagination ("I have made no progress") are destructive if allowed to gain momentum.

Thought-form and their emotional-content reside in our awareness or *chitta* as mind-intellect-ego. Everyone needs to thrive and heal through self-acceptance from when we start our spiritual journey; on this journey, there is never any competition. This self-acceptance or self-love, is an acknowledgement we are connected to God. This sense of self-acceptance, leads man to acquire a non-judgmental and quiet mind, capable of having recurring precious gifts of intuition, which leads him to a renewed self-commitment. This process is called, "At-onement-with the Cosmic Mother."

An example of a "healthy doubt" is what follows. Early into my spiritual journey, I had become preoccupied with the elements—space, air, water, fire, and earth. If God was not a void, was he space?

> Again, I turned to my Master for guidance and he wrote back:
>
> "The Atman (Self) is likened to space.. only in some aspects:
>
> a. All-pervading;
>
> b. Envelops all but nothing envelops it;
>
> c. Everything exists in it;
>
> d. In fact everything is born, grown, decays, and dies in space.... but SPACE itself is neither born, grown, decays or dries. I am not PFT (perceiver-feeler-thinker); but I am *Atman - 'Aum'* and as 'sky' I am not born, (so undecaying, undying) Essence.."

Mind and Meditation

Once a seeker conquers sloth and sleep, he is able to meditate long and deeply. He can command his soul-identified being to focus into his own spiritual being within the divine cave of the brain and spinal cord. This is *spiritual perception*, and constitutes the *first stage of meditation.* The seeker is gradually separating himself from his sense-inflamed outgoing mind that once dragged him towards the world of objects, emotions, and things (OET).

Even sporadic attempts at deep meditation can lead the seeker to feel a deep sense of peace and joy. The frequency, length, and depth of his meditation determine the magnitude and duration of this spiritual perception. This constitutes the *second stage of meditation.*

The seeker, now keenly aware of the importance of *yama* [restraints] *and niyama* [adherence to restraints], has arrived at the middle point of his *sadhana.* He begins to have glimpses of *ananda* or Bliss. This experience leads him to the realisation that all awareness exists within himself, within his own centralised beingness, in the divine cave. With faith, he works even harder at his meditation because *he knows how it must be done.* (Please refer to Figure 14).

> "Without faith it is impossible to please Him: for he that cometh to God must believe that He is, and that He is a rewarder of them that diligently seek Him" . Hebrews 11:6.

In the last stage of his meditation, the seeker takes his spiritual perception right into the halls of perfect Awareness and Consciousness where he awaits final union of the soul with the Spirit. He is now beyond being influenced by his personal and family desires, his likes-and-dislikes, and habits that bind him to sense tendencies. He is beyond disease and health, and beyond the power of *maya (*delusions triggered by matter-qualities) and Her qualities or *gunas*.

Yet, the greatest battle still awaits him: he must erase the ego by merging *Shakti* or Energy of Awareness *with Shiva* or Light of Consciousness. The duality of awareness-consciousness can only be fought through spiritual determination and self-control.

The knowledgeable seeker is extremely aware of this quandary. While charting out the next step in his *sadhana* or spiritual journey, he knows he must invoke deep dispassion. The instinct of survival of the ego is born of Nature. He knows he must re-examine all the material he has studied throughout his life so that he will not face the inevitable opposition of the ego.

The seeker needs a *guru's* or Master's guidance and encouragement for his own self-evolution. The student has an instinctive tendency to become very dependent upon the Master. The student must dig deep into himself. All the knowledge has already been uncovered through austerity and meditation.

> When I sought him for support, my Master was quick to admonish:
>
> "...seek me for guidance and direction. I am the window and I will show you the way... Look through me... do not lean on me for support because you must fly on your own wings."

Ego is the grandfather (*Bheeshma of the epic Mahabharat)* of all habits and tendencies. Only by keen dispassion and sublimation of ingrained habits and tendencies, can the outward flow of the sense mind be reversed. This is the only way the life-force can be coaxed to flow towards the Spirit.

Through the *sushumna* or central channel of the divine cave, the life-force gradually rises through all the subtle spiritual centres (*chakras).* The upward direction of the flow triggers not only an intense desire for God-communion but also a distaste for materialism. (Please refer to Figure 17)

The act of deep meditation reawakens all slumbering habits and tendencies that have previously been ignored. Their strength increases the force of ego=s fierce resistance.

The knowledgeable seeker must now replace these tendencies and habits with newer, positive habits of peace, calmness, and concentration *(dharana).* Despite a growing power of awareness and discrimination, the seeker will continue to be distressed with the tendencies of bad habits such as gloominess, moodiness, or anger. These, and the old eternal questions about Matter and Spirit must also be re-answered. There will always be flaws in a seeker's understanding. He will ask the same troubling questions from a different level of understanding. Each level of questioning is an evolution of the previous one, during a previous discussion.

and the Master explains these same issues [using an *Upanishadic* text] at one of his ten-day *yagnas :*

"***Prasnopanishad*** is written in a questions and answers format. Six *shishyas* or seekers of the sage *Pippalada* ask six often repeated questions:

"**The first question** is: 'From what are these beings [manifestations in the Universe] born?' The answer is: 'The Lord of all creatures, *Prajapati* performed penance and produced a couple *Rayi* or matter and *Prana* who is the enjoyer of food or Spirit. They are the origin of Creation'.

"**The second question** is an inquiry about the relationship of the five senses *[indriyas]* and the physiological functions or vital-airs of the body. *Pippalada* affirms that *prana* or life-force as breath, is the most supreme of all the vital-airs [physiological systems: respiration *[pranaya]*, digestion-elimination *[[apanaya]*, circulation *[vyanaya]*, crystallisation or metabolism *[samanaya]*, and awakening through the neurological organs in the divine cave *[udanaya]*. He confirms that it is through the senses that objects of sense-desires are offered to the vital-airs for assimilation.

"**The third question** is: "How does this *prana* [as one life-force] enter the body? From where does it come? How does it exist by dividing itself [into five vital-airs]? How does it depart [as mind-intellect-ego or *chitta*]?"

..and *Pippalada* answers:' *Prana* is born of the self [Aum], is fixed in the self just as a shadow is fixed to the man; the self comes into the body because of the actions [deires] of the mind [causal being]. *Prana* [as life-force AUM} engages other organ-systems [five vital-airs] just as a king employs his officers. *Prana* [as *chitta]* passes a north-bound path [exiting from the physical body at the time of death] leading to the world of the virtuous [higher astral world or heaven] or the southern path to a sinful world [lower astral world or hell].

"**The fourth question** refers to the world of dreams [subtle body or *sukshma* sharira} and is: 'What organs sleep and what is awake? Who experiences the dream and happiness?

"and *Pippalada* answers: "Just as the setting sun unifies and absorbs all the rays and disperses them again with the rising sun, so too the senses merge with the mind when the mortal is asleep. At this time only the *prana* [awareness] is awake. In the dream-state the *jivatman* or individualised soul sees the dream [as mind-intellect] but in the deep-sleep state [causal state of existence], the *jivatman* [individual soul] *and paratman* [Universal Soul] merge and there is none to see the dream.

"**The fifth question** asks about the gains made by meditating upon AUM. *Pippalada* asserts that this is the most important means of meditation upon *Brahman* [God].

"**The final and sixth question** is 'Where does *Brahman* exist' and *Pippalada* answers "Inside the body, in the lotus of the heart [*anahaata chakra]*.."

When the life-force withdraws from the senses and is transferred to the divine cave in the brain, the seeker senses victory over the inferior bodily sensations that are becoming gradually dissolved. The seeker does his daily rounds of outward routine work, but is inwardly united in supreme bliss. The pictures of life suddenly acquire a new meaning: the intricately organised scenes (plays of the Lord or *lila)* are all services to Mother Nature. In the whirlpool of activity, the seeker sees the vibration-less infinitude of eternal bliss: the many from the One.

Mind and Knowledge verses Wisdom

There is power in knowledge. This knowledge from sterile *book-knowledge* must be transformed into a *personal knowing* which evolves into an inner *wisdom.* If this does not happen, the young seeker of the Path may become an intolerable caricature of arrogance, born of ego.

The Path to attaining such wisdom is long and arduous, requiring walking on a knife's edge in order to create absolute self-reliance.

The Path requires *concentration on the following ideals*:

- Daily reflections;
- Breaking away from the *herd* (the need to belong or rule a group);
- Freeing oneself from one's upbringing;
- Standing *alone* on one's two feet;
- Becoming responsible only to one's inner authority; and *Practising straight-thinking*, that is:

  getting straight to the point in speech and thought;

  reflecting on daily events and analysing each day; and

  keeping a spiritual diary to record observations.

All spiritual endeavours are aimed at fine-tuning the gross body to the finer inner forces that are aware and know that there is a greater power than themselves: "ME" the ego, who wishes to know "I"!

In sleep, these finer-inner-forces record perceptions that are presented to awareness at different levels. Spiritual practices sensitise these levels to become aware of the finer forces!

> At a time when girls were considered as only mothers and wives to be, we had a father who wanted all his six daughters to become educated and wise "mothers and wives". He warned us all with the following story:
>
> "*...Sarasvati* is the goddess of "knowledge"...She carries in Her hands the trident of wisdom and concentration, a pestle of refinement, a bow of determination, an arrow of speech, the radiance of the full moon, the discus of revolving time, and the book of knowledge.
>
> "She is the Infinite Creative Energy that preserves Eternal Knowledge and

upholds the Universe, in all Her aspects of change, perfection and dissolution. You are to salute Her in humility while you acquire her Grace.

"arogance about your education will lead to lack of discrimination, devolution, and narrow vision. Use your education wisely. It would pain me to discover my children sank to materialism, conceit, and self-deprecation because of the privilege of 'education' your parents allowed you!"

Knowledge

Man's intellect depends upon the senses and their contact with the world of objects to create inferred data. He interprets everything according to facts and figures he has in his memory. This, to the materialist is Knowledge.

Each aspect of Man's being is involved in all that he does. His body obeys the instructions it receives through the image he holds in his mind. His emotions are triggered by the images and stoke the fires of his life-force that fuel the body towards his images. The body only gives form to the chosen images. The mind patterns the thinking and gives shape to his mind-stuff.

These images speak to him constantly. His inner voice tells him the shape and form of these images from his past actions. The evolving script becomes his present life.

Meditation has the ability to change these images until the body, mind, and intellect (BMI) changes. What then transpires is that everything outside himself (OET: objects-emotions-thoughts) also a perceptual undergoes change, until it becomes a reflection of his own inner being. Man now realises that he is connected to all things big and small. He now has the choice to change for the good of the whole! Man now takes steps towards what is good for his own life.

When man concentrates *(dharana)* and meditates *(dhyana)* deeply, he goes beyond the realms of reasoning thoughts. He perceives and witnesses thought from the standpoint of awareness, until thought dies away. He becomes aware of a personal knowing, which is free of all accumulated data of past knowledge. This is intuitive knowing and involves a deep understanding that man's intelligence is the light of the intellect. Intuitive knowing works in a limited way through the mind and intellect, but is independent of them. Intelligence cannot work without the power of intuition behind it.

Therefore,

- Mind co-ordinates the senses;
- Intellect is reasoning thought;
- Intelligence is the awareness of thought; and
- Intuition is the consciousness behind intelligence. It is the Power behind all mental phenomenon: thought, attention, will, sensation, perception, memory, feelings, and impulses.

Intelligence, guided by intuition in meditation, disciplines the ego and takes it to the revelation of Truth. Intuition inspires the ego to forsake desires in favour of soul-happiness.

He may have heard words of wisdom many a time, but man's attention is limited to persons and things. He denies his *wholeness.* He denies he is connected to all life. He understands that his physical essence or *ojas* fuels his life-forces' creativity or *prana.* His heart knows the purpose of his manifestation and his spiritual light of awareness or *tejas* directs him towards the right relationship with all beings.

Memory

Physical self-control without mental self-control will temporarily distance Man from the attractions of senses, but his mind will continue to dwell upon the temptations until he once more becomes their victim. The road to safety is the supreme experience of soul-happiness. Once the seeker has experienced the bliss of the Spirit, he loses interest in sense pleasures.

Renunciants must become *yogis*, lest they lose sight of the divine goal of soul-Spirit union. Outward renunciation without learning to withdraw life-force from the senses *(pratyahara)* is unlikely to lead the seeker to spiritual benefits; rather, it will cause inner torments of temptations. The memory of sense-pleasures lies dormant and hibernating within the seeker's subconscious mind; their tentacles have lured even wise men.

> and the Master wrote:
>
> "A man firmly established in wisdom is tranquil. His equipoise is never broken even when he is investing his entire energies in the world outside for the service of mankind.."

The wise man must forever guard against signs of greed, sex temptations, the love for physical beauty, and the desire for flattery, or for indulgences. His wisdom should have the ability to slay such tendencies. No seeker should underestimate the power of the subconscious mind.

He must be able to withdraw the life-force from the senses and possess the ability to keep the mind united in devotion to his *guru,* or deity, or ideal of his own choice. His intellect should not become a victim of his sense-indulgences. He must make discriminating judgements in all decisions and actions.

Even in the wise, unfulfilled desires cause anger and cloud the intellect. The seeker loses memory of his own self-respect and develops righteous indignation. Egoistic anger compels him to become increasingly irrational. He loses his inner balance and develops physiological and psychological changes that are spiritually lethal. He loses memory of what he must do and how he must behave. Normal feelings of good sentiments fade, his discrimination disappears and he loses contact with his own awareness.

Sense attractions must be sublimated so that all desires are discriminated and the motivating force of all actions is right. The discriminating intellect's thoughts must be the steering force of all sensory-mind's demands; only then can the intelligence be clear of any clouds.

Many have difficulty thinking beyond their past habits, grievances, mistakes. hardships, and trauma. A positive way to deal with past memories is to appreciate that it served as compost for what is growing inside the seeker on his present-day spiritual journey. Nurturing the garden of present delights transforms the mind and empowers the aspirant who now lives his new memory.

He is freed of past memories and looks at it from a new perspective. The new rich life-experience now guides his present. This re-arranging, and re-programming not only supports him, but becomes subjected to subtle commands from his subconsciousness. He becomes a ruler of his own reality.

Wisdom

The new image feels his abilities of leadership and has the qualities of kindness and generosity. He can assume the roles of peacemaker, diplomat, or counsellor. His visions become manifest for all to see. He does not command anything, but he has the wisdom to walk with the flow of the life-force.

He recognises inclinations and abilities of all those around him. He has the wisdom to encourage self-expression of these innate qualities and tendencies. He makes them feel fulfilled by utilising the energy they were called for. Using such potential is ancient wisdom because it gives momentum to what is already happening anyway.

This seeker has attained control of his senses through discrimination. He abandons all tendencies and entanglements while performing his duties. He possesses soul-happiness, and his discrimination acquires a soul-force of intuition. Intuitive guidance becomes his wisdom and it is this that guides the intellect to reason correctly.

Those who refuse to live according to the inner dictates of meditation-born peace of the soul become entangled with the senses and lose their direction away from the goal of life as Man. The discriminating intellect is misused. Instead, there develops pride and a sense of accomplishment that are the hallmarks of the ego.

Only a few wise ones understand that this soul-happiness is an expression of his own *intelligence* that is also the Universal Intelligence experienced at the *kutastha chaitanya* or Christ centre. The yogi reasons that his conviction is instinctive and latent in him: he knows he must awaken his total intuition.

The *sadhak* or seeker who has known both sense-inclinations and soul-happiness possesses a standard of comparison that is non-existent for the worldly man.

A deeply meditating *sadhak* understands that he first must practice *physically to withdraw* from his senses and arrive at the altar of the divine cave. Next he must be able to watch the breath while connected to the Cosmic Vision. Next he must listen to the Cosmic Vibration of Aum within himself. He must enter both the eye of the Cosmic Vision as well as the sound of the Cosmic Sound until he ceases to hear the voice of the senses.

Finally, he must rise above the astral sounds of his astral spine *(chakras*). Only then will he hear the Cosmic Aum within and without and see the Cosmic Light that he must penetrate. Once he enters the Light, he contacts Cosmic Consciousness.

Harnessing Wisdom

Money is power and therefore never enough, to the modern man. To a wise man it is a force to make wise choices with, to maximise its potential to create benefits for a common good.

To the modern man *time* is for indulgences and pleasure. The wise man every moment counts to love, create, to enhance his will-power, and search for the Self.

The creative-force of *thought* manifests the outer world. The wise man takes command of his thoughts in meditation and changes the inner patterns of his thinking so that they may manifest in the outer world.

He treats every *loss and failure* as a new freedom. He considers it a gain of a new life-opportunity to perfect his renewed effort at self-perfection. The perfected skill allows Mother Nature to re-channel the energy for a greater common good. He teaches all those around, that taking command of the life-force is better than embracing struggles! He bridges his perceptions of the outer world and supports it with his *guru's* and Nature's wholeness.

To increase perceptions of wholeness and learn to create a path between you and your ideal; Mother Nature will open the Universe before you:

- *Bring the guru into the divine cave behind the eyebrows and remain focused at the Cosmic Guru or Teacher.*
- *Fill the cave with Light and watch your gross breathing. Adjust its regularity using the Ham...Saa...So...Ham technique, for some time.*
- *Watch the breath coursing through the nostrils: (it will become less frequent and more subtle over time), look at the guru with the tongue rolled back. Feel his presence in the divine cave.*
- *Now invoke the guru (by mentally taking his emotion-charged image) into*

your Fourth Chakra of the Heart which is situated in the spine just above the level of the physical heart.

As Universal Teacher and Guide, he understands all protocols of every life-situation and every life-changes, both in darkness and in dawn. He will guide you through every life-dance and reveal all things sacred. He will call your inner being to make the necessary changes. Your spiritual heart will know you have made the right changes and choices.

The Light of the Universal Teacher removes the "personality" of the *guru* who has been physically known to the seeker. There is, instead, an inner intuitive perception. The seeker perceives all that emanates out of the Light as the Total *Guru*, the *Sada-Shiva* as *Shiva-Shakti.*

The Sun is considered by many as the Total *Guru, the Sada Shiva-Shakti* manifesting as Light and Energy (Consciousness and Awareness all in one). Heightened sensitisation of this oneness with the Light gives the aspirant the ability to become invisible to a passer-by: the energy field created by the seeker blocks the energy field of the passer-by's sight. The energy field around the body is maximised by control of the senses. The result is the ability to control the mind!

Even he who has progressed far on the spiritual path may suddenly find some sense attraction distracting his awareness. Discrimination of the intellect and self-control through more intense efforts at deeper meditation will help the seeker maintain an iron grip on his thoughts. He who conquers the blind emotional mind abandons all entanglements in materialism. The attractions and aversions of the senses are abandoned and he continues to perform all his duties in the world.

> and the Master wrote: "End all spirit of antagonism with the outer world of things and beings. Hate none. Love all. And with this love conquer even the most brutal of forces around you. As Sri Aurobindo [early twentieth century saint] says: 'Live with Him; do not be shaken by the outward happenings'.
>
> "The Gospel of *Vedanta* thunders, 'Man, you are of one nature, the substance of God, one soul with you fellow-men. Awake and progress towards your utter divinity. Live for God in yourself and in others". This secret Gospel that was given till now only to the few must be preached openly and freely for all mankind...immediately, urgently, and ardently!.."

The seeker's reasoning becomes fixed in the soul. He acquires the light of soul-happiness and enjoys the Bliss while in meditation, as well as, while serving the world. He has educated his intellect with knowledge, but his intelligence (awareness) needs the light of intuition (consciousness). Intuitive guidance manifests as wisdom that now guides the intellect to perform correct actions. The seeker acquires peace or stillness of the body and mind. He is free to enjoy the stillness and silence in meditation.

During this period of your spiritual journey, keep a diary of the messages of the *guru's* guiding voice. Watch what you in fact do, in the outer world. Meditate at the *Kutastha;* touch what you have previously been afraid to touch; love from where anger once lived and feel the changes in your own being and then in the world outside!

Analysis of Mind Control

Thoughts and ideas may dwell on fantasies and idealism which gives the seeker hope and inspiration for future health and wealth! These are seeds of images and imaginations. They need nurturing with inner resourcefulness and responsibility until they blossom.

Now comes the real work. All ideals must be harvested for distribution for a common good in areas of peace and service. The seeker needs to understand the changes that have taken place in himself. He must learn to re-package himself, free from past conflicts and opinions of his ego.

While doing service, he remains silent and watchful. He waits for the right opportunity and opening to speak just enough to trigger interest and respect. He has learnt thought-control and steadily makes minor advances at a time until he has expanding co-operation.

Control of the Mind means control of thoughts and therefore also of all outer actions:
- Can patterns of thinking be changed and subdued?
- How does this occur?

Thoughts are reproductive. Their creative energy allows their seeds to grow if they are to be planted in the mind.

Note coincidences of "similar" thoughts in others.

Record how these happen and if they can be done at one's own behest.

Mind has a drawing power:
- When is one best able to will a thought into another.
- Is this a particular time of day when this occurs most easily?
- To influence another with blessings and benediction, focus on the *ajnaa* center of the recipient [reflected at the *kutastha*]. Now invoke your will while the recipient of your wishes is asleep.

Do I keep promises to others?

Do I do the same when making promises to myself?

Observe dreams pertaining to past, present and future:
- Recall all dreams over the past three or six months.
- Compare your recollections with the original notes on dreams you have made earlier.

Dreamless states are not unusual.

- Watch yourself falling asleep.
- Can I take part in the process of falling asleep?
- Can I redirect a dream to become more pleasant or even stop one?

Daily moods need observations:

- Record moods at three times of the day: morning, noon, and evening.
- Note if there are cycles of highs and lows.

Make similar observations about thoughts versus moods and habits.

- Note differences in habitual and spontaneous responses to these triggering factors, for example sleepiness, times of day, your conscience.
- Are they connected to moods?
- How does it happen?

The unenlightened *chitta* (mind-intellect-ego complex) is responsible for moods or feelings of Man. They are the foundation structure of man's soul personality. Mind manifests as emotions and in the intellect, it manifests as thought.

The result of this combination, is an ego personality that mirrors the underlying structural health of the person. A refined structural basic foundation (causal-astral level) leaves the mind-intellect silent. A silent mind is capable of receiving the first gift of *sadhana* or austerities of spiritual journeys - to Love and to Intuitively Know in interactions with OET and in dreams.

Mind Energy

Energy, when **unmanifest** is classified male or *deva or alinga*: **Manifested** energy is a *devi* or female. The manifested Universe is Awareness or *Prakriti or Shakti*, the powerful Mother Nature; She physically vibrates as the Energy *Aum*. The unmanifest counterpart is *Shakta, the Purusha*, whose characteristic is Consciousness, which vibrates Its Light as *Aum*.

In glory and splendor, She or *Shakti* surpasses the Master. *Shakti* allows the seeker to be born in Her Womb, to play the games of enjoyment for His pleasure. While the mortal plays, She keeps him hypnotized by Her delusive powers of *raaga-dvesha* or likes-and-dislikes and veiled under the spell of Her *Maya* or Her innate qualities of matter or *gunas*. She nourishes the seeker and the non-seekers alike, with Her Divine Nectar of peace, joy, and satisfaction.

The seeker now aspires to become one with the Mother. All efforts by the seeker are therefore adulation to *Devi Shakti*, also called the energy of *Kundalini or Devi*, by some schools. All Creation is Her manifestation, in so many names and forms.

and the Master wrote:

> "A sincere devotee sees the whole universe as the very form of his beloved. The *gopis* [milkmaids] saw the Lord *[Krishna]* everywhere; even in the chirping of the birds in *Brindavan [Krishna's* hometown] they [the milk-maids] heard but the chanting of His glories. To be thus in Him, with all of one's mind, so that even the sense organs cannot land upon anything, without bringing the association of the Lord to one's experience is called 'whole heartedness' or *ananyatha*."

Light and electricity are visible energy forms of Her *Shakti* or Power. The physical body is a vibration of the same energy, crystallizing into the physical form in so many shapes. Mind also is this same energy manifesting as *thought*. Similarly, the Total Universe is this Energy manifesting at different vibration frequencies to give it name, shape, and form — the Total Energy of *Prakriti*. She is in every atom and in every cell as *Aum*, the Holy Spirit!

Each of Her manifestations has been endowed with His Consciousness. Together, they form the Total Cosmic Conscious Energy: the *Shakti-Shakta or Prakriti-Purusha* or Universe-God.

The thinking process is an energy process capable of producing thought. When thought is converted to *action*, there is an expenditure of energy. When action is combined with emotion, there is an emotional investment of energy. This Energy expenditure is measured by the degree of fatigue-of-separation or joy-of- oneness, experienced.

> and the Master wrote: "We can discover our joy in the precision and perfection of the work that we turn out. Whether others recognize it or not, we have the satisfaction that we did our work as best as we could, and a silent stream of joy sings a secret song at all times in our hearts.."

Freeing the Mind

This love song of the heart entices the inner person into relationship with the outer world. The within and the without become lovers, the two halves of the one whole! Within lives a perfect Self which has manifested through atoms, energy, and thought ideas. The Self needs to dwell in harmony by existing a balanced existence, attending to the needs of Mother Nature. Here he finds his own equilibrium. His mind attains rationality and intuitiveness both as the seeker works and plays.

This heightened perceptions of the mind requires freeing the mind from unnecessary preoccupation, running in different directions from the body structure. These *rays* of mental energy have to be drawn back into their *source*.

Anything that manifests as a *ray of thought energy*, takes on a *life of its own*. Therefore, we are responsible for every thought, word, and action; each is an increment of energy vibrations, depending upon the organs involved in the act.

Consequently, a *sadhak* meditating upon God, should not allow himself to think about material objects. He should be able to renounce all desires born of egoistic mental plans. His mind should be withdrawn from all objects that give rise to sensations and their resultant thoughts and desires. Through concentrating in the act of meditation, all distractions are arrested.

Until the *sadhak* has mastered such interiorization, he must practice mind control and minimize the invasion of external stimuli. In the beginning, the *sadhak* is asked to close his eyes during meditation, in quiet surroundings. All sounds must be eliminated by listening attentively to the *Aum* through the inner ear. When sight and hearing are eliminated, all other senses are quietened and distracting thoughts are silenced. When thoughts recede, subconscious thoughts are also laid to rest.

Freed from both external and internal distractions, intellectual thinking also recedes. Intelligence now stands witness to the stillness and the silence and the *sadhak* or seeker is advised to guide his intuitive intelligence to perceive *soul-happiness*. With patience and daily effort, he succeeds in establishing his mind-intellect on this *bliss*. By gradually identifying himself with his own intuitive discrimination, he attains divine tranquillity.

By repeated and prolonged efforts at concentration and meditation, the seeker is able to destroy restlessness. Only interiorized concentration can still the mind and disconnect it from sensory stimuli. Since only *rajas (*activity) has the ability of mental and material creation, it can lead the *sadhak* or seeker to nature-born duality in the mind (good-and-evil, likes-and-dislikes).

When all thought activities are stilled and silenced, the *sadhak* or seeker attains an interiorized state of *samadhi* or oneness with self, *even while the body is fixated.* This is an 'enforced' arrest of the mind in a state of soul-happiness through which the seeker becomes the enjoyer of universal bliss. During normal activity, his mind returns to external functions. Eventually he learns to retain his quietude during the performance of all actions, both inner and outer.

> and the Master wrote:
>
> "The purer the mind and intellect, the brighter will be the beams of consciousness that shoot out from the individual. The saint or the prophet is one who has the maximum awareness manifest in him. The *sruti* says*:"Brahmavit Brahmaive Bhavati"* or the 'Knower of *Brahman* becomes *Brahman'*.
>
> "To realize the pure awareness, which is *Atman*, or the Life Center, is the goal of life, the culmination of evolution, the fulfillment of supermanhood. Rediscovery of the Self is not only the ending of all confusions and our sense of imperfections, but it is also the ascent into a state of supermanhood and Godhood!..."

Once the *sadhak* or seeker is able to hold his concentration (*dharana)* in a steady state of inner calmness, he is able to perceive his soul. Through further perseverance, he enters the hall of Bliss and **realizes** the "touch" of the Spirit. The longer he stays *there,* the longer he **experiences** the blissful state of awareness-consciousness as *Aum* in Existence.

Thought and Speech in Worship of Mother Nature

We presently live in a world that is unbalanced. The resources have been mined relentlessly with no thought of restoration and replenishment. Mother Nature knows how to readjust to such cruelty. She has the option of destroying exhausted land masses and creating new ones through dissolution. Most destruction occurs where man has harmed Her most.

Her natural laws are powerful. Mother Nature abides by Her own divine plan, but Man continues to work against them. Her greatest generosity to mankind is with seeds of re-creation. They must be replanted in spaces of Her own body which She has readied and converted to compost.

Mother Nature will not regenerate what Man poisons. She will transform the poison and will kill the poisoned areas of Her with Her powers of phenomenon. Here the Law of Justice or *Karma* or the 'rod' is impeccable.

> "Their houses are safe from fear, neither is the rod of God upon them"
>
> "How oft is the candle of the wicked put out! and how oft cometh their destruction upon them! God distributeth sorrows in His anger"..Job 21: 9, 17.

Man continues to destroy Nature. Little does he realize that the Universe is a living, breathing, moving whole, like any other body. She will heal what Man injures and amputate what is irretrievably injured. She will respond in kind when Her subjects are collectively injured. She will destroy Nations, if the need arises!

Alll scriptures claim that when Awareness in Matter [*Prakriti* or Energy] and Consciousness [*Purusha* or Light] unite, the power of action and manifestation takes place. This is Creation. The Light of Consciousness is the Eternal Witness and incapable of functioning without the help of Her Energy.

Many stories are told to children about the might of this Cosmic Homemaker! The Trinity of *Brahma* [Creator], *Vishnu* [Preserver], and *Shiva* [Dissolver] of the Universe must also first prostrate to the Cosmic Homemaker.

Even if They wished it, without the presence of Her Energy, the Trinity would be incapable of singing to Her their praises,. Who is She? She is the Divine Mother, the *Durga Devi*, Mother of all thought, word, speech, and action.

It is She who is the homemaker of the Universe. She carries a thousand names, each describing Her quality. First She is *Mahamaya,* the wonderful secretive mother-of-mankind. She is the consort of each of the Trinity as *Sarasvati* of Knowledge*, Lakshmi* of True Wealth*, and Parvati* of Power and Energy. She is also the transcendent: the fourth and most difficult form to realize. She is the repository of the great magical Wisdom who allows the Universe to revolve. She is the Power *Aum* of the Ultimate Reality or God - *Brahman.*

Shakti or Devi or Mother manifests in both the microcosm and the macrocosm

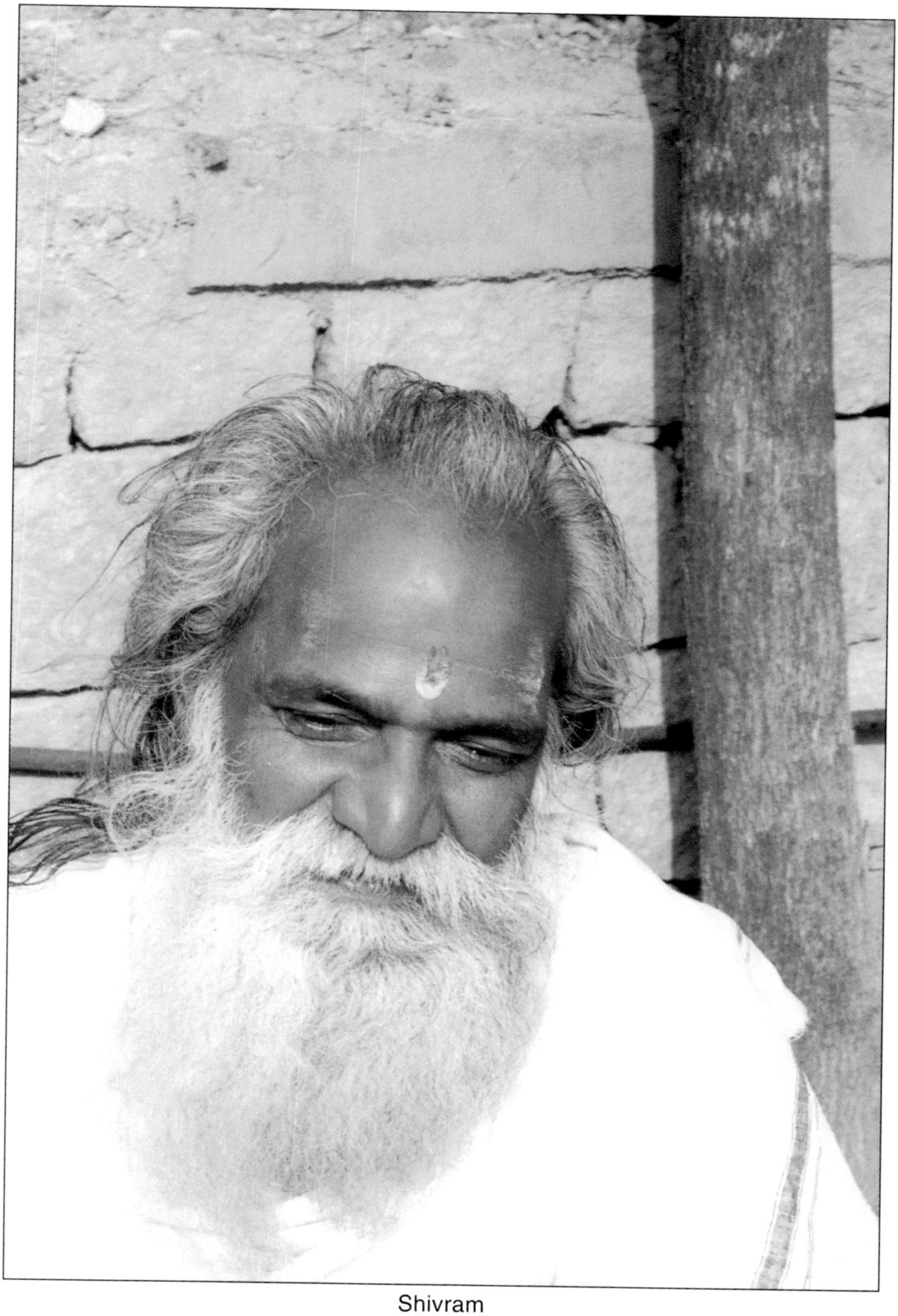

Shivram

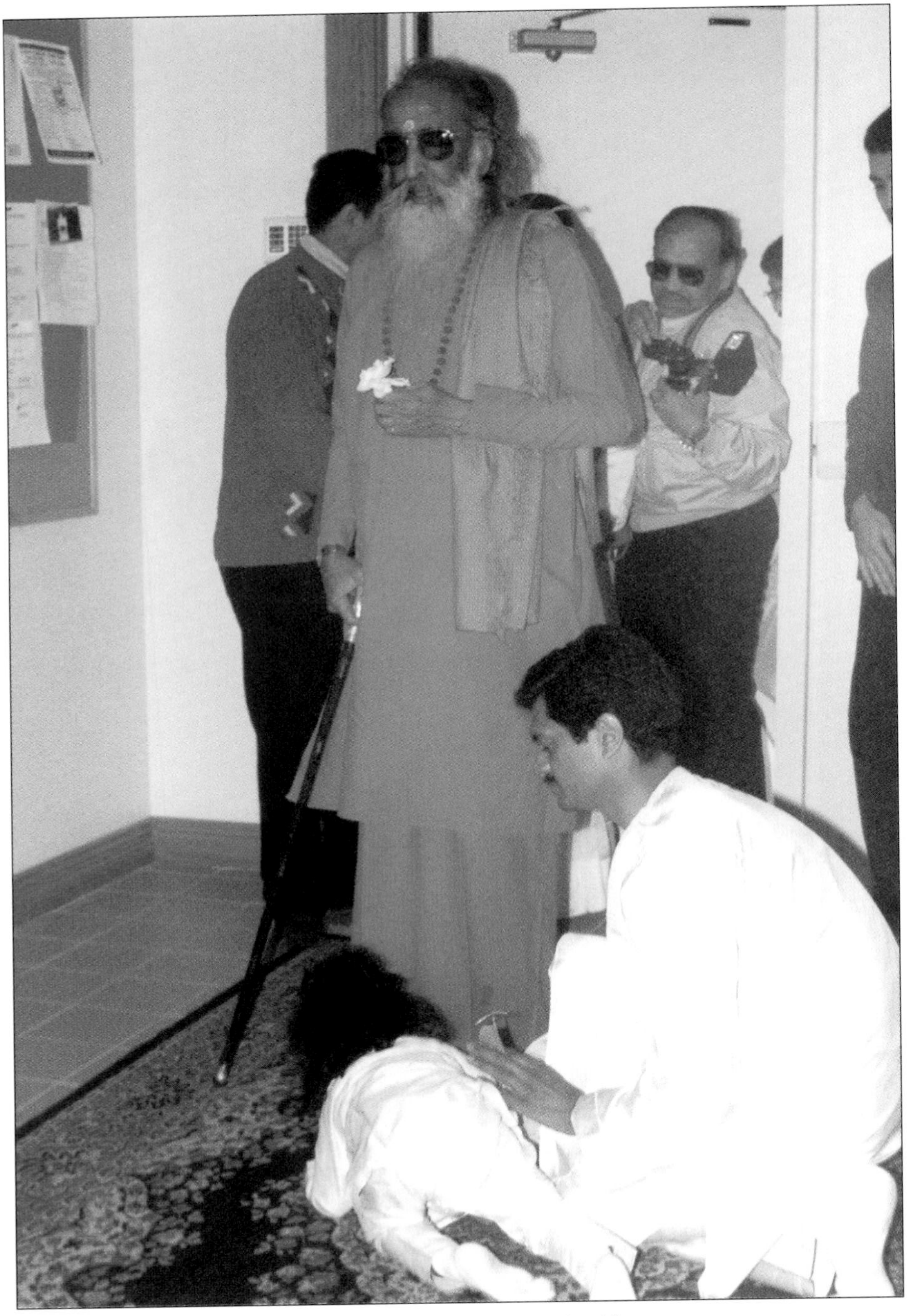

The Third Generation follows the Master

as Awareness, functioning both inwardly and outwardly. She is formless and with form; terrible as well as beautiful; human as well as inhuman. It is She, the Holy Spirit who expresses Herself in all levels of creation. She permeates every atom and molecule in the animate and the inanimate. She is the Holy Spirit.

The Holy Spirit is the repository of the Ten Wisdoms that reveal themselves in the Universe and in Man's own psyche as word, thought, and speech. While Her teachings are about the beings and things, wise Men remain attached to Her messages about deeper Truths.

These uncontrollable forces of Cosmic Energy are mysterious and difficult to tolerate or control, despite scientific advances made to date. Her forms are frightening, provocative, and also contradictory; their purpose is to neutralize the thought processes which bind Man to the world of objects, emotions, and thoughts (OET). The life of Man is also mysterious: although he knows he was born to die, he struggles as if he is going to live forever, continuing to desire, to possess, and enjoy his possessions and status. All cultures therefore instinctively remain connected to this very giving Cosmic Mother.

In every country in the different countries of South East Asia, *devi worship* [of Mother Nature] has its own tradition. Worship of the Cosmic Mother practiced in *Mahayana Buddhism* [Tibet, China, and in Japan] has a great deal in common with Hinduism. They both utilize images of *devis (goddesses*) and their female powers *(yoginis)*. *Tara* and *Chhinnamasta* are names that are common to both.

Both traditions have the same descriptions to identify the ten Wisdom goddesses. The ten forms of *Mahamaya* are Her Cosmic Forces. All traditions agree that they cannot be manipulated in the Universe. They all also agree that they cannot be controlled within one's own psyche. All traditions know that She can be surrendered to: for Her grace. Her motherhood will allow Her power to work in the true seeker.

In the Hindu tradition, goddesses possess three forms: Knowledge, Power, and Beauty *(Sarasvati-Kali-Lakshmi),* which are adored separately. The Three are also adored together as One. Since they are *Vidyas* or knowledge, the ten goddesses enlighten, save, protect, love, render compassion, and give beauty. The Cosmic Homemaker renders Her grace as one special grace or as ten graces in one.

Ten Functions and Images of One Mother

In *Svetasvatara Upanishad* (scriptural text) there is a stanza which translates as: "You are man; You are lad and You are maiden too; You are the old man who totters with a cane; You are born with Your face turned in all four directions".

God appears to Man in a million forms. It appears in the strength of a man and the gracefulness of a woman. Ii is in the abandon of youth and in the wisdom of the aged. He or She creates all things and sustains them too. In the end, She withdraws it all into Herself. Motherhood is an old concept and evidence of Her worship are found in old relics of every civilization. Mother-worship in India has been the most potent force for spiritual regeneration of the Hindus.

The metaphysical position of *Advaita* [philosophy of non-dualism], is often replaced by Mother Worship of *Dvaita* [philosophy of dualism] . The fact that *Shakti-Shakta* (Matter-Spirit) is the foundational theme of the ultimate Reality, both forms of worship reach the same conclusion: God as He or as She or both as One is *sat-chit-anand* or existence-knowledge-bliss.

Worshipers of Mother Universe or *Mahamaya or Durga or Shakti* acknowledge that She the Holy Spirit. She is *sabda brahman* or the Word-God: *Aum.* The ten Wisdoms She signifies are the ten *devis* or Mothers-of-Wisdom, described by sages.

The Mother's functional characteristics start with *Kali* and ends with *Kamalaa-Ambika-Gauri.* They emerge from *Mahamaya* and merge back into Her as well. They all reside in the divine cave of man. Man works at the first five spiritual centres or *chakras* in his spiritual *sadhana.* Having acquired the first five wisdoms, he must keep working away, until he acquires the remaining five wisdoms.

Each of the *devis* or mothers is assigned a *yantra* or triangle for the nine continents of the earth, in a *chakra* or circle representing the orb of the earth. The combined *yantra-chakra* is now called *Shri-Chakra of Shiva-Shakti* of forty-three triangles - the mansion of the Mother. In this mansion reside *Vishnu, Brahma, and Loka-palas* or all Her assigned protectors of the Universe.

My husband and I grew up together as children. My background was that of an idol-free worship of the *Pranava: Aum.* My husband's family have been worshippers of the Divine Mother for over seven generations.

As a child and a teenager my sisters and I watched their intense devotional practices. To my husband She still is the Mother of the Universe with whom he is totally identified. There are no prayers, no demands, just a trusting loving relationship that She will do what is best for him. To him there is no need for any other Knowledge.

For a long time, She invoked alarm in me by virtue of Her Fierce Strength and the dreadful powers of annihilation. She was capable of invoking intense Fear in me. At that time, She seemed impossible to perceive or comprehend. This state of disequilibrium rendered me unprotected.

My father encouraged me to paint Her, read about Her, invoke Her...after all I married into one of Her's! I knew She sat heavily on my ignorant Inert Consciousness.

While I spent years trying to 'understand' Her, my husband taught the children and the grandchildren a powerful *mantra* invoking Her in all Her ten forms. I gradually realised that it is She who is the *Chhandi* in the *Devi Mahatmayam* [the text my daughter recited over my grandson's still and inert body] who destroys all thoughts while I am awake or in meditation. It is She who is the Slayer of all thoughts, passions, and anger. Many years later, She gave me the intuitive vision of Herself as the Cosmic Mother who destroys all negativity in thought, speech, and action!

Shakti as *Aum* has ten sound manifestations starting as a *dhvani* or murmuring in the *muladhara* or base *chakra.* A sincere seeker can hear these astral vibrations emanating from these astral *chakras.* As their *chitta* or awareness evolves, the seeker ascends the ladder of astral sounds. The seeker is finally united to the roar of the ocean: here he hears, sees, and feels *Aum* in all Its mystical manifestations within the divine cave. Man reaches the highest centre of manifestation in Consciousness, in his own body temple.

> "Heaven is My throne, and earth is My footstool: What house will ye build Me? saith the Lord: or what is the place of My rest? Hath not My hand made all these things?" Acts 7: 49-50.

She alone can lead the seeker down the garden path of *Maya* or delusion and also liberate him by awakening the Life Force *Shakti* of increasing "awareness" during *sadhana* or self-effort. Man's experiences lie between *Maya* and Liberation, causing the intertwining of thousands of possibilities between the two extremes. When interconnecting with Her manifestations of the Universe, She moves, revolves, and buffets in a dizzying illusion.

When on the Path of Liberation, the relationship with Her must be based upon an impeccable character, self-discipline, and faith. When the seeker feels Her presence within the heart, there follows an intimate play of Forces, described as Living in Her Grace!

As long as the seeker lives directly in contact with Her, She will care for Her child with love and tenderness rarely ever felt anywhere before. The seeker now grows within Her Light in a spirit of surrender, desiring only to be led by Her. She lets one live a life, not rejected, but transformed in love.

> and the Master commented:
>
> "To love truly is to add to one's life. One who is in love expands to function from two points...from oneself and from one's beloved. To love the whole Universe is to experience the All."

Healing

The body holds all knowledge of lives lived before and has the experience and template of a memory bank of every information of the seeker's spiritual journey over time. His physical atoms seek pleasure of indulgences and sensuality; his life-force or *prana* in the subtle body, functions through the power of creativity;

and his causal body emit light of matter essence and ideation.

He becomes aware that his body is a temple and it must not only be a place of peace but also be healthy. Here dwells the Self in all its effulgence. Identified with the three outer coverings of the Self, Man's spiritual journey is obstructed by an unhealthy body, uncontrolled emotion-ridden mind, and an unenlightened causal body or *chitta*.

Bodies have the ability to heal themselves, unless abused for over twenty years at a stretch. By this time the body is filled with the stresses and temptations that have led man to ignore the body's wisdom. The recovery period now requires an accumulated time period, which is denied to Man.

Cosmic Awareness is a powerful energy that far surpasses the power of the human mind. Man can *channel* life-force or *the creative pranic energy (*reiki) and induce healing through the healer's will power, concentration, faith, reason, and common sense. Healing is also possible through transfer of astral energy from evolved astral beings to mortals on earth.

> I fell at the home of a friend in New Delhi. As soon as I hit my left knee on the marble floor and felt the shearing pain, I knew I had done something terrible to it. My hostess who is old enough to be my own mother was so alarmed that I had to hide the pain from her. We walked all around the city for hours and I returned to her home exhausted. Now I had this painfully throbbing swollen knee, which remained a 'friend' for the rest of our trip. We left by train for *Sidhabari* that night with my pregnant second daughter and her husband, to pay homage at the shrine of the physically departed Master.
>
> I limped up and down the hills of the *ashram* or hermitage at the foothills of the Himalayas. Our hearts lamented that the Master was not there physically. What a fuss he would have made over this pregnancy! We were discussing this, when my husband and I were called to the final resting place of the Master. As if from the other world, the Master's batsman *Shivram* was there with the 'children' doing the *seemantam* rites. We were delighted at the 'fussing' that was taking place. We all knew the Master must have triggered this!
>
> We left for Delhi the following evening by land-rover and then by train from *Pathankot.* My knee was throbbing with intolerable pain. I was exhausted. Once we were in the train compartment, sleep erased all the awareness of pain! I awakened at 4 a.m. and walked to the bathroom and back and suddenly realised that there was no pain in the massively swollen knee. Even from his astral world, the Master's compassion posed no barriers!

Diseases, especially chronic disease, have deep roots in the subconscious mind. The healer makes positive affirmations to the subconscious mind until it reaches the superconscious mind. It is here that the magical powers of cure reside. The healer and the healee must both be free of doubts. Patience is required for will, faith, and attention to remain focused until the desire to heal or affirmation reaches the superconscious state of beingness.

Only pranic energy heals directly as is done in *pratyahara* or withdrawal of life-force through the senses into the divine cave. The seeker wilfully withdraws from his senses and infuses the astral body with the ***Aum;*** through intense contraction and relaxation, the body undergoes changes, including healing.

External practices like 'touching of the hands' *cooperate with the healing capabilities of the life-force.* If the mind has the power to produce disease, it also has the power to effect cures. *Autosuggestion* is also *powerless without the* power of the will and the power of affirmation.

Disease habits of the subconscious must be uprooted by deeper and repeated efforts at affirmation for healing. *The effort of the healer is the seed of a cure.* The healer understands how to control this healing energy that is being projected into the patient, who for his part must have the faith to receive it.

Laws of Nature must be obeyed so that there is no bodily disharmony caused by unbridled desires, fear, rage, intolerance, greed, and overindulgence. Cultivation of peace and faith in God frees the mind from all disturbing thoughts that trigger disease, decay, and death. Mental cures are superior to physical cures because will, imagination, faith, and reason are states of awareness which act from within.

The healing is a psycho-physiological technique of directing life energy to the superconscious mind, by the power of will. Harnessing the will is a learned technique.

A healing crisis is an event that simulates an actual illness. It is triggered by an act of health which is both naturally ad nutritionally sound. The acts may take the form of fasting, refraining from stimulants, eating natural foods for a few days, meeting an exceptionally advanced spiritual soul, or solitude for prolonged periods. The discomfort of the healing crisis can be many times more distressing if the seeker does not take steps to improve his health. Pay attention to your body's needs and select a proper diet of fresh fruits and vegetables or fasting.

Healing through Mind Power

Seekers, who follow the path seriously, gain control over emotions (sensory indulgence or desiring *manas)* and cultivate them to become refined inner feelings of compassion. Compassion has a desire for self-expression. When one yearns to help others, healing will occur, especially when motivated by the nobility of compassion.

Meditation processes and the invocation of the Divine Light, assist in dealing with issues such as opinions, concepts and beliefs. Their hold on the seeker dissolves, leaving him with more flexibility and subtlety. The seeker is able to reach more meaningful relationships with the Universe such as in healing.

Diseases: Are these Karmic Effects?

Diseases are the result of willful, long-term physical self-abuse, through indulgences for the sake of pleasure. Disease can be healed spiritually only once - if at all. The patient must have the will to correct his habits of daily living, if healing is to work and continue. There must be a desire to get well, and the will to live a purposeful life.

Matter exists as a cosmic delusion, but it cannot be ignored, except by learning the Laws of Nature and Truth. Creation involves the transformation process of Consciousness into Awareness, leading to the crystallization of matter. The Infinite becomes finite. Awareness is the vibration of Its subjective Consciousness, and Matter, is Its objective vibration, giving rise to names and forms. The difference between Matter and Spirit, is in the speed of its vibration frequency.

Each person is stamped with their own special signature, reflecting their own special awareness. The seeker can include disease by his own thought vibrations, but can also undo the damage through the power of his own will.

The Art of Healing

Healing is an interplay of forces between the healer and the sick:

- The healer, who is a mere channel for the life-force, must possess cultivated emotions and feelings of gratitude for this ability to heal, through the grace of Divine Will.
- The healed must want to get better and be willing to change his life-style.
- Spiritual forces transfer extra healing energy from the healer to the sick.

The underlying process of healing is the power of the mind that makes powerful suggestions; the healer merges his own self-image with the Higher Healer and infuses new life into an afflicted-life and induces healing. This is the type of healing-power that generates confidence, trust, hope, and a will to live.

Look-Watch-Listen-Feel Aum and Transfer

Assume meditation posture with back straight, shoulders together, abdomen in, eyes to the east between eyebrows, and tongue rolled back.

Enter the divine cave and become aware of your own inner silence.

Watch the breath and look at the Cosmic Vision in the Kutastha Chaitanya between the eyebrows.

Listen to the Cosmic Sound of Aum; if there is a problem with "hearing", lightly close the ears with the thumbs and hear the roar of Aum.

Contract the whole body from head to toe and feel the Energy and Light of Aum fill your divine cave. It has all the combinations for healing to occur, despite distances involved.

- *Having invoked the Light, transfer the Light to the needy who is deeply relaxed or is asleep. Allow the Light to do its work. For best results, focus on the recipient's kutastha or Christ-Krishana centre between the eyebrows. Repeat the request daily for one to three months or always.*

Understanding Humility and Gratitude

Gratitude is an attitude of the body and mind, wherein there is an awareness of being grateful for all we have received. Most must learn to be grateful by balancing their tendencies to criticize and by controlling strong emotions. Cultivation of gratitude or appreciation leads to humility. The mind, then, stops its constant scheming.

We were summoned to arrive in Bombay when our first daughter was twelve weeks pregnant. Our second daughter had by then been traveling with the Master for two years. My husband who was in Indonesia was asked to meet us in Mysore. Our arrival in Bombay was met with the loss of our suitcases and we were forced to have new clothes made in a hurry!

The *ashram* or hermitage in Bombay was buzzing! The Master was returning to Bombay from Bangalore to chaperon us both back to Bangalore. We were both shocked and embarrassed with all the fuss, while he waited for our clothes to arrive from the tailor!

The Master knew we were unaccustomed to traveling unchaperoned. I was overwhelmed with gratitude with the Master's love and sensitivity!

Humility is mental surrender which expresses as bodily prostration, often occurring spontaneously: it is a bodily expression of the mind feeling absolute trust and gratitude.

We were now in Mysore. I was furious and complained vehemently at the treatment my un-chaperoned daughter and I had received. The Master listened patiently! My younger daughter walked into the room with a tray of lit lamps and burning incense. The Master quietly said: ADrop it!" and without a What or a Why she dropped it! My mind worried about setting the carpet on fire while my husband watched the scene!

And the Master admonished: "Now this is a perfect *shishya* [student]. She is endowed with perfect obedience and trust in her *guru*.. do you?"

Helpers and Givers have expectations of "how" they need to be thanked for favours rendered. It is important to realize that perhaps they do not "see" how the other expresses gratitude.

It was a hot morning when we arrived in Mysore. The *Yagna* host drove us to the home where the Master and his companion, my younger daughter, were to be staying. My husband had still not arrived from Indonesia. We sat on the front steps as the sun reached its zenith. I began worrying about the pregnant daughter, who had had nothing to drink for over four hours. When there was no acknowledgment of our presence, we both took a taxi in search of a Hotel. All the Hotels were booked with visitors attending a Conference and we were therefore grateful for the Hotel we finally got.

By 4 a.m. we [my daughter and I] began feeling unsafe in the Hotel. We decided to take the only taxi we could find - the scooter taxi. It was a bitterly cold tropical morning and the driver could not locate the residence of the Master's host in the new development section of Mysore! We must have been in the taxi for nearly two hours before we summoned help at a police station.

We were both [mother and daughter] in tears and I blurted out my complaints. The Master again listened patiently. That morning the Master dealt with the subject of the 'Divinity of a Guest' and the code of ethics involved. In the meantime, I had resolved not to accompany the Master wherever he was being invited for his meals! I dragged my husband to window-shop for my younger daughter's trousseau. The Master despaired at my action. I could not understand why he did not see that my actions were 'justified'!

Years later and long after the Master had left us, my husband and I overheard a sneering derogatory statement about a very successful *yagna* arranged by my daughter *for Swami Tejomayananda,* the present head of the organization. The attendee of the Conference did not know that we were the parents of the person she was talking about. We were our daughter's guest and had to just tolerate the insult and pain showered on us about our daughter!

Then came the realization why the Master was so disappointed with me: Pride of one's own imagined materialistic self-worth, self-importance, and self-evaluation is the sinister presence of an injured ego who justifies his bad manners with self-serving pontifical justifications! I was the Master's guest. I should have submitted to whatever his host wished to gift to us! The ego presents itself with many faces.

There is a natural desire to admire and worship. The *admiration of an ideal* can be to false-gods, such as food, sex, position, possessions, success, beliefs, convictions, and concepts.

Worship of guru needs analysis: Does it ever fill one with a sense of emptiness when he is not around? When love is established between you and your Guiding

Master, the bond is permanently established.

"Close your eyes and I will always be there" the Master promised.

You may give the Master a face. Some recognize his presence by feelings of vibration coursing through the body. Others actually smell him or see him.

My younger daughter was asked to become engaged to her future husband-to-be before the Master would allow her to travel with him during his lecture obligations all over the world. She was with him for two years and there was in her a gradually increasing dispassion for the worldly ways of living. She registered for admission into the Bombay Seminary and was accepted.

Her in-laws-to-be were fussing over the wedding arrangements and she became angry! She started to use this as an excuse to avoid marrying. The Master refused to get drawn into the issue and said: "How else will I return to express myself?"

On their way to Singapore, where the wedding was to take place, the Master gave her a *rudraksh* ring and said: 'With this ring, I thee wed". Into spirituality, she was wed *before* she married her spouse!

An egoistic mind busy scheming is the birthplace of habit formations. These *habits* are experienced later in life as pain, which may be interpreted as miseries-of-our-destiny. Instead, appreciate the daily *little miracles* in our lives. This is the best form of humility and gratitude.

Attachment to the sense objects we possess is a natural tendency of the blind mind. Enormous energy expenditure is involved in this *pleasure of possession* (emotional mind). It is better to intertwine your personal desires with those of Mother Nature's, with whom you are already compatible. The beast in you is then finally tamed. Deep longings of the soul need both of you to work hand-in-hand for a collective good. Bad habits, self-serving attitudes of self-worth, are transmuted into the power of caring ways, powered by the energy of inner convictions that the purpose of one's life is the upliftment of yourself and others. This is service to the One Cosmic Mother.

The seeker finally reaches the shores of his own inner freedom. Instead of a search for name, fame, and fortune, he has laid the foundation for a search of his own Self. The inner guide will take you along the path to spirituality. The first part of the journey is a 'walking alone'. The second part of the journey draws the guide deep into your inner being where the two meet in divine inspiration.

Those who have experienced the communion of the Self with the Spirit are secure within themselves. They know they have been instinctively led to the right people, the right books, and the right situations. They can remain silent in their deep understanding. Such sharing of information is not with those who would never understand!

Studentship and Celibacy

Man has the resources for creating, sustaining, and dissolving in accordance with the Divine Plan of Mother Nature. Man makes deliberate choices of action. The Creator living in man gives him stewardship and the tools with which to do the work. He is given a physical body of Matter substances of the earth from which he creates. He is also given a psychological-physiological body of life-force or energy through which is channeled the creative-energy or *prana.* His third body of clear shining thought-ideas allows him perfect understanding of his role in the stewardship under Nature. His causal being offers him love and blessings of sharing Natures gifts with man. He is made aware that he is connected to all life through the flow of sexual energy fueling all of creation.

Man understands that this life-force is to be respected and conserved. It can only be directed towards right relationship with all beings whom you care for. They in return must have the ability to comfort, help, and support according to their purpose in Her Divine Plan. All tools given to man are powers that create the world of a higher vision.

The blending of energies in a sexual encounter is an intimate gift to one another with whom you become one in wholeness. That is the ultimate mystery of the primal spiritual forces inside life. They are energies to be reckoned with and not for ignorant squandering. Ancient cultures acknowledge this and have devised rules of conduct for mankind.

The first twenty five years of life is that of a student who must conserve the life-force energy by observing *brahmacharya* or celibacy-during-studentship. If a sexual encounter is for the purpose of procreation, then whether studying, playing, or healing there is energy expenditure. Every thought and action is an expression of energy-expenditure through the senses. Analysis of an irresponsible sexual encounter reveals it is an emotional attachment for the pleasures felt. Habitual thought preoccupations with '*sex*' translate themselves into action. The expenditure of energy is enormous.

To investigate this, one must analyze why there is a need for this type of pleasure: In all institutions (seminaries), the renunciate student or *brahmachari* must be comfortable with celibacy. It takes three to four years to become entrenched in *yama* (restraints), *niyama* (adherence to restraints), *asana* (postures of meditation), *pranayama* (first stabilizing and then watching breath), *pratyahara* (withdrawal of senses into the divine cave), *and dharana* (concentration).

The renunciate is on a journey to experience the bliss of self with Self union. He now conserves his creative energy for *dhyana* (meditation) *and samadhi* (oneness in super-sonsciousness). He comes to a personal conclusion that is his own. There are no institutional rules dictating that he must be a celibate; rather celibacy becomes his own personal conviction.

There is a great deal of confusion about the word *brahmacharya* (celibacy): It is the first stage of a mortal's life, namely a celibate student's life. Hindu custom demands that the first quarter of a person's life be a pure celibate student's life.

In the life of a serious renunciate, ***brahmacharya*** (celibacy) must be practiced by having the patience to allot three to four years to study the old teachings. After this, the seeker must do a self-assessment — whether the life as a celibate and *brahmacharya* is for him.

The refinement of desires and imagination in regard to *sex* is a pre-requisite groundwork that must be dealt with for those seeking a spiritual life as a monk or renunciate. Attaining control is possible only through correct investigations. Only then can a renunciate have the correct goals for which to aspire.

One must be sure that the ecstasy of *oneness* with Spirit is the Ultimate Goal. Intense efforts in meditation are the only way to discover this ecstasy of pleasure and happiness. Unless this is personally *experienced*, the goal remains esoteric and the practitioner lives in the "imagined realms of the act of sex:".

> and the Master wrote:
>
> "*Brahmacharya* means living in self-control with respect to all our sense enjoyments and does not mean their total denial. The world-of-objects is meant for enjoyment and the scriptures do not deny us the freedom to enjoy them. They merely advise us to be masters of our enjoyments and not allow them to dominate and enslave us. You may eat food, but let not the food eat you!"

Ecstasy of Oneness of Soul and Spirit

Concerted effort at daily deep, and prolonged meditation leads the practitioner towards "oneness" of soul and Spirit.

- At such moments of attainment of psychic-energy, continue to refine the senses.
- Experiences of partial-oneness will serve as boosts of encouragement to overcome natural trials on the path of *sadhana.*

A *guru's* authority may be needed at first, but the seeker engaged in spiritual practice can become self-reliant and free from the pleasure attachments of the senses.

She had just finished her degree at University. She had only a month to be with the Master! While still in the aeroplane, she wrote him a tiny note that told him: she had now finished her basic education as directed and would be with him a very short time. She had no time to waste! He was to make sure that he took her 'There!'

He wrote back to me 'complaining' about my daughter's demands of 'short-cuts' into spirituality! Before she returned back home, the Master took her to the realms where there is no race, no creed, no name, no fame, no Master, no *sishya* (student)..only the experience of *Sat-Chit-Anand!* The seeker becomes one with Krishna-Christ Consciousness, the reflected Consciousness in creation and inherent in the Word *Aum,* the Cosmic Vibration.

> "Upon whom thou shalt see the Spirit descending, and remaining on him, the same is he which baptizeth with the Holy Ghost" ..John 1:33

Dangers of Mechanicalness in Spiritual Practice

Mechanicalness is the most common reason for failure in spiritual practice:

- Routineness of action must be watched for as the first sign of "breakdown"! All actions, no matter how mundane, must be a worship at the feet of the ideal:
- The mind must constantly be aware of the Cosmic Energy flow.
- This results in *the "escalation and empowerment of the mind" to achieve greater perceptions.* Therein lies the discovery of the Divine within oneself.

In different faiths, *the symbols and rituals may differ,* but the acts of gratitude and humility are stepping stones to ones acceptance of God. Eventually, the refinement of the senses takes the seeker to accept God as Cosmic Intelligence who is without shape or form.

Analysis of the Heart Chakra

All the *sadhana* is now synthesized on the heart *chakra.* The seeker becomes increasingly aware of the meaning of the changes he has experienced and is experiencing.

This is a point of crossroads: Ideals now require review and refinement so that one can escalate and intensively apply what has been learnt so far. *A daily diary now becomes the measure of one's progress and development.* Constant re-evaluation is the foundation upon which more work is done.

Awareness of the subtle changes has to be applied to daily life. One's self-image is and has changed, and there is growing recognition that one has the ability to develop in the direction decided upon, which is itself a source of encouragement and inspiration. *There is a change in the seeker's Energy field that tends to attract persons of like minds to oneself:*

Friendships develop and perhaps one needs to deal with this "new" issue. In the Path, friends may have problems of their own and, in their moments of doubt, may drag you down with them. Evaluate your friend walking the spiritual path. Friends must have the ability to accept, discuss, and support you during periods of doubt and of uncertainty in spiritual life.

During these periods of temporary instability, a friend must have the depth of character and understanding not to drag you away from your chosen path in life. The seeker must steer his commitment to life in a direction that is best for himself. A wise teacher must remain a friend who will give his student the right advice above all else.

She had just come out of a very painful relationship with a young physician she was engaged to while still at University. She was now befriended by a classmate. We, the parents felt uncomfortable with the direction taken by this new relationship. We decided to let her serve the Master on his travels.

The Master studied her well, over the following few months. She remained clear and adamant and decided to marry her new friend. Her interest in spirituality had temporarily taken second place.

And the Master said: "Return home and ask your parents to make preparations for the wedding!"

The Master initiated the engagement and was with this daughter until the morning of the wedding. She cried and begged him to stay back. The laws of a renunciate did not allow him to stay with us that morning.

That evening, we were told by his host that the Master had deliberately missed his flight to Boston and remained at the Toronto airport until the Vedic wedding ceremony was complete at noon.

There was an unexplicable orange glare over whole mugo-pine during the wedding for four hours. Was he there in his astral form witnessing the wedding? Did his unselfish love and friendship for this daughter prevent him from leaving the area?

Years later, after the birth of our second grandson, the Master said: "Your years of preoccupation with *maya* are now over! You will return to me [God] again. Spirituality will take centre-place in your life once more..!" And it did.

When Man enters the spiritual world, he becomes a 'son of God' (or daughter). He or she understands the "Word" or Holy Spirit *Aum.* There is a realization that the individual is a mere idea resting on a firmament of *Aum.* The seeker now enters the divine cave and sacrifices himself in the altar of God. He now sheds all ideas of separateness and becomes part of the whole.

> "To him that overcometh will I grant to sit with me in my throne, even as I also overcame, and am set down with my Father in his throne"..Revelation 3:21.

Those fortunate ones will find their guru, their best friend. Moments of "painful awareness" are real! It takes a good friend to bring about the best in the one toiling along the path.

Invoking the Divine Light or Cosmic Energy is the best way to overcome obstacles. Aum is the embodiment of Its Power and Truth. It is a powerful tool for attracting higher forces until, one day, It sparks a "flame" deep inside the practitioner. Once lit, it is a self-generating force of continued benediction.

> She was with the Master at the foothills of the Himalayas. He instructed her to go out into the evergreen forests to listen to the sounds of the early morning and report to him. She returned to tell him she had heard: the rustle of the trees, the wind, and the birds as the sun rose at dawn. "No! Go back tomorrow and listen again.."
>
> She returned to the woods the following morning and came back with another list: the distant gurgling brook, the cars, the cows... "No! Go back again!" and she did.
>
> The next time she reported that she had heard the calm and silence of the dawn. "You are getting there... go back again!"
>
> She returned into the woods on another morning, one last time during the 'teaching'. It took her a very long time to return this time: 'I heard the silence within myself', she told the Master. "You've got It... now identify it and become one with It!"

When negative qualities recur, replace them with the opposite positive quality. List them in a diary to ensure the feelings become more aware. When emotions arise, catch them, look at them, and eradicate their power by no longer identifying with them. In this way, disarm the emotion. If the emotion erupts before awareness can be enlisted, assume the role of witness of the erupted emotion and detach from it.

Desires arise from experiences of the past which are now projecting into the present and future. Selfish desires are outgrowths of competition and comparisons. Whatever the source, they must be sublimated after careful evaluation. *Leaving a desire to the faculty of emotion becomes a burden of attachment.*

> and the Master wrote:
>
> "Let us develop a sense of gratitude to the Lord, by focusing our attention on what we have, which a good many less fortunate have not and are yearning for. By refusing to crave for objects which we do not have, we shall be conserving a lot of energy which alone can give us the peace within and a capacity to act rightly in the world.."

Negative thoughts must be disarmed by following the rules of sense and speech control. Avoid discussions about sex, money, various pleasures, or any other indulgences.

Investigate all "beliefs": Pay attention to what people "think of me". Listen to what people say and assess what they perhaps mean. Correct the mistakes detected.

Question "pain and pleasure" and how it is experienced. Perhaps they are values given in terms of what you like and dislike?

What concepts have I now formed of Energy and where do I feel pain?

- What about Light? Is it a concept?
- What are my daily "attitudes"?

This state of mind must be perfected in preparation for thoughtless meditations. The mind can control breath and therefore mind must surrender to the greater sensitivity of refined senses. Once the Mind is carried on the waves of breath, (starting with *Ham' aa - Soo' ham* and then by watching breath), it reaches the shores of Awareness: the Self as Aum.

Purpose of Stabilising Breath

Prana is Awareness in Consciousness, the Total Cosmic Energy in the Universe (both manifest and unmanifest). *Pranayama* is also the practice of breath-stabilizing and watching, that enables the seeker to attune to the Cosmic Breath of the Universe that expands and collapses, exactly as one does while breathing. The same Life Force radiates to all parts of the physical body from the divine cave with inspiration and collapses back into it with each expiration—both in awareness.

The practice of breath-stabilization and watching allows the inner self to become "isolated" from the influx of thoughts. Through pranayama, the seeker gradually gains control over the mind, intellect, and ego as chitta. This process involves the control of inspiration, pause, expiration and pause with actualization of the soul for the purpose of concentration, meditation, and ecstasy in oneness. All of this happens while one watches, looks, feels, and listens to the rhythm of breathing.

Pranayama and character-building go hand in hand. With a purified character the *Guru* leads the seeker to awaken the dormant creative life-force or *Shakti.* The seeker is able to feel the energy or *prana* spread and retract from the divine cave and travel along the nerve channels and spinal cord, where Divine Energy flows.

Pranayama leads to control of emotions and limits selfish desires, so that the mind is prepared for meditation. This happens by increasing alpha waves in the brain that have calming effects on both emotion and mind.

Pranayama cures "nervous disorders" and refines sense perception. First, though the body must relax and employ energizing exercises as preparatory techniques to deep meditation.

The brain is divided into two hemispheres; the left controlling the right side of the body and vice versa. The brain has two parts. The more primitive or posterior brain at the base of the skull is the contemplative brain, the seat of wisdom. The frontal lobe is the active and calculating brain that deals with the external world.

Yogis realized the various disparities in the structure of the brain, lungs and other parts of the body. They adopted *asanas* (postures) and *pranayamas* (breath-watching techniques) to promote even development, equal extension and attention to both sides of the body. They do this by introducing the *prana* (breath) in and out to pass through each nostril in turn, thus revitalizing the two hemispheres as well as the front and back of the brain.

By changing sides for inhalation and exhalation, the energy reaches the remotest parts of the brain through the *nadis* (tracts) criss-crossing the *chakras.* The seeker gains the secret of even and balanced action in all four quarters of the brain, and through this experiences peace, poise, and harmony.

This technique requires meticulous attention and firm determination. Energies are channeled to discipline the breath for the purpose of eventual spiritualizing of the body and mind. The brain and the fingers must learn to channel the in and out breaths while in constant communication with each other. When this is refined, it takes the seeker to the innermost self where *dharana* or concentration is directed to the *mantra "Ham'Saa - So'Ham."*

The fingers are kept on the nostrils throughout the ***grounding breathing exercise***. The head is moved in different positions. When the head is dropped on the chest, the frontal lobes become silent and the posterior contemplative brain becomes active.

- *Practice this pranayama on an empty stomach or at least four hours after the last meal.*
- *Sit in the asana (sitting posture) of your choice and breathe normally through the nostrils.*
  Gently contract the lower abdominal muscles by pulling in the abdomen as if towards the navel.
  Pull the shoulder blades back until they both meet with shoulders pulled back. Hold the chin up parallel to the floor with the breast plate lifted in line with the tip of the chin.
- *Focus your attention into the divine cave behind the kutastha between the eyebrows and roll your tongue back: keep* ***looking*** *at the Cosmic Vision in the east.*
- *Be conscious and aware of the breath going in and out of the lungs. Watch the breath. Continue* ***watching*** *in this way with eyes closed, for at least five minutes.*
- *Practice pranayama or breath-stabilizing with the abdominal muscles contracted. Watch inspiration (4 seconds) and then a pause (4 seconds); next watch expiration (4 seconds) and then a pause (4 seconds).*

*Each time, remember to look at the Cosmic Vision in the east, roll the tongue back, watch the breathing, **listen** to the Cosmic Inner Sound, and **feel** the lower abdominal muscles pulled into the spine and towards the navel, thereby releasing the diaphragm for breathing.*

- *Close the eyes without tensing the eyeballs; the looking should be passive, receptive and assuming an inward gaze into the divine cave. The ears are alert to the Cosmic Sound of Aum and the receptive 'witness' watches the breathing with the tongue rolled back.*
- *First exhale maximally until the lungs are comfortably empty.*
  Now enter the preparatory stages of maintaining even breath durations throughout the four components of breathing (Inspiration-pause-Expiration-pause), all the time maintaining a contracted lower abdominal muscle. Watch the harmonized breathing.
  Fill the lungs maximally without exerting too much effort.
  Pause for four seconds by immobilizing the diaphragm and contracting the lower abdominal muscles.
  Now exhale slowly until the lungs are empty; then pause.
  Continue in the same manner for five minutes until the rhythm is smooth.
- *Withdraw into the divine cave by willfully withdrawing fron the body and the senses. Contract and relax the twelve muscle groups until you sense the energy alone. Rest in the divine cave in Awareness.*
  Now ensure that the tongue is rolled back, and the gaze lifted upwards and into the kutastha, looking at the Cosmic Mother of Infinity.
- *You are now in the astral phase of the divine cave. Listen to the Cosmic Sound through the right ear. Watch the breath.*
- *To increase devotion, contract and relax body parts and acknowledge the presence of His Power in you.*

At the end of expiration, adjust the fingers to block first the right nostril and then the left.

- *Block the right nostril and narrow the left nostril with thumb and index finger and exhale until the lung is empty;*
- *Then readjust the fingers to block the left nostril for inspiration through the right nostril followed by a pause;*
- *Readjust the fingers and repeat by blocking the right nostril and expire through the left nostril followed by a pause.*
- *Continue for five to ten minutes.*

Imagine the ida (parasympathetic channel) rising from the base of the spine towards the left eye and transfer the current to the right eye. At the same time, shut the left nostril and open the right nostril and exhale through it:

- *Exhale through the pingala (sympathetic channel) which courses from the right eye to the tail of the spine;*
- *With left nostril closed (with index finger), inhale the pingala channel towards the right eye and shut the right nostril as you transfer the current to the left eye;*

- *Shut the right nostril and exhale through the left nostril while the ida current falls towards the tail;*
- *Repeat the sequence for 15 times until the body is relaxed and the mind and body grounded.*
- *This exercise stabilizes the autonomic nervous system and the endocrine glands of the sukshma sharira (physiological-psychological astral body). Practice strengthens nerves and prepares the seeker for dhyana (meditation).*
- *This pranayama allows the deep penetration of oxygen.*
- *The nerves are calmed and purified, and the mind becomes still and lucid.*
- *It keeps the body warm, destroys disease and gives serenity.*
- *The vital energy is drawn from cosmic energy through inhalation and passes the chakras, autonomic nervous system, as well as the endocrine glands which control the whole of the body.*
- *The respiratory center is stimulated to be tranquil.*
- *The intellect leads the mind to right living, right thinking, quick actions and sound adjustments.*

This is because the "rhythm" of life is breath, which is characterized by the expansion and contraction of the chest or inspiration and expiration. It is the umbilical cord through which the mortal connects with the Cosmic Mother.

The ***mind*** *has a polarity that draws upon itself a nexus of its own: it has the characteristic of* ***stillness*** *experienced within the divine cave.*

Establishing one's breath with dharana (concentration), using the mantra "Ham'saa - So'ham," binds the rhythm of the breath to the rhythm of pulsating life everywhere.

Such harmony with surrounding life forces will bring about an inner stillness; indeed, prolonged periods of such concentration can lead to loss of awareness of the body.

This mantra can be used before the invocation of the Divine Light or Aum.

Continue this dharana (concentration) for as long as you can, until centralized.

This exercise can be continued silently before going to sleep or in the din of things and beings; however, when used in these situations, the spine need not be straight.

Pranic Pranayama

Concentrate on the Muladhara Chakra (at the base of the spine) after the necessary preparations of asana, pranayama and dharana.

- ***Look*** *at the Cosmic Vision in the divine cave behind the two eyebrows and roll your tongue back.*
- ***Watch*** *the breath and* ***listen*** *to the Cosmic Sound.*
- *Once the mind has been* ***silenced*** *and is tranquil, raise the pranic shakti or*

"life force" as a cool inspiratory breath up to the base of the skull and then forward towards the kutastha chaitanya.
After a pause of four seconds, expire a warm current down to the base chakra. Immediately *re-start inspiration without a pause* *between inspiration and expiration. (This is different from the Ham'saa So'ham Technique)*

This exercise is done by concentrating and ***feeling*** *the currents in the divine cave of the brain and spinal cord.*

- *Observe all changes.*

This is the most difficult yogic practice to perfect but is also the most refreshing and rewarding, requiring perfect discipline.

- *The breath moves like a string holding pearls of a rosary (mala). The chakras are the pearls and the breath is the string.*
- *The body, breath, mind, and intellect (chitta) move towards the Self like a spider returning to the center of its web.*

In the beginning, the breath is rough and the mind and intellect waver. There must be unity of the *chitta* (mind, intellect, ego) and the breath, so that the self ("Me") can reign it in to **secure stillness** to become "I" in the **silence.**

This state can only be achieved through controlled discipline of the body, senses and the mind *(yama* or universal commandments and *niyama* or rules of self-purification). *Chitta* is kept still through *pratyahara* (withdrawal from the senses) and *dharana* (concentration). Prolonged withdrawal with concentration or *dharana* allows the attention to **expand into silence**. It now becomes released in meditation *(dhyana).* It is here that the Will becomes submerged in the Self.

This subtle difference between stillness and silence has to be experienced. Stillnes is achieved by quietening the koshas (sheaths) that envelop the body from the skin to the self. This is done by *pratyahara* or withdrawing from the senses.

These sheaths are the: *annamaya* (anatomical), *pranamaya* (physiological), *manomaya* (emotional mind), *vignanamaya* (intellectual), and *anandamaya* (causal) sheaths. (Please refer to Figure 4).

Once stillness of the body is secured, learn to control and watch the breath. *Next, silence the mind and the intellect* by watching the breath and listening to the Cosmic Sound. *Finally, walk into the silence of the bliss sheath and become one with It.*

- Imagine drawing up of the *Devi Shakti* (also called *Kundalini* by some schools of thought) or Life Force up the divine cave, with a cold breath experienced during inspiration and felt at the back of the throat.
- Direct the current into the spiritual eye in the East between the eyebrows, as if making a forward sweep from the back of the head into the *kutastha-chaitanya,* between the eyebrows; retain the breath for a count of four seconds.
- Now exhale, sending down a warm energy current down the spine into the

Muladhara Chakra again felt as a warmth in the back of the throat. Re-inspire immediately without a pause.

The seeker should begin with 14 breaths and gradually increase the number until he becomes centered in the divine cave of the spinal cord and brain, free of all the sense interference.

The state experienced is that of deep-sleep, but the dimension is one of acute awareness and profound stillness and silence.

Here Watch - Look - Listen - Feel all Changes taking place in every cell of the body during *Sadhana* or spiritual austerities.

Reiki is Channeling Prana

Prana or Aum, enters the physical body through the "mouth of God" in the medulla. It can be stored within the medulla oblongata and released at will towards the part of the body or person requiring healing.

- The "healer" is *Aum.*
- The will to heal is also individualized *shakti* desiring.
- The body is only a medium "through" which healing energy is transferred to the diseased or afflicted.

"Laying of the hand" or a gentle massage can be used while the energy is channeled into the body of the afflicted. Maintain a positive attitude of success, free of criticism and concentrate deeply within the shell of the healing Divine Light of *Aum.*

Let the Light flow "through" you and NOT from you! See yourself as a channel giving the energy as a laser beam. If the mind begins to chatter, divert its activity by talking to the part of the body requiring healing.

Reverence for Life

There is an American Indian story that describes the first people on earth had the Powers of Mother Nature but *had no respect for Her Wholeness*. It was apparent that if these powers were abused for self-service, the Universe would be destroyed. The Knowledge of the Laws of Nature were therefore kept hidden from them. Mother Nature would reveal them only to those that loved Her.

As they traveled life, She passed Her truths to receptive minds through images. They were inspired to walk the spiritual paths of harmony with all of creation. Over time, there were tribes of people with this knowledge and She called them *whole people.* The *whole people* spoke of the Circle of Life for all to hear. Yet, there were many who just could not *see* this wholeness!

Saying grace before meals is an acknowledgment of a reverence for the wholeness of life! After grace most of us resume chatter. To overcome this, cultivate the sense of taste, smell, and sight as regards the meal.

Ask if I am hungry and want to eat?

Analyze why I wish to eat.

Does my body require nourishment, and if so, why?

For survival or indulgence or perhaps for the pleasure of self gratification?

Review the process of food gathering:

How much did I kill and rudely acquire off the earth's surface?

Did what I collected have a life?

How did I cook it?

Did I require the energy of fire?

Who coordinated these actions of collecting, cooking and even the process of eating and digestion so that I may be nourished?

How many had to sacrifice their life so that I may eat?

Do I recall this sacrifice while I sit down to eat?

Why do I need to eat?

If I need the human body as an instrument in my search for the Most High, all life that I had to kill in the processing of my nourishment must benefit from the energy vibrations of sacrificial thoughts.

Analyze the "Grace" said at tables before meals:

brahma-arpanam-brahma-havir
brahma-agnau brahmanaa hutam
brahm-aiva-tena-ganta-vyam
brahma-karma-samaa-dhinaa

Brahman (God) is the oblation; *Brahman* is the clarified butter; the oblation offered is by *Brahman*; it is offered into the fire which is also *Brahman*; *Brahman* shall be reached by him who sees *Brahman* in all actions.

Constant Awareness of one's connected-ness with the Cosmic Mother is a self-healing and self-communicating pulsation emitting from one's foundational level. This creates an "interconnected complex" resulting in resolutions despite the push and pulls, twists and turns of all our external, mental, physiological and intellectual activities.

Physiology and Psychology of the Meditative State

The practitioner, at this stage, can discern the difference of experience in the state of concentration *(dharana)* and the state of meditation *(dhyana).*

In the early stages of concentration, wandering thoughts disturb consciousness as:

- Memories of recent events;
- Emotions of these memories (anger, joy or sorrow); and
- Overwhelming feelings of suppressed desires.

These thoughts must be allowed to surface, then gradually dispelled from the crevices of the past. Even after attaining silence in concentration, the experience may be disturbed by sudden, unusual vivid experiences from the past. These are usually memories of the unconscious that have not yet been purged.

Even after such forceful memories have been purged and dispelled, the silence may be disturbed by "neutral thoughts" of experiences of "nothingness" or body-lessness. These, too, must be allowed to fade away by the vigilant mind as an unattached witness.

The practitioner at this stage has gained advanced control over the technique of *pranayama, pratyahara, and dharana* and is able to assume *asana* for prolonged periods of time. In this state, the mind is at complete rest, as is the body.

In this state of meditative rest, the physiological processes allow:

- The heart rate to decrease; and
- The breathing to become slow and periodic.

Pranayama now charges the lower half of the body with vital energy (felt as a tightening of the lower abdominal muscles) and the upper half of the body feels feather light. The practitioner is ready to start meditation seriously. He becomes aware of the astral dimension of his being. In this meditative state, the practitioner is sure there exists only consciousness.

This is a state of the "sixth sense" which operates within the "physiological and psychological functions" of the body. This is different from the operation through the physical body. It is an acute awareness that this state is enormous, powerful, transparent, and radiant. The EEG records a baseline only of continuous alpha waves at this level of meditation.

This physiological slowing of the heart and respiration may persist even in the awake state of the practitioner's life, causing physiological changes in the body.

Spiritual Potentials of Intense Meditative State:

Every stage in the practitioner's progress towards deeper meditation is a small step towards increased understanding of one's own spiritual potential. The depth of meditation is an indication of success the seeker is making in his *sadhana* to erase the ego as *chitta* (mind-intellect-ego complex) and becoming one with the Universe.

The practitioner must acknowledge that (the experience) the entry into the astral dimension is only a "stopover" on the long journey of *sadhana* (spiritual self-effort). It is not the destination. This state of partial union has a psychic potential. There may be out-of-body experiences. The practitioner may see that there is an exact counterpart of the physical world in the astral or energy-world in the "form" of thoughts and emotions.

This disembodied being or "spirit" possesses all the emotional and intellectual characteristics of the previously embodied being, even though the physical body has died. If this being had very strong attachments to the material world, this interest remains and will manifest in another future physical existence.

However, if the practitioner's spirit has reached a higher plane of astral dimension through spiritual growth (meditation while in a physical state), at physical death, the disembodied being will transcend the lower regions of the astral dimension or Lesser Heaven.

If the practitioner is able to transcend the lower levels of body and mind, he enters the causal-state of being. This is a superior spiritual state of *karana.* It is the root-state of all previous manifestations of the practitioner's long journey of manifestations over thousands and perhaps millions of years.

The causal or *karanic* state of being has only one quality. It has the quality of transparency. Its shape and color are beyond the realms of description. Characteristics of the physical world (color, shape, smell, sight, texture) are unable to extend beyond the astral dimension.

If the practitioner awakens to the *pranic* energy of the astral plane, he can transmit energy to another person for goodwill and healing. If the recipient of such energies is also a practitioner of meditation, he may experience the presence of the person's astral being (mental and emotional) as a distinctive presence. The presence may be sensed as a characteristic odor of the person, similar to what is experienced in a dream state.

> My eyes lifted to the photograph above the computer. The last word of this material was typed as my chin rested on my right hand. A beautiful scent of sandal-wood emitted from my right hand. There was an instinctive awareness of the Master's presence. He had given his approval!

Once the practitioner transcends the lower astral plane (mental and emotional beingness), he enters the higher state of intellectual *karana.* This transparent state (physical deep sleep) consists only of knowledge and intellectual "ideas" of the ego.

Here, in the *karana* or causal dimension, the practitioner attains a spiritual awakening of extreme depth that permeates even his awake state of beingness. This is a continuation of the experience in the seat of meditation.

Once the practitioner gains entrance into the *higher astral planes*, he develops paranormal abilities that he can transport into the physical world. He no longer requires the physical senses and organs of actions to assist him in acts carried out in the physical dimension.

The psychokinetic energy expended at every stage of advancement is a function of the Will of the practitioner. *Attachment to a "stage of development*" is a function of the practitioner's purity. He has preconceived images in his memory. This determines his will to continue with *sadhana* or become stagnant at this level. The memory of this determines his future rebirth environment where he will continue his evolution towards perfection.

Physical attachments restrain the being and compel him to return to the physical plane. *Astral attachments* may occur because he values the emotional and mental dimensions of beingness. This leads to confinement in the astral plane, which may persist until the astral being desires an alternative and renewed awareness of himself.

He may seek to be reborn physically for further evolution. If this happens, he is born again as a mortal and evolves from where he left off. In meditation, he ascends his physical, physiological, psychological, and intellectual beingness *and enters the causal state of beingness*. The realization that there is a greater spiritual benefit with higher identification allows the practitioner to abandon the restrictive attachments to the lower levels and ascend towards the *karana* or causal dimension. Here he awaits the grace of final oneness with the Cosmic Self.

Ascending Life Force in Meditation as Chitta

When as *chitta* or mind-intellect-ego, the practitioner enters the astral dimension in meditation, the dormant life-force is awakened and begins functioning through the altar of God in the divine cave. It courses through the five spiritual centers or *chakras*, each time entering deeper into its increasingly subtler astral dimension. Disharmonies may be felt as electrical" sensations such as chills, shivers or heat.

Discomfort may be experienced due to impurities in the up-surging energy that take the form of mental images of possessive emotions. Unless these are purged, they return into the astral dimension as heat or similar sensations. (Please refer to Figure 11)

Once the practitioner has succeeded in purging this trapped heat, he experiences freedom of movement in the life energy through the opened channels of the spinal cord *(sushumna, vajra, chitrini, and finally, brahmanadi).* (see Figure 15)

If the experience is associated with apprehension (manifestation of a fearing dissolving ego), the practitioner is asked to start the *"Ham'saa - So'ham"* breathing exercises. The teacher usually assists in this by tapping the student on the head.

Unless the ego relaxes its hold on the mind, greater consciousness cannot manifest. Concentration, meditation, and *samadhi* are processes for shattering the ego. With each partial union of "Me" with the "I", the grip of the ego gradually weakens. Once the greater awakening occurs in the awake state, one does not need to enter meditation to achieve the state of union. (see Figure 14.)

It must be noted that the *svadhisthana chakra* (sacral plexus) is an unconscious center. It cannot withdraw at will; instead, the practitioner must persist in *yama and niyama* and allow a spontaneous state of evolution to occur. As he evolves towards a greater awareness, the practitioner feels a "moving" sensation up and down the spine: this sensation is a sign of progress in *sadhana.* (see Figure 18 and 19)

> *Pranayama of Kriya Yoga* was shown to me by a friend and colleague who was visiting me from India. So exhilarating was the experience of this meditation technique that I began spending long hours at it. On one Saturday, this exercise led me to a very painful astral experience. I resolved to 'feel' [the pain] it through until I could break this barrier. I persisted for nearly thirty minutes until I could bear it no longer and I ended the exercise.
>
> The Master was no more. Since the younger *Swamis* could not help, I turned to the *Yogini, Swamini Sharadapriyananda...* "There is nothing to be concerned about. You need not be in such a hurry to get there! Take the mind slowly there into the silence without shaking yourself!"

The writings of a Japanese mystic described the movement of the *chitta* through the various depths of one's astral being. He described the technique of stabilizing oneself when faced with similar disequilibrium. The need of an experienced *guru* is necessary and advisable! This is not to say that a sincere *sadhak* will not receive help when it is wanted!

Conclusion

Material well-being and adjusted thinking allows creative expression of the Spirit. Not only must man reflect upon the Light but manifest as the Light of Consciousness. To do that he must pass into the sphere of the *kutastha.* Once Man abandons his vain ideas of a separate existence, he attains the world of the Ultimate Truth. Here he is released in the embrace of Oneness with the Spirit.

> "Jesus saith unto him, I am the way [meditating through Christ Center}, the truth, and the life: no man cometh unto the Father, but by me." .. John 14.6

SECTION FIVE

Topics in Section Five

Spiritual Journey is Harmonizing Forces of Opposite Polarities

The Spiritual Journey starts with dealing with both negative *[tamas]* and positive *[rajas]* forces. Neither are bad or good. They are the two polarities of existence *[sattva]*. Existence is both Bliss and Truth. Existence is Awareness. Awareness is Knowledge. This physical manifestation is because of It. She or He is *sat-chit-anand* or Existence-Knowledge-Bliss.

The journey takes the seeker towards God. By focusing on the two opposing forces, the seeker travels a pathless path towards Changelessness. *Raja Yoga* accelerates the speed of this spiritual journey.

Like a research scientist, the seeker should have no expectations. He must concentrate on the harmonizing the polarities *[sattva]* and reducing the distance between *Kurukshetra* [in the spinal cord] and *Dharmakshetra* [in the crown of the head].

His meditation should be to stabilize the gaze, the breath, the position of the tongue and the feel of the divine cave and its coverings.

Vishuddha Chakra

Preamble

The *Vishuddha Chakra* is symbolically the final adjustment site. Personal powers of ability to love the Cosmic Universe are intuitively understood. Her whispers come from a state of one's own grounding. The changes and adjustments through *sadhana* render the causal-astral-physical foundations almost healed and free of pain of maladjustment. The seeker is now able to validate himself in his connectedness. The seeker is moving upwards into his own self-healing and self-expansion.

> "Know ye not that ye are the temple of God, and that the Spirit [soul] dwelleth in you?" Corinthians 3:16

Vishuddha Chakra
Fifth or Throat Chakra or Cervical Plexus

The Law of Karma or Justice works within the seeker by eliminating all that is unnecessary in his thoughts. He walks knowing that the Universe will grant him what is best for him. He is able to consider and judge the effects of his actions, on future opportunities capable of benefiting the many around him. He begins to work in the present. His inner convictions carry him to acting for a collective goodness. He starts to validate all the theories presented to him up to this point. The responses give him the necessary balance and harmony. He is freed of thoughts and desires that previously limited him. He becomes a hermit and breaks away from crowds and festivities that do not allow him further inner growth.

The seeker is now able to self-direct through self-discipline. He feels accountable to Mother Nature. He instinctively knows his mistakes affect the whole! This awareness that 'I am in Her' allows him to rise as well as expand in Her gift of peace and tranquillity.

The symbol of the throat or *vishuddha chakra* is a circle in a flat plane; it is a circumambulation of completion, a circle of balanced understanding. It is both a disc and a sphere, which signifies that there is room for growth and expansion into the infinite sphere, from all the directions. It is at this fifth step of evolution that one is meant to express the joy of the Spirit, in music, and in poetry. There is a sense that he possesses something at last, that he can give back to Mother Earth.

In the undeveloped state, this *chakra* becomes an instrument of the ego, instead of being the flute to sing His tune of surrender, for a greater good. The ego absorbs all human attention and blocks the flow of Divine Consciousness. Nonetheless, his egoistic creative-force has taken Man to new heights of achievement. Unfortunately, Man has identified with these achievements and has arrogantly assumed the role of the "doer".

There is no pain in sacrificing the ego. He is the monster that promotes separation and suffering from a loss-of-connectedness with Mother Nature. He can become one with the overturned Tree-of-Life. He can rise vertically up to his roots and align with God and also expand horizontally working with Her on Earth. Both are acts of Love!

> and the Master wrote:
>
> "Love is the heart of religions, the theme of all classical works of art and literature, the song of all devotees. Scientists know only what love does...not what love is. Love can indeed empty our asylums, perhaps all our prisons, may be all our hospitals. People suffer in life due to lack of love. Love is to human hearts what the sun is to flower!"

Instinctive knowing and a pursuit of the Path of Meditation have led some aspirants to the conclusion that they are really not the doers: this realization of their true identity with the Spirit is perhaps the only way that "Me" can identify and disappear into the "I". In the calm inner light of divine perception, the seeker recognizes an awakening intuition. As the seeker gets into the habit of meditation he comes to accept that this is the only way to harness the spiritual forces and guard against the restless forces of sense inclinations and past habits.

The fifth *chakra* is the first filter of the body and as such is very sensitive to pollutants, viruses, and bacteria. Diffidence to the laws of living impedes the normal functioning of this center. This center is also very sensitive to any illusions of separation from the forces of nature and all life.

Persons who assume responsibility for the behaviour of others create in themselves anxiety and guilt, only aggravating the crisis being faced. These situations are characterized by "I said.. and you said... why was it said". Efforts at self-justification are only stress overloads for this center and eventually will cause blockages at this level, especially on the left side of the autonomic nervous system in the *Ida.*

Surrender with absolute faith and letting go of things and beings that you formerly depended upon is the spiritual effort or *sadhana* of this center. Surrendering includes giving up self-doubt, self-embarrassment, self-guilt, and the old self-image.

The seeker is urged to dive deeper into his divine cave until his inner divine being becomes the image of the Universe: this is the marriage of surrender and true love *with the other half!*

Love in Committed Partnership

The soul thinks in images and nourishes itself on images which materialize in reality. Dwelling in love on these images in the mind and soul, allows man to identify with his inner and outer life partner. Accept and take the time to listen to the images of your life partner. Observe and appreciate the image. Give and receive the message of these images gracefully. Let them empower you to become reminders of a divine relationship of two halves of one soul. Expand into the image of love's giving and receiving.

Most marital problems centre around wanting to 'change' your partner to fit into the mold of one's own liking or exerting power over the other! No spouse can change or nor can any of them take the responsibility for the behaviour of the other. The wise tell us to allow each one to grow in the Light of the other. There is no need to block the Light .

Dwelling on images of harmony in marriage and friendship become flesh, and begin to live among partners. Preconceived ideas learnt from parents block the sunshine from entering relationships. Each friendship is unique. Each marriage has a structure and a unique potential to work with. Together, friends must figure out how they will mutually face the world. Before that is possible, the couple must become equal halves of one whole in love. This love becomes the inner strength in the heart *chakra*.

Blocks at this level in the *vishuddha chakra* result in guilt and pent-up anger which can explode into harsh words. One partner may not have the wisdom of the *sadhak* or seeker. The seeker must surrender to his inner guide, the innate *guru* or teacher. Together with the inner guide, they can assume the role or image of a *"saakshi"* or witness. Together they can see things as they really are and in the correct perspective!

The seeker must remain centred in the higher awareness. The vision of a Higher Power prompts all future actions which guide the seeker with a promise self-renewal. Perpetual stress loads at this level create cynics and critics prone to outbursts of frustration and pseudo-intellectualism. Man finds himself helpless in impossible situations because the ego hits back with the tongue. Responses made in anger or cynicism pollute the deep blue sea of meditation.

Provocation of the ego only sparks reaction, not correction. In the realm of the fifth cervical or *vishuddha chakra,* the subtle activities of the ego cause man to constantly *role-play* in his interaction with others. He appears a caricature of pride or *mada*. The solution to the whole game is to transcend it.

The fifth *chakra* is also the centre of diplomacy which is brought to play to overcome adversity. Even *Krishna* preferred the use of diplomacy over force, turning to force only as a last resort to uphold *dharma* or righteousness.

The ***Mahabharata*** is one of the world's greatest books and the longest poem ever written. It is fifteen times the length of the Bible. Written in *Sanskrit,* it is composed of ancient stories which date back to the fifth century B.C. In a hundred thousand stanzas, the poem gives tangible origins to the many Indian beliefs, teachings, thoughts, and legends which even today are part of the Indian thought and culture.

The story teller arrests the mainstream of the action of *Mahabharata* for a short while to tell different stories to illustrate a comment made in the main story. In one short story, *Krishna* visits the two sets of cousins [*Kauravas and Panadavas*] to counsel them on the preference of dialogue over war between them. [harmonising the polarities in the War of *Kurukshetra*]

In the ***Bhagavad Gita*** (Holiest book of the Hindus), which occupies a central part of the written epic, the conversation between *Arjuna* and *Krishna* emphasizes the roles of human Conscience and Consciousness. The epic is the royal initiation of mankind into political, social, moral, and spiritual codes of ethics!

The *fifth chakra is the flute expressing the sweetness of the heart to delight* oneself first and then the others. Many nerves pass through this centre and end up in the sub-plexus, the *hamsa,* just before the sixth *chakra.* The *mantra hamsa-soham* is the involuntary utterance of the soul or *jiva* with every act of inspiration and expiration.

Conditioning can be built into this *chakra* by training the mind which has been exposed to education, programming, and society. Only wise parents and teachers have the ability to program a growing child and youth with the *dharmic* or righteous attitudes to life and living. *Adharmic or contrary conditioning* teaches us to react to things and issues that are dead and meaningless.

Upon assuming the role of a *saakshi*, the witness psychically opens the *chakra* and sees it as it truly is. *Discretion and constant vigilance coupled with self-correction matures discretion* during the mind's pilgrim through evolution.

The Primordial Being, the *Prakriti,* then gives us the collective consciousness to become One with the Whole. This collective consciousness becomes actualized in an experience of enlightenment which is felt acutely within the divine cave of the central nervous system.

While working with this center, the vibrations may be felt in the index finger of the left hand or in the second left toe. This *chakra* controls the sense of hearing and is concerned with *feelings for others* and understanding through discrimination.

With mind and emotions controlled and surrender achieved, the fifth *chakra* promises constant, steady peace of mind. One sees the present, past and future with courage and forgiveness. There is freedom from greed, malice, and pride.

Intuitive Awareness and Sensory Mind

When a strong-willed ego meditates upon the blessedness of the soul, it is consumed by the soul's superior joy and begins to lose its desire for sense pleasures. The seeker now has a standard of comparison between the two joys. Even while engaged in sense pleasures, the deluded intellect cannot forget the joy experienced in meditation.

Once the incorruptible nature of the soul is discovered, the seeker can restrain and discipline his sense desires by spiritual means. Those who embrace the inner calmness of self-control, discrimination, and meditation remain on the plane of intuitive soul perception; this is a stable state and those who meditate deeply and daily seldom fall.

The only reliable self-disciplinarian is the true self. Once it has acquired soul-wisdom, intuition leads the seeker to soul-perception of the truth, where there is no accumulation of objective knowledge through the intellect. Intuitive intelligence's perception is that of the witness alone.

At this stage, the seeker becomes extremely aware that even his refined speech is restricted to *words*. Perceptions take the form of *thoughts*, but even this faculty is limited. The seeker knows that the highest experience must be *perception beyond words and thoughts*; that is, beyond mind. Perception beyond the mind is the knowing of the heart, which is under the control of the *Devi* of Speech. It is beyond words, senses, and concepts. It is ethereal and radiates like the sun's rays.

> We had been summoned to Mysore while my first grandchild was entombed in the mother's womb. Every evening, the pregnant mother was asked to sit with the Master for a snack. He intermittently and nonchalantly spoke to the unborn child and fed him birth advice and citrus fruit. We were all amused with the goings-on! This grandchild has the precious gift of always speaking the truth and standing by righteousness...and he loves citrus fruit!
>
> When the same mother carried our second grandchild, the Master fed him stories of bravery and valor while the mother was fed grapes. This child is a little soldier who withstands intolerable physical pain [he underwent surgery for a congenital heart condition during the first few months of his life].. and he loves grapes.

This perception of an inner knowing is felt by awareness and experienced as the manifestations of grace of *Gauri* and *Guru* or Mother and Teacher. It is heard as an experience in the resonance of *Aum*. It evokes an intense emotional response in the recipient of grace.

Physical words are felt on the eardrum which receives the vibrations of sound, and interpreted by consciousness by its resonance.

- *Beware of using words as traps for others and yourself, by asking leading questions: Analyze when I have used the technique to bolster my ego and emotion "to make a point"!*

Similarly, the tone of voice itself can serve as a magnet capable of attracting seekers on a similar path. When a seeker is in contact with the ascending Life Force (now symbolically represented by the *Devi* of Speech as *Sarasvati* or the Goddess of Learning), She clears the way and gives the seeker the persistence, courage, wisdom, and circumstances to achieve the goal of *sadhana* or self-effort.

Recognition of the presence of this Creative Energy or Life Force or *Shakti or Aum* (also called *Kundalini* by some schools) is to bow to Her Motherhood (Nature). She is the Eternal Cosmic Intelligence, expressing Herself as the Universal Intelligence in the *Kutastha Chaitanya* or Christ-Krishna Center between the eyebrows and manifesting as a personal, secret experience.

Intuition

The soul is unmanifest and awake in the Spirit, as unthinkable thought, undisturbed by change. When the Spirit dreams, It dreams of Universes; when the soul dreams, it dreams of covers of bodies, physical, mental, and intellectual. Even while the Spirit and soul dream, they remain the same: on a substratum of Awareness and Consciousness.

The unmanifest soul manifests as the waker, dreamer, and deep sleeper. *Thought and sensations* are not part of the soul, but are experiences of the ego in a *dream.* Thinking under the influence of conditioned neurotransmitters and neurohormones, thought and thinker become inseparable components of the dream of an individualized egoistic soul or unenlightened *chitta.* This ego is identifying itself as "Me".

Thought and feeling do not exist is *deep sleep*, but there is awareness in unconsciousness. The seeker knows he exists: this moment of truth is *intuition.* It reveals the presence of the soul without the instruments of thought and feeling. Intuition is the Light capable of revealing itself as well as the thoughts and sensations projected by the ego.

Intuition is the bridge between the soul and ego's thoughts and sensations. If the seeker can remain without thoughts and sensations in the awake state (not in the unconscious deep sleep state), he can develop intuition, which is the inherent nature of the soul. Here he knows that knower, known, and knowing are one in their awareness of the soul.

Meditation is the means to keep your children good. She [the mother of the family] awakens well before the rest stir. In her meditation she focuses her goodwill by aligning her Centre of Will with that of her child's between the eyebrows in the *Kutastha*. She advises him his *dharma* or duties in life. She *loves* him for the sake of loving alone. She *feeds* him good thoughts of truthfulness, valor, kindness to others, good health, and charity. She envelops him with blessing and good cheer for the struggles he must face as he grows. This is what my Master taught me!

Sadhaks or seekers who meditate deeply until all thoughts are dissolved enter the halls of intuition, in the divine cave of meditation. He perceives the soul as created in the same image of Spirit.

Intuition or the awakening of awareness expresses itself in five forms, as determined by the effects of the five *koshas* or sheaths (*annamaya* or gross body, *pranamaya* or life force, *manomaya* or mind, *gyanamaya* or intellect, and *anandamaya* or bliss) inherent in awareness:

- Intuition of *annamaya kosha* as: "I exist with body and mind". This sheath is intuitive because in it there is a feeling of "myness"; It is experienced in the early stages of *asana*.
- *Pranic* energy of the *pranamaya kosha* coursing through every cell in the body, has an immediate intuitive knowledge of its own. Its ability to sustain itself through seeing, hearing, feeling subtle sensations, smelling, and tasting is intuitive. Its existence is intuitively felt in *pranayama* or breath-control *and pratyahara* withdrawal from the senses.
- The intuitive knowing of the mind or the *manomaya kosha* is the effect of combined perception and cognition through the senses, intermingled with some *prana* as well. This is again acknowledged through *pratyahara* or willful withdrawal from the senses *and dharana* or concentration.
- The intuition of the *gyanamaya kosha* is a function of the *buddhi* or thought itself. It is an expression of direct knowledge of the ego and the discriminative intellect, and is not disturbed by the turbulence of the mind. When fully developed through meditation, it gives birth to wisdom. This is experienced in successful *pratyahara* when the seeker who now resides within the divine cave is immersed in *dhyana* or meditation.
- The *anandamaya kosha* knows bliss as an all fulfilling divine experience of ultimate satisfaction. This is experienced in *dhyana* or thoughtless meditation *and samadhi* or thoughtless oneness.

While everyone has the first form of intuition, the remaining four have to be developed through meditation. Pure intuition is soul intuition: the knowing of the Soul by the soul.

She was leaving for Washington and called me for any messages for the Master. Apologies were sent. I would not be visiting him this year. On my way to work, my heart reveled in the beauty of the orange [the colour of his robes] sunset and a feeling love soared in my being. My heart whispered to envelop him in me: 'Oh I love you *Swamiji*'!

My daughter reached her destination and the Master's first question was: "..How is your Mummy? Will you please call her at once and give her this message: 'I love you more than you ever can'!"

My daughter was perplexed and protested that I should not be disturbed at work. He insisted and she complied. "I am sorry to disturb you but I have a message from *Swamiji....*" My heart missed a beat.. Our hearts had met in the soul-Soul experience of *shishya-guru* oneness!

Antardhvani — the Inner Sound of Aum

The *Devi (Aum)* may be experienced *as both a spiritual and a psychic experience:*

- The *spiritual experience* is a self-transformation felt as a Cosmic Fire on the horizon: It cannot be repeated at will. It is a profound realization of awareness of constantly living in a blissful state.
- The *psychic experience* is felt in the senses and powers of the mind.

In quiet moments of peace and reflection during meditation, a mood emerges to cause a stillness of the mind. Lights of the color of a rainbow are experienced in hues of yellows and blues, merging into each other like the splendor of the Northern Lights.

These experiences should encourage the seeker, but he should not indulge in the experience. The logical significance of these "lights" is that the mind was free of thoughts at the time. It is imperative that these "lights" should not be interpreted as anything beyond the *Guru* encouraging you to "keep going, as you are on the right path".

The light of the Cosmic Fire is a gift from the inner Mother-who-Removes-all-Difficulties or *Durga*, encouraging the seeker to pursue newer dimensions of spiritual experience, through *sadhana*. It is a very personal experience, and must not be subjected to interpretation.

The evolved seeker relates the experience to Energy of a Cosmic Vision of Cosmic Light beyond name, shape, or form. During such visual experiences in the inner gaze, the seeker also hears the Cosmic Sound of Aum. During deep meditation, the seeker experiences a sudden insight or a state of acute awareness, wherein all mistakes are realized and all things are seen as they really are. These are moments of "change" in oneself, and the seeker abandons habits of mechanical thinking, habitual responses, and reactions.

Eighteen months before he physically left us, the Master summoned me for the last time. I intended to go for two weeks and stayed with him for six weeks. Although we had spent a life-time together and his influence on the family including myself was profound, my ego and pride had refused to 'submit' to him in the open! Over the years, my inner self had been chiseled and molded mercilessly! His piercing gaze would remove every last shreds of my false personality 'coverings'! I spent a lot of time in the hermitage at the Himalayan foothills in meditation and profound regrets. There was no doubt in my mind that he had relentlessly hammered away at me for twentyfive years!

When it was all over I dared to ask: "What took you so long? Why did you not call me earlier?"

and the Master said:

"...You neither had the time nor the inclination for such a submission! You were too busy with your desires! Blinded by pride and egotism, you blazed the world! You analyzed my teachings and dissected them with your intellectualism and pragmatism! I wanted your heart! You gave me your heart this time: for the first time after so many years!"

Hearing

Vishuddha chakra serves the sense of hearing, the last of the physical five senses. Mind is the interpreter and consequently is the sixth sense.

The sense of hearing is represented by the element of Air: powerful, ethereal, and elusive. To hear the Inner Mother or *Devi* speak the Cosmic *Aum* is the ethereal experience, the crown of all powerful experiences.

Much energy is wasted listening to thoughts of mental speculation, self-defense, and self-justification. These interfering voices prevent one from hearing what another says, let alone what one should be hearing: *Aum.*

I attended many lectures over many *yagnas.* My mind would wander, contradict, analyze, accept, reject, and unconsciously assimilate! The Master followed every one of my unspoken thoughts and courted them with compassion during the lecture or after! He had this uncanny ability to pick every thought in the audience, a sign of a true teacher! Others voiced the same experience and opinion! Amazing grace!

Listening

Listening is an art and requires refinement. True messages have to be heard through all the veils of what the speaker is really trying to say. It requires subtlety of character to hear the inner voice. The power of hearing depends upon the ability to concentrate and the mind's willingness to relax completely and receive the word meaning of messages received. The ability to be a good listener is extremely important, and to be successful, one needs a depth of understanding and an ability to recall.

In order to sharpen the sense of hearing, one must stop listening to the chatter of thoughts in the mind. The seeker must become 'dead' or nonreactive to all extraneous actions and completely surrender to what is going on. In this way, the seeker ends all mental and physical arguments.

Replace all thought-reactions with positive sentences. Stop taking responsibility for the actions of others by reacting and responding to their hurt and insulted egos.

Exerting Will

Assertions of self-will, which are responses to spoken messages of another, have no validity beyond the individual. We may delude ourselves that the need for reaction will yield good results. Responses such as speaking loudly in the hope of arousing comprehension in another are false, and motivated by pushiness. Such dominance is a manifestation of an uncultivated Will. Sweet soft voices can also be a sign of deception: hearing, therefore, can be *sattvic* or harmonious, *rajasic* or restless, *and tamasic* or ignorant in quality.

Control of Speech

Speech has no relevance if there is no listener. At this fifth *chakra,* there is increasing interaction of the energies of the body and mind which come out as speech. There is a lack of awareness that control of speech comes from the mind.

To refine speech, one needs direct commitments, clear goals, and straight-forward thinking. The target must be clearly defined and tackled head on, with refinement and control of all the five senses.

Manipura or the navel or third *chakra* will make its last attempt to ensnare the seeker in its fire-wheel of emotions. It will flare up with all its power and imagination to prevent the surrender of the self-will. This fire of emotional struggle can be made to shift gear into the fire of enthusiasm, where ignorance is burned in the fire of wisdom.

Analysis of Speech

The seeker by this time recognizes intuitively that the Law of *Karma* or Justice unites every thought, word, and deed with all of Creation: 'What goes around comes around'! He also has the ability to return to the rooftops of his inner Self and look back at the footprints on the path of his spiritual journey. He should be able to see and ensure that his heart centre has no anger and no judgments. It should be empty and have the space for love to occupy the void created.

The body can be taught and molded into a spiritual tool which pushes ever onward in the pursuit of self-development:

- Listen to the small voice within urging me to listen to the inner ear;
- Keep a daily dairy to the discover old traps and habits which we often ignore;
- Surrender self-will.

Watch out for the lurking personality of the ego which may be trying to re-assert its old power:

- Sharpened discrimination and razor keen awareness are required; without these, the seeker is in serious danger of slipping.

Deterrents to spiritual efforts come from varying sources:

- Desires and doubts are major deterrents, and one must disempower them by will and discrimination.
- Watch out for the influence of friends and relatives who view monetary, political, and social gain as the only objects worthy of aspiration.

The road to spirituality is at first a lonely one: targets must be clear. Seeing the heart free of all judgments symbolizes resurrection above the separation from Creation. Co operation with things and beings is to accept the unity of all interactions in the Circle of Life. This intuitive experience gives the seeker the wisdom to make the right decisions in action and speech without the interfering emotion of guilt.

Speech is the final aberration. It reflects and manifests as judgmental thoughts, opinions and concepts, already embedded in his causal-psychological levels, where it is unmanifest. Limited concepts about ourselves also limit his freedom to move or speak. His personal expressions appear as distortions of the Real Self. Even those who do make gains through *sadhana*, may have a vulnerable system, where he stores his stresses that are triggered into activity, under intense stressful conditions.

The goal of *sadhana* is to increase options, by removing inner demands, negative thoughts and distorted images of self and others. Older tendencies can be seen in a new light. They can be used as experiences necessary for the awakening to come through spiritual study.

Analysis of Hearing

Sadhana or self-effort for self-improvement through the first three *chakras* (coccygeal, sacral, and lumbar) and the *anahaata chakra* (thoracic) are prerequisites for evolution. The base and sacral *chakras* are concerned with restraint and adherence for *yama* and *niyama*. The *navel chakra* is about sustained self-control. When the flow of negative energies from these *chakras* have been reversed towards the divine cave, the seeker connects with the life force in the heart *chakra*. This in common parlance is walking towards spirituality versus walking towards desires and indulgences.

True listening requires surrendering physical speech and mental talking so that one can be heard clearly. The *Devi* of Speech as *Sarasvati* (Life Force-Energy manifesting as knowledge and speech) appears at each *chakra*, because speech is man's greatest performance.

Man has an insatiable need to speak of his own self-importance

- Keep a diary of your surrender to another's talking in order to achieve quality listening.
- Most who have **"authority complexes",** are dictated by the ego.
- When the ego listens, what does it listen to? Hurts, criticisms, compliments, or praise?
- Become aware that the ears listens only to things they wish to hear. Is what is being heard twisted?.
- Who is listening: I or my ego?

Short negative sentences also originate from the ego: "I always make the same mistakes" or "I would rather die than to" are verbalized sentences of the mind ego. These approaches must be turned to the opposite ("I have never done this but will try"); so there can be a positive foundation for greater inner security.

Insecurities arising from emotional, physical, and mental levels must be dealt with. Habitual actions and reactions need investigation and shifted to higher ideals. Discrimination requires refinement and the control of self-will.

Our senses and ego do exactly what need to keep functioning. A constant vigilance on what the body is storing in his foundation is the first step to understanding the implications of energy deficits and emotional tolerances. To prevent instinctive reactions to what is heard, alertness and information scanning must be the seeker's initial response, especially during the formative period of *sadhana.*

Speed of Self-Growth and Will

Speed does not reflect efficiency in self-growth; rather, one needs time to discriminate will from self-will which is an expression of ego. *Self-will* is the daily battle of human relationships for dominance, a choice I make by submitting someone to my influence. It is also an admission, that I cannot listen to others.

Observation reveals that self-will is a response to the egoistic chattering of the mind which prevents one from listening to others. Will is the pursuit of the best in oneself for the benefit of others.

This *chakra* is the throne of both *Gauri*, manifesting as Life Force-Energy of awareness and *Sadashiva* as unmanifest consciousness. They are separate but one and in balance in a spiritual marriage of the two halves: Matter with Spirit or the without with the within or Awareness *(Prakriti)* with Consciousness *(Purusha).*

The perceptions of each, the irrational and the rational, must be heard by listening to the intuitive ear – **the "third ear".** To prevent the interfering influences of other senses, listen by shutting the eyes, or listen to pure sound without the emotions.

Analysis on Hearing

The influence of this positive rebirth fills the seeker with a renewed vitality to continue seeking. This is a turning point in his regeneration, free from all limitations of *raaga-dvesha* or likes-and-dislikes and judgments. He is finally connected to *Durga,* the Mother-who-Removes-all-Difficulties. He now expresses himself with a renewed creative energy. There is new meaning to flippant assertions: 'God be with you'! He IS with you; keep listening!

When **hearing,** clarify what it means.
- What am I listening to and what am I really hearing?
- Is it a sound or am I hearing what I am thinking?
- Are these garbled thoughts or are they just noises of the mind?
- Why am I listening to the garble?
- Am I avoiding hearing what I should be?
- Am I afraid to be confronted with a decision I must make?
- Am I listening?

What is the message?

- Are these just words or am I blocking out something? Can I hear my own voice?
- What does the listener get from the tone of my voice?
- When I listen, who listens? The ego?
- If it can be removed, do I dis-empower it?
- Is the ego a manifestation of the self-will?

Is there a difference in the perception of hearing and listening?

- Do I "give" of myself when I listen? Does that give me "insights"?
- Does self-will require surrendering?
- To what? To Divine Will?

Can I discriminate between:

- reason and emotion;
- logic and intuition;
- fear and courage;
- softness and strength;
- clumsiness and deftness?

Do I have the courage to surrender to Divine Will when the ego puts up a fight?

- Listen to what is being physically heard.
- Do I have a tendency to screen out what I do not wish to hear?
- Persistence in these exercises will release me from self-centered-ness.

Watch music evoke emotional responses and trigger memories of forgotten events.

- Listen to nature, and see how chanting bubbles from within yourself.

Distortions of hearing is reflective of non-integration with what is going on outside oneself. The result is an unbalanced energy, costing restriction through emotion and action.

If the *saddhak* or seeker should align his foundational inner half with the needs of the Cosmic Mother. If he hears Her attentively and in devotion, without expressing the Self-Will for the sake of Ego, She will allow him the vision of the Light at the end of the tunnel!

Analysis on Speaking and Listening

Intuitive knowledge lives within the body in the heart center. Trusting the sixth sense allows the seeker to react correctly to all situations because it gives the seeker the ability to make the right decisions for the moment.

Every new thought, speech, and action stemming from the intuitive platform reorganizes the bodily cells, starting at the DNA molecule! Old cells embodying old ideas die and the creative energy uses its talent to create new knowledge gained in the reflective state of meditation. In the processes of meditation, Man drops all past personalities, past education, past desires, and walks through the valleys of spiritual wisdom. This walk is towards that ultimate wisdom.

Choose one person to investigate and watch the way you speak and listen to this person:

i. Recall what you said;
   - How you said it;
   - The tone with which you spoke with;
   - Do you like what you hear yourself say to this person?

ii. Tape yourself to allow for self-assessment:
   - Now try and convince the other person what you want heard.
   - Do you get emotional and how do you sound?
   - Now record the conversation and see if you hear the other talk:
   - Are you listening to the person?
   - Now list all the emotions being evoked during the conversation.

- Is there begging, joy, elation, power, strength, anxiety, pain, confusion, or tears?

iii. Listen to the noises of the body and record them.

iv. Listen to mental conversations:
- What are you listening to?
- Can you stop the mental chatter?
- If you can, how do you do it?
- If you cannot, how can you learn to control the mind?

v. Focus into the divine cave and gaze into the east (in front within the Christ-Krishna Centre); now watch the breath and chant a mantra for 60 minutes and watch the mind:
- Record what happens for any 15 minute quarters of each 30 minutes.

vi. Listen to music for 15 minutes both while sitting and lying:
- Note the difference.

vii. Listen to an unpleasant sound like scratching for a few minutes:
- Record your reactions.

viii. Listen to different musical sounds for five to seven minutes each:
- Record the reactions evoked.
- Is there a difference in what is heard when the eyes are open and when they are closed?

The Light of meditation reveals the wisdom of Reality. Old patterns of thinking, listening, and hearing have been followed to their very roots through meditation. The seeker must now walk through life with one foot in his inner world and the other one connected to the Universe. The seeker now has the ability to lift himself to focus on the relationship of the inner and outer halves.

Another look at Hearing and Listening

Vishuddha chakra (cervical plexus) controls the sense of hearing and listening. Observe what we do to filter out what we do not wish to hear: This is why we do not communicate effectively. To follow the *sadhana* of progressive and inner development, one must listen carefully.

Learning through practical application is the best way to do *sadhana* or spiritual self-effort. Now it is time to incorporate colours and see how we colour our mind with symbolism. For example, purple comes from mixing blue with red. The colour red or *rajasic* activity is how we live life while blue represents Infinity and Depth and is therefore spiritual. In the field of images, *Gauri* or Life Force-Energy or *Prakriti,* is seated on a lotus whose petals look smoky. This is because our listening, clarity of thought, and understanding are unclear even at this stage of *sadhana* or spiritual practice.

The noose *Gauri* or Mother Nature carries in one of Her hands is a warning against intellectualization and the mechanicalness of actions and reactions. The fire of emotion is rebellious and opposition easily flares in us when confronted and cornered. The gourd urges us to keep walking the journey. There is water in it for refreshment after a long walk on the spiritual journey.

Shiva is Spirit and *Gauri-Shakti* is Her Power. She represents awareness in matter or *prakriti.* She is also the power of delusion or *Maya* of Mother Nature. Together they signify the balance the seeker must aspire for. The seeker needs to acquire perfection in areas of:

- emotion and reason;
- intuition and logic; and
- tension and letting go.

These pairs of opposites must be balanced so that the practitioner can become a unit of sensitivity. The seeker should now be able to unite "Me" and "I". In this "union", the seeker is capable now of hearing the overwhelming experience of *Aum.*

Maya

Maya (Gauri or *Prakriti* or Life Force-Energy or Awareness) governs the Law of Qualities or *Gunas (sattva, rajas,* and *tamas)* which are incorporated into the Law of Relativity (likes-and-dislikes or *raaga-dvesha* stemming from my causal being*).* Mortals are constantly attracted towards the senses and their objects of pleasure. *Tamas (inertia)* and *rajas (activity)* are the two polarities of our existence: both are dynamic states of being. The seeker must balance the two in *sattva* or stillness and silence.

The seeker does not have to strive for this balance; it comes automatically. He needs only to prepare himself through:

- *yama* (restraint) */niyama* (adherence) */asana*(posture) */pranayama* (breath-regulation) */pratyahara* (sense withdrawal) and */dharana* (concentration).

He must then surrender and wait for that Incredible *darshan* (insightful-vision) in meditation. *Sadashiva* or Consciousness, is ever at the beck and call of the devotee who calls for the *Guru* of all *gurus* in the third eye of wisdom. This symbolic *guru* is the *Bholanath*, the Compassionate Lord who, while sitting on the tiger skin (to insulate Him from the magnetic vibrations of the earth), will preserve our energy *(Shakti)* from the pull of earth-bound influences attracting us outwards along the senses and towards the fruits of life's activities.

By controlling the mind and the life-force, the seeker develops wisdom and becomes familiar with inner calmness and aloofness from identification with the body. Compelled by his past *karma*, he remains imprisoned in the chambers of births and deaths. Caught in the powers of *maya* or delusion, he must fulfill his desires and pay the debts incurred by his own actions. Meditation and identification with the Spirit are the only means of gaining eternal freedom from the delusion of *maya.*

Keeping a Diary

A journal of an inner spiritual journey serves to remind the seeker of the different stages of growth and transformation he has undergone, starting with the beginning to the progress he has made. It is a process of re educating oneself.

It is a review of how the seeker used his tools: his body, his creative energy, his mind and emotions; and also how he offered his past or causal being to his 'other half' for connectedness with Mother Nature.

It serves as an understanding of how man gains his happiness by transferring his physical sexual energy or *ojas* to fuel Creation for purposes the seeker holds most dear to his heart. The seeker channels this as life-force or *prana* towards right relationships with all of Her Creation through a deep sense of conviction and knowing. This inexplicable inner knowing gives him the highest shining wisdom or *tejas* in his psyche. The seeker now has his own library of knowledge accessed through meditation and attainment with the Universal Memory.

Keeping a diary helps one identify whether wishful thinking is intuition or wisdom. It assists in the effort of constant readjustment, stressing areas which require refinement and development.

Life undergoes seven year cycles and the brain cells change every eight years. Keeping track of the cycles and the changes allows the seeker to see whether he has accomplished what he intended to do.

When listening to others

- See what memories of past events are triggered;
- Take into account that the mind tends to replay past events and memories, whether heard, seen or inferred.

In dream-sleep, images are seen and voices heard:

- Recall only those which carry messages to encourage the aspirant to embrace gentleness, peace of mind, courage, forgiveness: these are voices of the Self.

The still mind has the ability to hear messages and orders issued by the "rightful ruler" of my being.

- It is like listening to the ocean in the conch in a spirit of surrender; one cannot tell the shell what to speak for it only speaks what it must.

Wandering thought processes must next be investigated to identify thought associations with past memories and for mechanicalness or habits:

- If they are a nuisance, get rid of them by using audible mantras or practicing pranayama (Ham'saa - So'ham technique).
- Once subdued, they should be discouraged from reappearing and finally eliminated by becoming witness or *saakshi* to the thought processes.

Voices from the past have a habit of re-surfacing as "wandering thoughts":

- They arise from "Me", the *chitta* or the mind, intellect, and ego complex, trying to re establish itself in the realm of ego.
- The brain (lower astral dimension of mind and emotions or sensory manas and the higher astral dimension of ideas and knowledge or unenlightened *chitta)* needs to empty itself.
- Each purging of present and past lives must be dealt with until there is only increased consciousness left in the silence of meditation.

The duration of this thoughtless awareness allows the seeker to enter the next stage of development.

Birth and Death

Birth and death are actions born of desire. Birth occurs in response to desires unfulfilled in a previous birth. Death is for the creation of a New Me or *Chitta* in the future.

> and the Master said:
>
> "That is your final procession in which you are absent!"

The causal being has the wisdom of many previous lives in its womb. The seeker's spiritual journey in this life, combined with the talents acquired from previous lives become a resource of expertise in many books on his many spiritual journeys. The seeds are planted with every thought Man dwell upon. It may not manifest at that moment, but the body has the creative resources to create the permanent images in the seeker's mind-womb.

A purified-*chitta*-birth for a more evolved individual requires that the *chitta* becomes further enlightened for the purpose of eradicating the ego. All the past, as astral and causal beings, is dealt with and a new "Me" is created from the ashes of burnt desire and egoistic actions of past and present. His thought power will lead him to manifest in an environment where his visualized desires have every range of possibility necessary for realization.

Dreams play an important role in experiencing past lives, revealing agendas left unfinished and mistakes requiring correction. The body and mind need respect. The only way to achieve this is to subdue the ego, sharpen perceptions, and balance living away from *"raaga-dvesha"* or likes-and-dislikes. It is only the ego that experiences pain and pleasure.

The Life Force Energy of Matter as BMI or Body-Mind-Intellect, is a neutral power. Mind's senses and emotions colour the BMI when it expresses as perceiver, feeler, and thinker (PFT). Self-will for indulgences motivate emotions which feel the pain of wrong actions, manifesting as physical or mental illness. All problems and anxieties must be dealt with directly and unemotionally. (Please refer to the BMI chart).

Negative emotions take the form of hostility, resentment, and jealousy. They must be dealt with by analyzing the what, where, when, why, and how of the problem. Suppression of emotion will only result in it raising its head again as an expression in another person, by which time the ego will have been strengthened rather than disempowered.

The Ego judges, condemns, and criticizes not only others but also oneself. It is a hard taskmaster. It must be dealt with from the spring-source of the negative emotion.

Negative emotion may arise from ego, lacking in awareness. There is a not knowing the intrinsic worth of the Divinity lying hidden within "Me". Thoughts such as "my opinion does not matter" or "who wants to hear me" stem from an ego which feels worthless and helpless.

Ego may express itself as a possessiveness, preventing the true emotion of love. Most of us accept the concept of love as we feel ourselves in it. This usually ends up preventing us loving as we should. "The giving and letting go" emotion of expansion and release is a function of "Me" trying to unite with the "I".

Ego Expresses as "Me" in Chitta

The old "Me" can be taught. New concepts can be substituted for old values. Indulgences can be sublimated through the awareness of giving choice. Energy can be utilized through fostering an awareness of one's habits, mechanical actions, thought processes, and evaluations.

Ego or *ahankar* is a rope of many threads entwined involving:

pride;	greed;	self-importance;
cravings.	illusions;	passions;
and desires		

Pride or *mada* can exist in ten areas:

physical strength;	intellect;	morals and virtues;
psychic powers;	spirituality;	noble birth and status;
wealth and possessions;	physical beauty;	talents;
and powers of command.		

The interdependence of body and mind and ego must be recognized. Although the body is materialistic, the mind is an abstract emotion capable of spiritual understanding: the practitioner must be able to bring the desiring of the body and the emotions of the mind together. For example, "refined speech" takes the form of a audible *mantra* which over time becomes inaudible and is heard and listened to by the inner ear. The mental capacity for listening can now become a self-generating dynamo of chanting and listening in the mind, free from all mental chattering.

Man Crystallizes what Mind Thinks

Every thought constitutes a mental image of what the aspirant wants to be and what he wants to achieve as a goal. Auto-suggestion uses positive messages starting with:"I will... and I am going to ..". It is an indication of clear thinking and discrimination. This influence on the power of suggestion, is just a start. An awareness of the identity you wish to embrace must be mirror-clear.

> and the Master said:
>
> "...Life is not what you Think it is. Life is what you make of it!"

If there are problems on the Path, invoke the Divine Light and identify with the Source of All Beings, who created us perfect. Because we identify with our physical nature, our "Me" identity remains as the source of our ego. "Me" needs re-orientation as "I". "I" can only be seen to emanate from the creative energy, the source of all, *That Aum.*

> and the Master said: "Caesar would not be wolf, if the Romans were not sheep. It is we who give might and power to objects to persecute us with their joys and sorrows! Situations can hurt us only if the mind is weak enough to be hurt. It is desire and cravings for something that create this weakness of the mind.."

Who Am I?

The problem with seekers on the Path of *sadhana*, is that of identification: How do we identity with the body, the mind, and the mind's multitudinous personalities? Which personality do we identify with most and what are the insecurities underlying this identification?

How can we identify with the Higher Self? Wrongful identifications which have been mechanical for generations in many of the previous births make unconscious parallels in new birth existence: together, they make for many personalities varying from moment to moment.

> and the Master said:
>
> "Read my discussions and be one with me in my thoughts. You will be transported into my world of joy and peace.."

A good way to identify oneself is to observe the acrobatics of others as they jump from personality to personality through jealousy, pride, and other emotions which denounce our truly Divine nature.

> The girls were very young. One had her first camera and the other had a Polaroid camera. The Master posed this way and then the other way. The older one returned with all her pictures developed. The younger one had nothing to show for her pains and she bawled!
>
> and the Master said: "Nothing came because you were jealous of your sister!"
>
> She was about to throw away the 'non-pictures' when the Master continued "...these pictures will never turn out unless you allow me to hug your sister too!"

At this stage of development, the seeker has to accept responsibility for himself. He becomes gentle and modest. His mind is under control, free from greed, malice, pride and anger, and he automatically becomes forgiving and courageous. Refined feelings can now become a stepping stone to compassion.

Need for a Guru

The need for a *guru* is an overwhelming feeling at this stage. Study and guidance leave the aspirant with a vibrant feeling, that the *guru* is speaking to you in the mind as an intuitive voice of Truth.

> and the Master wrote to one of his many seekers:
>
> "*Guru* is not a person, he is a personality, an institution. He is the radio through which the Lord contacts the student. When a student meets his Teacher, it is always a miracle. In fact it is love at first sight. He is immediately attracted to him and his words ring a bell. Another speaker may speak better but only his Teacher will attract him...
>
> "If, in case you get the rare privilege of meeting such a Master and you really happen to really understand a little of what he says — then progress has to happen. It is unfailingly [true]. It is very productive [the meeting]. Whenever anyone meets his Teacher it is always a miracle!....
>
> "If in case you are benefited [by this meeting], do not forget that the Teacher was brought to you by *Ishvara*, the total *vasanas,* of which a part was you, .. And remember, there is no difference between God and the *Guru,* the corporeal entity before you....
>
> "Therefore, be on the lookout when you meet a Master. Search! Seek!...and [get] fulfilled!!"

As discrimination and sense perception become more refined, intuition flows freely into the seeker who is able to hear the inner voice of guidance.

The seeker now is still and can cut away the myriad of personalities with the help of discrimination. The practitioner will make the necessary changes in response to this inner being. The goal should be clear. The ego, "Me", must not be allowed to distort the aim.

The seeker becomes spine-conscious of the various stages of his development within the divine cave of the brain and spinal cord. The circle is complete**:** the practitioner has understood that physical surrender requires the balancing of the body, mind, and intellect.

There is an awareness that the balancing of the body, mind, and intellect *(chitta)* manifests in speech. Straight-thinking, straight-forward actions, and directness are the physical manifestation of *chitta* and speech.

The aspirant must constantly balance the five senses-organs and the organs of action with thought and speech, through an awareness learnt and put to practice through the preceding study.

A true master teaches the seeker to open his inner eye of all-knowing soul intuition. The disciple who has by now become devoted to the teaching will submit to the teachings of the master.

Men who live by the dictates of meditation-born peace of the soul find themselves entangled also with the sensory perceptions of objects; confused, they lose their sense of direction towards a God-ward goal of life.

> A class of Philosophy students in a Canadian University asked the Master to 'define the need of a Guru in the Eastern tradition':
>
> "In the past, colonizers went to Africa with guns and returned with animal trophies of the hunt. These days animals, gold rushes, and new lands to conquer are difficult to come by; but the adventuring spirit of the West is difficult to contain. This adventurism exists even to this day.
>
> "The adventurous youth of today sport in India armed with cameras, tape-recorders, and microphones. They are hunting for 'gurus' : to 'bag and return home' with them! There is no need for 'guru-hunting'. He or she will come to you when you are ready.."

Development of the Intellect

The *intellect* consists of thoughts and ideas embedded in awareness; it is a progressive force by which objects and experiences of the phenomenal world are analyzed and explained. *Intelligence* involves discriminative thinking by the intellect permitting proper action which will nurture soul-wisdom. Intelligence is the witness of all thoughts and actions of the intellect.

Man's intellect, has been developed and evolved for its own sake: to satisfy pride and to infuse the ego with a sense of accomplishment . Those few individuals who through meditation develop their intellect to discover the wise intelligence, will nurture it consciously to reach the halls of intuition, which is the conscious hidden expression of intelligence.

Such a journey requires the power of reason as well as conviction derived from the instinctive intuition which is latent in us. Unless intuition is fully awakened and operative, the reasoning intelligence may reach a false conclusion. Therefore the development of the intellect and intelligence should be guided by intuition. Through meditation and devotional study of scriptural teachings, the soul's intuition, the *guru,* begins to guide the development.

> My daughters lamented the end of the *Yagna* and his fast approaching day of departure.
>
> "A guru arrives yearly to sow seeds; their germination and fruition is the responsibility of the cultivator.."
>
> At the Airport, the young girls were alarmed the Master was walking without his familiar cane: "Where is you walking stick?" she asked.
>
> "I needed it in the past. I have no need for it now. In fact, it walked away faster than me." he replied, with a twinkle in his eye.

Processing Knowledge

In order to know, we must experience a succession of changing thoughts. Each thought carries a sense of conviction or knowing which gradually grows old and is replaced by a new, convincing thought. Intellect made restless by sensory bombardment loses its power to focus and becomes an undirected process of mental change. The witnessing intelligence sees false, meaningless thoughts and ideas.

Unguided exuberant intellectual energy disrupts inner calmness and renders intuition impotent. Intuition only can manifest as calmness and clear thinking. Only then can one's actions be guided by right determination.

Under the influence of *Maya* or delusion, man possesses an imaginative personality capable of destroying the natural ability to perceive Truth. Even small suggestions can generate different images depending on the mood of the seeker. Full of bitterness, the seeker can neither enjoy the pleasures of the senses nor look forward to happiness in the future.

Unless these doubting habits and imaginations are eradicated, man remains a victim of this paralyzing habit. This tendency should be controlled and not transmitted to others through arguments and conjectures.

> On "justification" of wrong actions, the Master said "Our Intellect serves as an ever faithful hand-maiden to support and give a false look of respectability to the vulgarities of our baser Mind .."

Breaking Walls of Unconscious Habits

Habitual thinking is interconnected with emotion and consequently is never questioned by man. It reflects anxiety to protect unproved beliefs and to perpetuate the habitual word-games we play. The purpose is to gain a favourable position to defend our beliefs. An alert seeker will note that wild-statements are tricks to control the opponent for the sake of ego.

These take the form of:

- Irrelevant objections;
- Discussion of minute details;.
- Aggression and dishonest trickery;
- Ridiculing another in order to win at all cost; and
- Pretending to know what you do not know.

Conviction for emotional reasons is dangerous both spiritually and in general. Manipulations using one's magnetic personality are dishonest. Listening within to the *Devi* or Divine Mother Nature will change habitual thinking along the lines of ego.

One must take responsibility for speaking even inaudible thoughts, for all thoughts have a creative power and will seek manifestation in action. What is created is the responsibility of the owner of the soundless thought process.

Control of thought is important. The mind, with its collection of thoughts, needs clarification before it utters something that has the possibility of becoming conceived in the womb of conscious creation. There must be equal development not only of all the five senses which are under the control of mind, but also of the mind itself.

When fully evolved, the *Devi* (Mother Nature or Life Force/Energy or Awareness) manifests Herself as the stirring of Herself in dreams. The energy of the dream is derived from the wisdom of Universal and Cosmic Intelligence *(mahat).* Self-awakening now is pursued according to one's natural inclinations.

When all the ground work has been done, when this new quality is brought into other aspects of the practitioner's life, then a human potential develops, fringing on the threshold of renunciation, for the purpose of a Higher awakening.

The purpose of life is to become one with this Cosmic Energy. The human mind can study its manifestations, but it is only through meditation that It reveals Itself and in all things.

Meditation in Light

To review: Assume an asana of your choice, close your eyes and look into the divine cave in the east. Roll your tongue back. Do pranayama (regulating breathing using the Ham.saa So.ham mantra) for five to ten minutes or more. Now watch the breath while concentrating between the manipura chakra (navel or solar plexus) and the vishuddha chakra (throat chakra).

Make sure the spine is straight as described in previous lessons, vertebra on vertebra: to straighten back, have lower abdomen pulled in, shoulder blades pulled back to meet, chin parallel to the ground and perineum gently tightened.

- *Now, quietly and inwardly chant the Ham'saa - Soo'ham while watching the regularity of breath (4 seconds each for inspiration : pause : expiration : pause); next practice concentration or dharana by watching the breath; make sure the tongue is rolled back, the gaze is directed to the east between the eyebrows, and the inner ear is listening to the inner sounds within the divine cave.*
- *Next, contract and relax for ten to twenty minutes the twelve sites of the body to energize each part: feet, ankles, calves, thighs, four parts of the back, lower abdomen, chest, hands, forearms, upper arms, shoulders, neck and head. Gradually transfer this concentration of energy in the astral body into the spine until you become "spine conscious" and lose all awareness of the body and the senses. This leads to pratyhara or withdrawal from of the senses and into the divine cave. It is the inward journey to spirituality.*
- *Now, fill the divine cave with awareness as AUM, from the bhrumadhya (between eyebrows) to the end of the spinal cord.*
- *Next fill the divine cave with the Light of Awareness-Consciousness rising up the hollow of the divine cave in spine lighting all the centers of the chakras.*
- *At the site where the head joins the neck spine, make the light beam fill the brain section of the divine cave, while focusing on the bhrumadhya or kutastha or Christ Centre.*
- *Here the beam of light flashes to illuminate the whole brain. Pause to enjoy this bliss of illumination in the divine cave.*
- *Now, see the beam go back to the first center where the Light of extreme preciousness started.*
- *Stay still in the mains of the inner sound and allow whatever comes, in an intuition of delicate perception, which may be classified as a deep peace, harmony, and absorption.*
- *Patience and perseverance gives one a deep sense of knowing that one is on the right path. Only patience and humility allows one to gain That experience.*
- *Next, widen the "Beam of Light" at the base and then at the head until enveloped in Light. Now open the light beam at the kutastha, between the eyebrows and enter to merge with the Light of Infinity.*
- *Bless the Universe (Mother Nature) with mantras such as the "Gayatri", the "Mrityun jaya", and "Om namah shivaya". (Review these in Section Two). Feel the oneness of the practitioner with the Cosmic Mother for as long as you can.*
- *You will now feel the Light within the divine cave. Now spread it to all parts of the body. You should able feel the denseness of the bodily Light. The outer covering of Light is lighter. Dwell in this Light within and without for a while.*
- *The meditator experiences a common phenomenon which is "felt" as a "sensation", the ascending and descending, as well as expanding of Life Force/Energy or Shakti in the spine, first . This "sensation" may persist even into the "waking state".*

Psychology of Dhyana Samadhi

When the practitioner enters the state of Oneness (experienced in *dharana* or concentration and in *dhyana* or meditation), the "Me" (mind as the object) and "I" (the subject of my concentration) merges into the oneness of the subject and object.

In *samadhi* or the meditative ecstasy of oneness, the Oneness is a realization that the subject I am concentrating on is the Self; but there is also a realization that this Self is the Self everywhere. It is cosmic consciousness that I and All is the Self.

When the mind or object is concentrating as the physical body, the object and subject seem separate (that is, "Me" and "I" are separate). When the mind ("Me") enters the astral plane, a partial union occurs between the object ("Me") and the subject ("I"). When the mind ("Me" as object) is synchronized with the subject ("I"), this unity is sustained and supported at its base by a lack of differentiation. In this state, the base *Aum* is also surrounded by *Aum.* There is no distinction between the two.

Every being has its own "beingness". Even God or Spirit has His own "Beingness". Man's relationship with Him is a vertical ascension. The seeker's "beingness" ascends to His "Beingness". The mind state must be left behind as the being enters the astral planes where there is an automatic transformation. In that plane, differentiation, individuality, or distinctiveness do not exist. "Beingness", therefore, ceases, and the subject and object are one.

Once beingness ceases, the body is automatically abandoned, and its unique identity is suspended. This new identity now understands the meaning and source from which all beings emerge and manifest as objects.

The Being assumes various forms as objects. We cannot equate the acts that the being performs without acknowledging that all acts are in accordance with His Will. In devotion, man only acknowledges his acts as distinctive. When the meditator becomes one with the Absolute ("being" with all of the "Being"), distinctions are missing and the practitioner becomes One with It.

- "But seek ye first the kingdom of God [in Oneness], and His righteousness; and all these things shall be added unto you"..Mathew 6:33.

The meditator retains his body as long as he continues to live. He continues to suffer the effects of his past *karmas.* His actions are now not his own: they become acts of His Will, a prayer-to-serve. This is, however, still not the greatest achievement because the practitioner continues to live in the causal or *karana* plane. The deeper meditator lives within the realms of Awareness, always connected to His Mains.

> On prayer the Master had this to say: "...We pray for health, wealth and prosperity. Prayer has become an exercise in beggary. How can you allot a special time

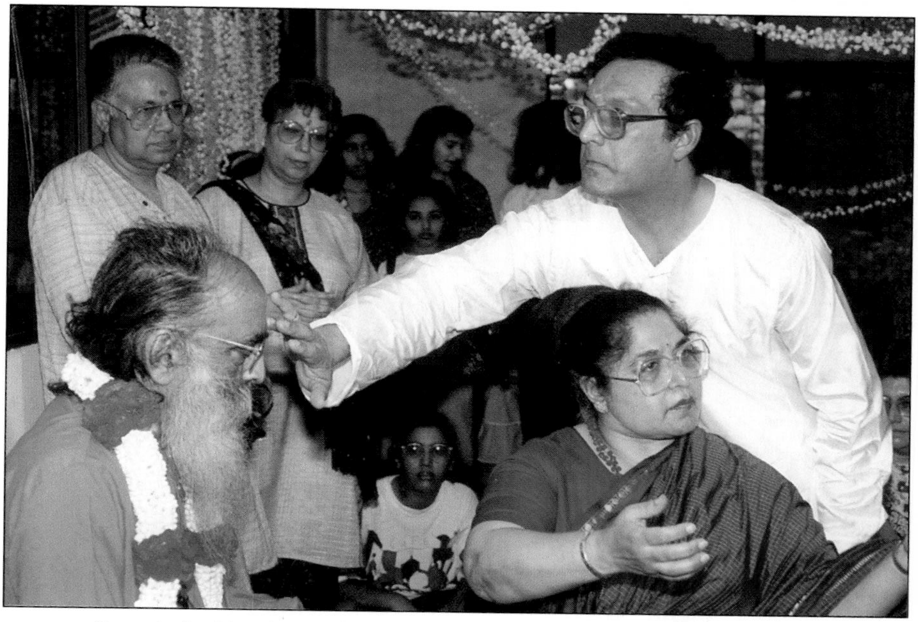

Parents looking forward to future generations to Honour the Master.

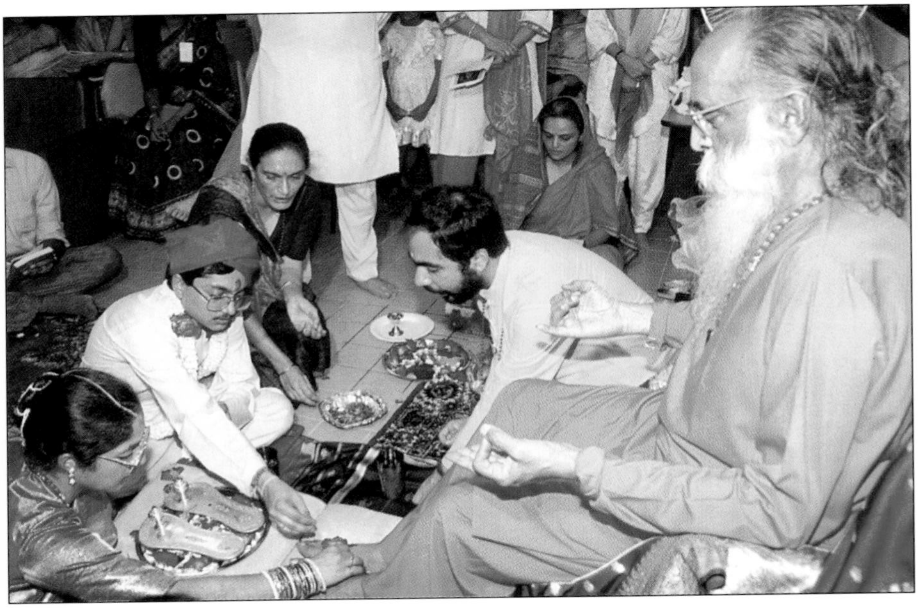

Thankyou for being with us

intervals for loving your spouse, your children, or your parents? Is not 'love' a continuous sense of identification with the beloved? Prayer is carrying Aum in your 'hip-pocket' or handbag at all times and in all actions..."

Truth

A *guru* is a repository of all wisdom and he lives free while living in the body. The serving *guru* incurs no effects of his actions in the world outside, because he serves Mother Nature for the love of it; he expects no fruits of his actions. The seeker who is aligned with a true teacher also has special characteristics

and the Master wrote:

"Opportunity [life with a true Master] comes to all of us. The diligent catch hold of it. The foolish let it pass. Therefore, let us be smart and awake to recognize our opportunity to serve, and while it is within our reach, let us seize it and make it yield to us the results we demand.."

Without awakening the faculty of intuition, the seeker cannot know the Truth behind appearances. Many schools of philosophy consider Truth a relative quantity, with no absolute value. A *guru* of divine realization has learnt to balance the rigidity of the intellect and the fluidity of intuition. He is able to discern in all the different circumstances of the relative world the course of action that is truthful, as judged from the standpoint of the Absolute Truth. Truth has been defined by different Masters over time but their conclusion was always the same.

It was in this context that the Master was asked about Schools of Hindu Philosophy: "*Vedanta* [Believers of the Vedas] is the philosophy of the *Upanishads* [knowledge Philosophy of the *Vedas*]. The Hindu seers were never satisfied unless they discussed every question to its logical irrefutable conclusion. It is this which led to different schools of philosophical thought, all claiming to be based on the teachings of the *Upanishads:*

Advaita of Shankaracharya
Vashishta-dvaita of Ramanuja
Dvaita of Madhavacharya
Sudha-advaita of Vallabhacharya
Dvaita-advaita of Nimbarka, and
Achintya Bhedabheda of Jiva Goswami

"There are no Schools of Philosophy. It would be correct to say that there are only different notions and interpretations about the same subject. All these teachers are struggling to express the inexpressible, and such differences in expressions are bound to be there. *Amruta-upanishad* helps us to understand: Cows are of different colours, yet the milk from all these cows is of the same colour, white.."

Every seeker has experienced intuitional glimpses of an inner feeling or conviction that has proved to be right. However, this power of knowing is developed by meditation and calmness into the pure intuition, he gains access to the library of all wisdom.

An advanced student of *Raja Yoga,* who knows how to withdraw his awareness and life force from the body and the senses, can enter the inner world of wisdom revelations. He receives all knowledge emanating out of the seven spiritual altars of the spine and the brain. Inner perceptions are realizations which may manifest as word thoughts or as distinctive intuitive feelings.

Concentrating on these sources of power, the seeker may be able to hear the vibratory variations of the sacred sound of Aum, and from within its sound-matrix hear, realize or experience truths.

> and the Master wrote:
>
> "As a teacher, I have given you all you need. Now it is for you to apply it all in life and learn to live accepting everything, rejecting nothing, reflecting all, yet keeping nothing. What is there in this world other than expression of His glory..."

Conclusion

Having acknowledged that every man functions from a foundational level of the unenlightened *chitta* (mind-intellect-ego manifesting as mood-feeling-personality or memory-of-past), he has by now, made every effort at modifying the structure to become connected with the Cosmic Mother.

The journey has just begun. The *Sadhak* or seeker is now wiser, and carries with him the shield of Wisdom, Intelligence, Love and Love-of-Service, emanating from an altered foundational level.

He uses his mind and intellect as the power to manifest itself within the womb of creation or causal or *vasanic* body. He has a clear concept of what he wishes to become while on his spiritual journey. He fills the womb with ideas of his own wished and willed perfection. Self-study, meditation, and service of Mother Nature becomes the gestation period of a new birth arising from within the core of the seeker's being: a transformed seeker, sought, and seeing.

SECTION SIX

Topics in Section Six

A Direct Perception of God

The Transformations have occurred in the senses which have now become free of encumbrances of old habits and concepts, and likes-and-dislikes. This evolution acknowledges that both pain and pleasure are but polarities of a single emotion. Neutralising the effect of these polarities is possible but change must be accepted. Rejection of any of the polarities would only magnify one or the other polarity. Once change is accepted as a blessing of God, the mind is able to rest within the divine cave where it feels Changelessness.

Pranayama or regulated breathing ensures that the influence of the life-force or *prana* expands and the aura is magnified over the medullary area. The astral fluid or *prana* of the divine cave flows more swiftly. The brain cells become super-charged with the divinised astral fluid. The seeker is free to continue on his onward journey into himself.

Ajnaa Chakra

Preamble

Efforts in meditation are self-healing processes to make corrections in whatever that was and is unbalanced in the practitioner. The seeker regains his equanimity by restoring balance within himself. He corrects his dealings with society and interactions with *Prakriti* or Creation. The inner voice of intuition knows all the right answers and guides the seeker on what to say, how to act and behave, and how to move. The seeker must only listen to this compelling life-force that takes you exactly where the seeker needs to be. His desires are aligned with the Collective Good for Mother Nature.

The seeker's body, mind, intellect, emotions, and *vasanas* (past-life tendencies), become a path that obeys all the Laws of Manifestation. The changes are recorded in every cell, up to the DNA structural level.

The centres are located in the Divine Cave**:** changes are received and it is here that the **experiencer** or *purusha* or *rishi* **watches;** changes are integrated in the causal *prakriti* (in the divine cave of the brain) where the *devata* **experiences** the changes and **looks** on attentively**;** new changes are transmitted (as experienced changed knowledge through the release of altered neurotransmitters and neurohormones)**;** they activate the autonomic nervous system to create triggers of **altered experiencing.**

The sum total of this sequence (meditation) is a changed awareness, compelling the seeker on the chosen Spiritual Path. He now sees the world of objects, emotions and thoughts (OET) with a different awareness! Meditation is the return journey of a mortal towards the lap of Mother Nature. Having made the necessary changes in his own divine cave, the seeker makes these adjustments in Mother Nature as well. He now serves Her.

The command station stems from this *ajnaa* centre at the base of the brain directly opposite to the *kutastha* which is located between and behind the eyebrows. This area is also where life-force or *prana* energizes the divine cave of the brain and the spinal cord with Cosmic Light and Energy.

Ajnaa Chakra
Sixth Chakra or Chakra of Mind (thought)

This is the brow *chakra* of the mind and therefore is connected to the senses. The spiritual center is in the base of the brain, opposite the eyebrow. The *bhrumadhya* behind the eyebrows is a reflection of the *kutastha chaitanya* (Christ-Krishna Center) in the *ajnaa chakra* at the base of the brain. The *ajnaa chakra* is entirely different from the previous five *chakras.* The two autonomic nervous system channels (*Ida and Pingala*) join in the *Sushumna* (astral spinal cord) opposite this point. For the purposes of concentration, meditation and contemplation, this is the main point where "I" resides, in and near the location of the "third eye" in the *bhrumadhya* between the eyebrows. (Please refer to Figure 13)

The sixth *chakra* is the differentiating faculty that has rays penetrating the four corners of the world. It is symbolized by two petals of the lotus, representing the mind as it functions in two halves of one world—the manifest and unmanifest. The intellect on this level, is symbolized in unity at the location between the pineal and pituitary glands.

It is the location of the enlightened "I" as well as the unenlightened "Me": it is the controller of the five previous *chakras,* unifying their five-foldedness. Through this control, "I" reigns supreme, having understood and appreciated all the pleasures and experiences of the five *chakras* while identified with "Me."

It also is where all the previous lives and their materialistic and spiritual pursuits have been recorded in the womb of all his previous manifestations. This exists as an essence. It is like a memory on a disc template of the *chitta* or a feeling of awareness manifesting in a very subtle form in the mind, intellect, and ego complex.

The seeker's efforts at *sadhana* have resulted in the tranquillity of the mind and silence of the intellect. The unenlightened *chitta* has come to terms with all the materialistic and spiritual results of the seeker's efforts outside himself and from within. He knows he is coming to the merging of his experiences and that the new experience will be much more than the individual parts experienced to date.

Transcendence of this *chakra* and enlightenment of the *chitta* leads to the secret thousand petalled lotus: the *sahasrahara chakra*. In this brow *chakra, Shiva-Shakti (Purusha-Prakriti)* finally meet in completion, at one point, like a star in space.

Faulty Human Endeavors

In Karma Yoga:

Human endeavor must be integrated into the mains of collective consciousness; otherwise, it slips back into serving the Ego: the "Me." Man must develop human faculties but not claim credit for the successes. One needs to be mindful that "I" and "Me" are both plugged into collectivity for the purposes of a collective good.

Evolutes of the sixth step and beyond such as Chinmaya, Baba, Christ, Buddha, Mahavir brought with them messages of compassion and non-violence. They taught man to be centered and to sublimate their egos for the purpose of a common good. Collective evolution, in the final analysis, works for others as well as for oneself.

> While traveling with the Master in India he instructed me to stop conducting "Value-based Classes" for children and youth I had been running for fifteen years. My ego lifted its ugly head and there was a feverish resentment brewing on my tongue. Before I could utter a word, the Master said
>
> > "Now that you have served your own children and those of your community, serve the 'world family' with the same love and dedication, for a collective good."

Anyone can serve his own family, his own friends, and his immediate society. Volunteering his services for an invisible larger family of his Cosmic Mother takes intuitive understanding and a personal inner growth and transformation.

Preoccupation with the Past

Often, aspirants on the Path of Meditation get stuck at this level. This occurs because of our preoccupation that we must atone for all the sins of our previous lives. Seekers who are unable to forgive themselves become, blocked here.

Whatever we harbour against others, hinders our progress. We project learned images, programmed into our psyche, onto the people we meet. We constantly play childish games of vengeance and demonstrate a need to punish others.

Wrong religious notions by dogmatic religious people also block the *ajnaa chakra.* Instead of ascending this *chakra also*, individuals may become side-tracked into the supernatural instead of evolution.

These old memories programmed into our psyche over many previous births have the ability to sustain us in the present. They become our own natural reservoir of past habits, and opinions in the mind; but the Self is beyond the mind. Our endeavors should therefore be directed at becoming the Self and responding to the Collective Conscious Self in the present and not projecting ourselves back to the past or into the future.

> and the Master wrote:
>
> "Silence the Mind and Listen. This is the final state of true meditation.."

Intellectual Blocks to Progress

In the present, life should not be pre-programmed and linked to your past. It should be governed by spontaneity. Life unfolds into a happy future only when the seeker is centred on the present.

Maya which defines and operates the delusory laws of qualities and quantities, may play games with the ego and rationalize with the logic of the intellect. Often, the logical deductions we make are based upon hypothesis, which are illusions themselves. Unless the ego is transcended, one cannot experience the truth which is available at this stage.

The skills of the intellect must be transcended. The *Devi* (Life Force-Energy) works from both within and without. Awareness of the Life Force-Energy enlivens the central nervous system. The seeker feels this Life Force-Energy manifesting itself as vibrations in the spine. There is an awareness of a Universal Presence.

Until now, this knowledge [of spiritual efforts] has been gained through personal inquiry. An inner perception and wisdom, comes from this knowledge. Speech now becomes the language to make known inner communications, intuitive perceptions, and increased awareness within the seeker.

Self-mastery - Progress in Spiritual Effort

The first and the sixth *chakras* are linked at this level. The astral *ida and the pingala* and the astral spine *(sushumna, vajra, chitrini)* combine here in an interplay of *pranic* or astral forces. The practitioner knows this through his intuitive personal experience. There is definitely NO intellectualization.

The astral spine is the channel through which the Divine Light can move quickly up and down the spine and deeper into the *brahmanadi.* Self-mastery now allows one to control even the brightness of this Light within.

During meditation at this level, all colour sense perceptions and images of past lives disappear. The mind or individual beingness, perceives only the White Light which is formless as a Universal-Beingness. It has learned to focus only towards this White Light of the Great Void. The mind now rests in It, in *samadhi* or meditative ecstasy of the Self with the Supreme Self, in a state of Oneness.

Once this perfection has been reached, a feeling of neutrality is felt about everything. What is life about *when there is no interest* in the pleasures of living? One may leave the body at will. Or, one may stay on to help others reach the state of non-attachment until the *exit time* occurs. Every help given is a seed to be nurtured for a successful evolution and future growth:

> It was the last day of the *Yagna* and the Master spoke:
>
> "A brand new department Store was had opened by the Lord in New Delhi. The angels fluttered towards me, the *swami,* and urged me to take anything I desired

from the store. I declined but this one angel was a persistent body! The *swami* finally relented and asked for an apple. The angel spread out her wings and fluttered around the store in search of an apple. She returned with a foil-wrapped packet and gave it to me. I opened the packet right there and was surprised to find in it seeds of the apple I had asked for. 'We only give seeds, not the 'fruits,' the angel told me sweetly..

"To ensure that you eat the apple, you must grow and nurture the seeds first. The Lord never gives happiness or joy. He only supplies the 'seeds'. We must have the knowledge to cultivate them and harvest our own happiness in life.."

Walking on a Rainbow

The mystery of life begins with the discovery of the life-force and its creative energy. It finds expression first as a physical being and then as a higher spiritual force. Discovering "I" leads to our final enlightenment.

As already described, our body contains seven primary spiritual energy centres, or *chakras.* Some schools of thought assign different colours of the rainbow to each *chakra.* This is of little consequence while on a spiritual journey. What is important is that each energy centre relates to a level of inner awareness. We traverse a known path as we walk-the-way towards spiritual enlightenment. Red starts with the *muladhara chakra* and progresses upwards through orange, yellow, green, blue, indigo, and violet. To some seekers who are focused into colours, each ascending centre represents a stage in their growth. They make a personal assessment of the work that still needs to be done.

The seeds of the basics-of-survival exist in the *muladhara chakra* or the coccygeal plexus. Here there are seeds of the resources required by seekers for further knowledge. The seeker only requires a vision. He discovers the purpose in life. With the help of the Cosmic Mother, he is given the tools to creates for himself a path of ascension and expansion of this image of intent and purpose.

At the *svadhisthana chakra,* the seeker acknowledges the fruits of his desires for manifestation. He has the outer gifts of kinship and comfort. These are now the seeker's tools of altruism, for a Collective Good. Having enjoyed his personal achievements, the seeker must attain spiritual gifts which he can share with others on a similar path.

At the *manipura chakra* he acknowledges his inner gifts of self-expression to achieve interaction with Mother Nature. In the process, the seeker lets go of all external dependence and becomes the Creation itself. At this stage, fear becomes manifest. It is a fear of letting go of his last personality as the self-serving ego.

At the *anhaata chakra* there is an awakening of the inner *guru* to encourage the seeker even further. His growth is an inner balancing of his inner half with the outer half of his connectedness with Mother Nature. At this level, fear of change becomes an incredible force blocking further growth on the spiritual path. The Inner Guide or *guru* is automatically available to help overcome the fear of death of the seeker's last personality. The guide's unselfish love assists in the seeker's reformation, transformation and evolution. Forgiving oneself and all others is a major ritual of this centre.

At the *vishuddha chakra,* intuitive creativity becomes manifest. There is now an inner and an outer balance. There is integration of the present, past, and future. The result is a perfect blending with the previous steps on his spiritual journey. He has experienced life as an extrovert and accepted every theory after testing its truth. He has the ability to evaluate, act, and direct all future activity in accordance with the Divine Will.

At the *ajnaa chakra,* there is profound imagery of thoughts of past births and their integration with the present birth. When manifest, the seeker is able to visualize all his beliefs, habits, likes-and-dislikes, and concepts. He has the wisdom to see the images as a protective shield, for the purpose of protecting him from Her Creation. With the loss of connectedness, he blocks off the connecting energy. Silencing and stilling the mind through meditation ensures an opportunity for a newer experience, with major perceptual changes.

This is now the *new shield* with a modified set of beliefs and concepts to separate the sensitive causal being from the onslaught of all encounters within Her creation. Each new shield protects only for a while. This allows spiritual growth to rise to a certain level of awareness.

At the *sahasrahara chakra* there is a final merging of Awareness with Consciousness in a revelation of Wisdom. The seeker has a sturdy foundation of a complete knowledge of all lives previously lived. Through meditation and experience of Oneness in *samadhi*, all old interference have been eradicated. The self is able to communicate and merge with the Self. The seeker can trace his steps backwards and can walk out into the beauty of his own connectedness with Creation.

The whole journey along the spiritual centers of the divine cave is like walking backwards into the divine cave on a step-ladder of the rainbow. A return journey into myself!

Exercise in Concentration or Dharana

Sit in the meditation posture of your choice and enter the divine cave.

- Look and gaze into the east between and behind the eyebrows;
- Imagine the divine cave to be a hollow void of light of awareness;
- Fill the tube with cold White Light, starting from the bottom up and hold the image as long as you can, until it becomes effortless with each inspiration;

- Now repeat the same exercise bringing down a **warm** Light with each expiration and focusing the feel of warm and cold in the back of the throat; gradually transfer this feeling into the divine cave.
- *Repeat this for the inner-sight at the kutastha, where it appears formless as a Mass of Light.*

At this stage, near perfection is *not yet achieved and not yet secured*; however, the mind has achieved subtlety and has power to receive the next stage of development. A feeling of independence is perceptible.

Reaching out more is the only way to walk-the-rainbow of the seven spiritual centers and the five *koshas* or sheaths, all within the three bodies or *shariras*. To achieve perfection, the seeker walks on an inward journey from the skin to the Self or *atma:*

i. *Annamaya kosha* (food sheath);
ii. *Pranamaya kosha* (physiological sheath);
iii. *Manomaya kosha* (psychological sheath);
iv. *Vignanamaya kosha* (intellectual sheath);
v. *Anandamaya kosha* (causal bliss sheath);
vi. *Chittamaya kosha* (awareness sheath);
vii. *Atmamaya kosha* (consciousness sheath). (Please refer to Figure 7)

Help from a Teacher

Through controlled thought and speech, the seeker has now acquired the ability to speak with Mother Nature, and intuitively perceives an increased awareness *of things as they really are.* Everything begins to fall into place. He must, however, have *faith that he is protected by his own sincerity.* He must trust the Greater Power of his *guru* who communicates with him mind-to-Mind.

> and the Master wrote:
>
> "If a seeker lacks *shraddha,* it is not worthwhile for him to continue his pilgrimage [spiritual journey]. Only faith has the guts to enter into the sacred realms where even the subtlest logic of the *Upanishadic* [of Reality] declarations falter in exhaustion. From such altitudes, faith secretly inspires the heart ...and rockets into the Absolute..."

Some may experience the *Guru* actually speaking to them through dreams or may see images, landscapes, people, and pictures in a dream. Each of these possibilities present advice to be followed. This experience can extend itself to the ability to see and hear in the waking state. When this occurs, physical speech must cease.

The practitioner speaks with his Higher Self from a bodiless consciousness, where the consciousness leaves the body to "see" in another place. Love becomes free from self-indulgence and possessiveness. The seeker now understands how much more needs to be done within his life. This is the period to incorporate into the mind the idea that "I am anchored, and am growing in the Light."

Having become all-knowing about himself, the seeker understands the vagaries of the mortal body. Through his scriptural study, he has understood intellectually why man is attracted towards desire and indulgence. He recognizes that the only difference between him and others is that he knows his weaknesses.

Shakti or the power of Mother Nature grants the seeker with Divine Knowledge and understanding of the message of the *shastras* or scriptures symbolized by the book the *Devi* or Mother Nature holds. The Creative power of the first or *Muladhara Chakra* has now reached the highest form of manifestation.

Meditation on the seven astral centres within the divine cave takes him into the causal string that strings all the centres in one garland. The seven astral flowers must also disappear. He must become the enlightened *chitta* [memory] or Awareness. The final step is to merge with *chit or atma* or Consciousness. He knows his journey as a mortal is complete. He may willfully exit from his mortal coil or remain in it to serve those mortals who also are struggling on the path of spirituality.

An enlightened Master will live as long as he or she is needed by his students. Even when he does exit, he promises to be there for you always.

> The Master was eating his breakfast opposite the window to the mountains. He began speaking to the snowline of the peaks of the Himalayan range: "Your skirt is higher this morning beautiful maiden. Stop flirting with me. I am prepared but not as yet ready to embrace you in my arms.."
>
> I was alarmed. I knew he was telling us [the devotees around him] that his frail body was preparing to shed itself of this existence. I protested under my breath.
>
> He looked directly into my eyes for a moment. The stare was unmistakable. He was reassuring me. He muttered back under his breath.
>
> "I will remain with you, with and without this body. I will continue to show you the way. It is you who will open the doors of opportunity.." He shed the body after fifteen months.

Progress at the Ajnaa Chakra

We are told that the *Great Void* before space is not empty. It is served by *devas* or angels, including magnetic forces of attraction, rays, and galaxies of the astral planes. The *devas* guide the aspirant beyond the realms of the three dimensions (physical, mental, and emotional).

Shakti or Mother Nature or the Holy Spirit has to keep the world going through the innate laws of manifestation *(karma,* relativity, and quality). The practitioner has only to offer one's Energy to do with it what She or *Prakriti* bids.

The mind must be cleared of memories of emotions. When we are stuck on the spiritual path, there is usually a need to release past moments of regret, hurt, anger, resentment, blame, revenge, fear, or deep sadness. These are old thoughts in the subconscious refusing to be forgiven. Love is the only way to dissolve them.

and the Master wrote:

"To Greet Another is to stretch our mind in love, to touch another heart. Let us expand to embrace each other, all things beautiful, useful and lovable."

- Sit in the meditation posture of your choice and focus your gaze into the east within your divine cave. Roll back your tongue.
- Imagine the space between the eyes in front of you is a stage;
- On the stage place the person or situation you resent or fear most;
- Visualize this until the image is clear on the stage and hold the image or feeling it rouses in you. Create a situation opposite to what has been your experience with the person or situation and hold the image or idea for as long as you can. This form of opposite imaging frees the seeker from guilt, resentment, and hurt about a thing or a person.
- Some images are difficult to let go and the exercise must be repeated many times.
- Put yourself up on the stage between the eyebrows and see yourself change. Mother Nature allows us to pluck whatever is desired, from Her abundance!
- You may allow the images or ideas of your loved ones descend into the heart chakra giving love and adoration to the person with each heart beat!

The Power of Concentration and Devotion to Shakti

The best method of such a submission is to create the Devi in the seeker's divine cave between the eyebrows within the centre of Will or Kutastha or Krishna/ Christ Centre. This exercise is an examination and an acceptance of one's Self. This allows for the eventualisation of the best in the seeker.

- See the Divine in everything and disregard the negative interference of our perceptions.
- Keep it alive by seeing the Divine Mother in everything that is beautiful, perfect, forgiving, or in all the faculties we desire in ourselves.
- Accept from Her the energy to destroy our vasana or past memory personality aspects of ourself.
- Offer this energy back to Her so that it may become bigger, more beautiful, and more real.

Soon this offering of an image or "creation" develops a life of its own.

A visiting *yogi* was heard saying this:

"Our thoughts of the present become embedded as beliefs in our subconscious and create both the best and the worst in our future life's situations and

> experiences. Mother Nature loves without judgment and will grant in accordance with the thought pattern...
>
> "You choose your thoughts and your beliefs and create patterns of failure or success in the future. Your reactions with your contacts is therefore shrouded with resentment and criticism which breeds painful guilt and fear..."
>
> "Change your thought pattern, dissolve the past and create a new future. Whatever we believe will become true for us!"

Exercises for Experiencing Auras of Shiva-Shakti

Auras can be seen by combining the power-of-creativity or *shakti* with the light-of-awareness or *shiva*. The two petals symbolized at this *chakra* are the link between the Light of Consciousness and the Energy of Life-force - the combined *Shiva-Shakti.*

The exercise helps what has been learnt to become a self-directed action. Visualization of images gives the body, mind, and intellect (BMI) the ability to enter into his own perfection. The perfected images empower the seeker with a perfect way to build from within his very own psyche. It has the power to at tune Universal Intelligence with Individual and Total Memory during meditation.

Stare at a grain of rice until the eyes water (without blinking), for a long time; then, project the image of the rice grain in the sky in space;

Through such processes, you will begin to see auras of white light (coloured auras are to be noted, but rejected).

Shiva is the *Shakta* or male power behind Her and She is *Shakti: He is the source and power of Light and* She is the *Shakti and the source of Energy.* The united *Brahman* or God is the mystery of form and without form. The concept is difficult to grasp. It is an intuitive knowing of the Ultimate Truth.

Both Shiva-Shakti emanate from Brahman or God before Creation and back into It at the end of each creative cycle.

Light and Energy

The source of power or the Light Itself, cannot be discovered, until It emanates Light by Itself and of Itself. It is one power of *Shiva-Shakti* from which streams from the unmanifest vibrating life energy *(Aum)* into the manifested life *(Aum)* of the seeker who wishes to understand the "mysteries of creation." It is the manifest and unmanifest power as one Power, of Divine Light Energy.

Persistence is Critical

Despite reaching this level of study, temptations still exist to drag the seeker back to where he started:

- Persuasions and temptations abound. The *Devi* or Mother, at this level of evolution, carries an empty skull to remind the seeker that the mind must be empty of all mundane thoughts at all times. The habit of interpreting everything is unnecessary.
- Absorb spiritual insights. There should be no more analysis or judgments.
- The *Devi* also carries a *mala* or rosary to remind the seeker that his efforts should be continuous, until the *mantra* acquires a self-generating capability of self benediction.

> "Enter ye in at the strait gate: for wide is the gate, and broad is the way, that leadeth to destruction, and many there be which go in thereat: Because strait is the gate, and narrow is the way, which leadeth unto life. and few there be that find it " ..Mathew 7:13-14.

Keep your efforts centered in order to move ever closer to the Divine Light of Consciousness, *beyond the mind.* The aim is to shed it totally. Excellence is now achieved through continued control of the mind. There will be gains and at times losses. The seeker is asked to remain focused on liberation.

> and the Master reprimanded about 'disappointments':
>
> "..This is 'life'! Yet we hold on to the fleeting meaningless and purposeless joys and value them more than the Lord and His Service! He alone is real, permanent, the sole Protector..."
>
> "Never give up your *Japa* and a short sweet meditation. This will help you to be quiet, self-confident, and effortlessly consistent. These are the ingredients of success..."

Mind

An evolving seeker sees the Self through every window of thought and space; the Cosmic Self sees the seeker through the window of His omnipresent Love. Locked in this love, he may remain united or maintain in a dual relationship, identifying with the Cosmic Self as his subject of adoration.

The emancipating *yogi* can remain merged or, if he wishes, retain his individuality. When the seeker learns to love all beings and through meditation, learns to love God, then and then only, is his longing for true love satisfied.

When the seeker *[sadhak]* realizes Unity everywhere, he understands not only that God dwells in all beings, but that all beings are His manifestations. The *yogi* dissolves all dual perceptions of matter and mind into a single perception of Universal Consciousness.

Whether the *yogi* is conscious and awake, asleep in his subconscious state, or in the superconscious state of ecstasy, he remains aware of the memory of God as his Creator and Dreamer.

The *yogi* who feels the Universe to be his own body, experiences the afflictions and joys of all beings as his own. His mind has expanded into Universal

Consciousness. He is free even while feeling the pleasures and pains of his own body.

The evolving *yogi* may have his peace shattered by the invasive restlessness of past existences but this will cease when the mind becomes fortified by the habit of meditation.

When restlessness is conquered by the stronger habit of tranquillity, the *sadhak* becomes even more watchful against the sudden appearance of desires and worldly moods. He learns to control his physical restlessness by *pranayama*; this is the only way to check the agitated mind.

Only through *abhyas* or constant striving in *pratyahara* for withdrawal of the senses from the organs of action, can the seeker keep his soul tranquil, within the domains of the divine cave. It is the only way he can achieve dispassion or *vairagya*.

Not all *yogis* realize this goal through meditation. Most begin enthusiastically but relax their efforts over time. Other *yogis* meditate regularly and with devotion; they may even attain a high degree of advancement, but because of past *karma* or his present continued indulgences, lose their concentration and fail to attain the divine union.

The sense mind or *manas* coordinates the five senses and five organs of action; it is the cause of all externalization. The mind remains superior. Without it, sensations cannot be received and activities cannot be performed in response to the thoughts arising from the ego. Even in dreams, the mind is able to sense without actually performing any actions. Only a discriminating intellect can persuade the mind to turn away from the pleasures of the senses and help it concentrate on soul-blessedness, so that liberation can be achieved.

A restrained *yogi* is easily identified. His actions express purity, honesty, and sincerity; he has no intention to harm anyone; he practices self-restraint by not acting on temptations and desires. His speech is empowered with the creative force of *Aum* and supported by the inner perception of truth through contact with his own true Self.

Concentrating on the Truth, his conscious mind penetrates the subconscious mind. If he goes deeper still, he is bound to reach the realms of superconsciousness - the soul. Truth becomes an experience of knowing, or it becomes a realization. Through regular meditation, the *yogi* increasingly becomes one with Truth.

Mental austerity is the only way to maintain tranquillity throughout the entire inner being. The habitually restless mind becomes placid and content through repeated ecstatic meditation. The sensory ego is fully restrained, and the ego is freed from the chatter of restless thoughts. The *yogi* basks in absolute quietude which, over time, purifies his whole nature.

Sattvic mental austerity strives for continued inner discipline in activity as well as in meditation. Freed from the aggression of likes, dislikes, and expectations, the seeker becomes accepting of all circumstances. A divine purity and virtue permeates in all his motivations. He understands the law of *karma* and endeavors to be without desire for the fruit of his actions, concentrating instead only on the fruits of meditation.

and the Master wrote: "Never complain about the number of hours you have put in to do a job. Your nobility must estimate how much of you was put into each hour of your daily work...

"Work is love made visible. To bring into vivid expression your love for others is *work.* To drag yourself through each day's schedule, morose, unhappy, miserable, is *labor.* Work alone brings achievement, never labor. Grow up to be a Man of sheer achievements through loving work..."

Psychology of the Midbrain

Some schools of thought consider the pineal gland to be the seat of the mind with its past memories as the causal or *karanic* body. Others say the causal being resides in the *ajnaa chakra.* All we know for sure is that everything in the mind is interpreted on the basis of past memories of images, especially of intellectual ideational thought. At this stage of development, the past may come into focus again and cause disturbances in meditation. This irritant can be disempowered by invoking Divine Light.

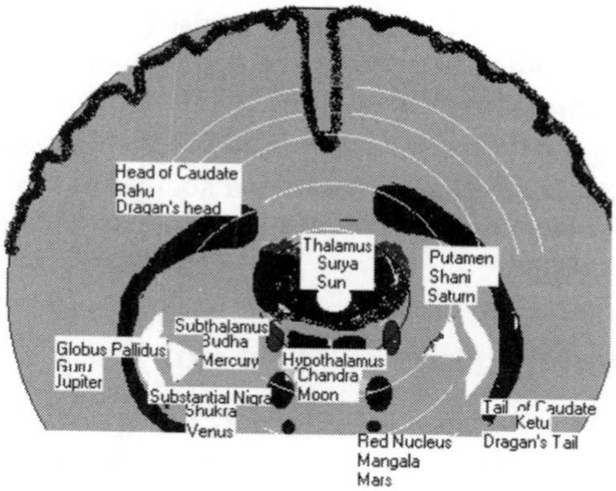

Figure 21. Planetary Centers in the Mid-brain

The hypothalamus [the moon in the planetary system] and the pituitary gland are considered the master-glands, capable of recharging the mind and transforming the entire body, through the release of neurotransmitters and neuro-hormones. It is here that *Shakti* or Mother Nature has poured the greatest amount of energy *(in the thalamus as Aum)* for the use of the seeker for his daily living.

The pituitary and the hypothalamus have an inherent system of all possibilities of good health, as well as bad health. These possibilities exist in the present life as memories [in the DNA molecules of the thalamus] from previous lives. The sensuous mind, governed by intellectual concepts about the world, forces the mortal to respond to his five senses demanding, pleasure. The mind does not have the power of discrimination, but the intellect can be reasoned with through *sadhana* or spiritual efforts.

The two, the thalamus [physical manifestation of the causal mind] and the master glands [moon-controlled health possibilities in the pituitary and the hypothalamus], are connected and balanced in a perfect circle. Neither one overrides the other. The control of these two centers is given to the self [individual person].

From the thalamus [sun which controls all movements of the planets and therefore the midbrain centres] all changes in the human psyche are permanently recorded. Changes match the individual's desires and needs. They are for spiritual gains [an inward journey] or for pleasure [an outward journey]. The thalamus [Light of Awareness or *Prakriti*] is increasingly perfected through inputs for desire for the Universal Self (Consciousness or *Purusha).*

All changes arise from this true centre of physical awareness [thalamus]. This is where the astral 'third eye' of the Sun is located. This is where the *Krishna* or Christ Centre or the reflection of the *Kutastha Chaitanya* is found, **behind the eyebrows**. This is where the *Shiva and Shakti* coalesce as "One Light with Energy," functioning perfectly, one with the other. Here, the mind-intellect-ego can achieve its most powerful indicator of perfect balance. The seeker who possesses a perfect health in body, mind, and intellect is the perfect vehicle for *sadhana* or spiritual journey.

> My father once explained to me the significance of the *tikka* or 'dot' on the forehead. "The ancient *rishis* knew that the seat of the soul resides in a cradle behind the forehead in [later identified as the sella turcica in my student days]. Therefore they honoured the spot with vermilion and sandalwood paste"

Achieving Perfect Balance of Mind not Easy

The objective mind or intellect requires a great deal of training through *sadhana* in order to be able to discriminate what the subjective mind of emotions or **experiencer or *rishi*** is *watching* from the altitudes of the *sahasrahara chakra.*

The **experiences** of the ***devata*** in the *chitta* [mind-intellect-ego] in the hypothalamus-pituitary axis are a continuous modification made during inputs of every new information, whether good or bad, into the thalamic 'microchip' template of the causal being.

All subsequent **experiencing** is now under the influence newly observed qualities. The new neurohormones and neurotransmitters have a changed quality and therefore their actions are in keeping with the new principles. They are therefore said to have a specific or ***chhandas*** quality. All new responses to the new information recorded into the *devata* [thalamus or awareness or *prakriti*] are now modified likes-and-dislikes or *raaga dvesha*, inclusive of past habits. The senses and the organs-of-action act in the world outside in accordance with the personality of this individual *devata.*

Every action and indulgence, if *repeated often enough,* becomes a habit and a part of an internal filing-system. Once they enter into the filing system, the experiences of past and present become the dossier of our next action (combined experiencer-experience-experiencing) in this life and in the next incarnation.

Governed by the Laws of *Karma* (action-and-reaction) and Relativity (likes-and-dislikes or *raaga dvesha*), his next brain recycle [every eight years] takes on a personality of the old and the new life-state, combined. This new personality is now the person's modified *vasana* or causal body.

It exists in the *karanic* or causal brain [thalamus as awareness of *prakriti*] as images of ideational thought. It contains every thought information lived through the body, mind-emotion, and intellect.

The objective mind or intellect must surrender through *sadhana* in order to make the correct changes, free from interpretations of the objective mind. Such a complete surrender of the objective mind, which instinctively interprets everything based upon past and present lives, is very difficult.

The functions of the controlling organ of all physical, physiological, and psychological functions of the body by the pineal-pituitary gland, can be negated gradually through the withdrawal of the creative life-force. In a *return-journey,* the seeker is able to reverse the out-going life-force through *pratyahara* (withdrawal from the senses and organs-of-action). Without the life-force or *prana*, the mind or *manas,* and the intellect or *buddhi*, the pituitary gland cannot discriminate. Once silenced, the life-force is silenced by becoming pure *prana* Itself. This is Awareness.

Pratyahara, thus, is the means for withdrawing life-force from:

- senses and organs of action *(annamaya kosha);*
- physiological functions of the body *(pranamaya kosha);*
- psychological functions of the mind *(manomaya kosha);* and
- intellect (*vignanamaya kosha).*

The objective mind (intellect) at this stage only intellectually understands the processes followed to date but requires further intense clarification and training:

- First, by laying and securing the foundations of character building or *yama;*
- Secondly, by laying and securing the foundations of spiritual character building or *niyama;* and

- Thirdly, by combining them through *gyana* or knowledge, *karma* or action, and *bhakti yoga* or devotion, to bring about wisdom or *vigyana.*

The objective mind or intellect as vasanas is a reservoir of collected material from past events and images of many lives.

The objective mind (intellect) which has stored all this material does not know what to do with it and this creates "personality" and psychological problems in the untrained mind.

For this reason, there must be perfect balance between the subjective ("I" the soul) and objective ("Me" or mortal). This is achieved when the objective mind or intellect is trained through *sadhana,* to modify the material extracted from this *devata or* causal mind where "Me-I" resides. Once the "Me" has been chiseled sufficiently, the "I" shines unencumbered as a subjective knowing!

Memory

The seeker is the High Priest of his own destiny. He can see his within and finds it as the cause of all that he sees outside himself. His world is an exact replica of what is taking place in his own inner psyche. His *karanic* self speaks to him in images of his thought desires. He has in it the knowledge of all his past lives. By meditation and attunement with the universal memory in the Cosmic Womb or *hiranyagarbha,* the seeker has access to all past information about himself and Creation.

He has the ability to lift the seven veils of his sheath-envelopments or *koshas* [food *or annamaya kosha*-physiological *or pranamaya kosha*-psychological *or manomaya kosha* -intellectual *or gyanamaya kosha* - bliss *or anandamaya kosha* -awareness *or chittamaya kosha* -consciousness *or atmamaya* or *chitmaya kosha*] (Please refer to Figure 7 and read 'Exercises in Dharana' in this section of the text).

He knows that the Light of Awareness *(Prakriti as chitta)* and Consciousness *(Purusha as atma)* permeates every atom and life's energy in his mind, senses, and ego. He is the power of feeling in his heart that determines how he will react to the contacts he makes with the objects of his senses. He empowers memory by which perceptions are held and connected with one another in the accumulation of knowledge. God is also the deluding cosmic hypnosis of *maya,* which has the ability to distort pure feelings, memory, and understanding.

Deluded by soul-humiliating emotional likes-and-dislikes, man becomes attached to his own bodily instruments and personalizes all his experiences, trying to bend them according to his inclinations. A seeker by now has learnt to say no to that which does not benefit him as a *sadhak* or seeker. His body has taught him lessons; his mind speaks to him through feelings and responses. He observes all his patterns of behavior and makes the necessary changes against a backdrop of past memories.

The *yogi* on the path of liberation strives to attune himself to mirror the Self and, through meditation, frees himself of the shackles of his mortality. He realizes his human perceptions and memories are entangled with the emotions of the heart. He is living in a *maya* (delusional) hypnotized existence as a physical being. He knows he must awaken the memory of his own divinity.

A *yogi* who becomes one with Him who is seated in all hearts, regains his memory of the Knowledge and Wisdom through meditation. He knows he has descended to become a mortal but must ascend back to His liberating presence. He knows that his sexuality or life-force, his creativity or *pranic* energy, and spirituality or *tejas* are all blossoms growing out of each other. It is a tough journey:

> and the Master wrote:
>
> "The divine path leading the pilgrim to the Temple of Truth, is not always even; it contains many a steep ascent. It winds through dangerous gorges, dark tunnels, fearful jungles, and precipitous steeps. To control the mind and to move steadily on, away from the fields of perception and thoughts, and ascend the tranquil peaks of the Infinite Consciousness, is not a pleasant travel!
>
> "Many a time the pilgrim feels waves of passions, gushes of despair, storms of despondency, and cyclones of hopelessness rocking his courage and shattering his serenity. To pursue the path in spite of these benumbing influences, the pilgrim must be a great hero, who has a private exchequer of inspiration and confidence from which to draw. He must indeed have an unlimited exchequer of power and strength. This exchequer of Infinite strength is called faith.."

Exercises for Ajnaa Chakra

At this stage, the seeker has become adept with the *pranayama* of timing his breathing with *Ham'saa - So'ham*. While his Consciousness 'watches' the quietened breath during *pratyahara,* his Awareness 'looks' at the changes taking place within himself (thalamus).

The seeker remains centred in the divine cave by rolling his tongue into the soft palate. His gaze is turned upwards and inwards to connect with the Cosmic Vision in the east between the eyebrows. He 'feels' the energy of his astral body. He 'hears' the vibrations of his own inner being as 'inner sounds' or *antardhvani.* Every sense-faculty is withdrawn into the stillness and silence of his astral divine cave. The seeker feels weightless while within himself and within the divine cave.

The effect of *pratyahara* is felt all over the body while doing 'energizing exercises' taught by Masters adept in *hatta yoga*. By watching the *prana* or life-force, first in the breath and then in the divine cave, the practitioner moves away from the out-going senses and into the shelter of the altar of the divine cave.

He acknowledges that his whole body is a mass of energy, through the processes of *pratyahara*. He now knows from a personal experience that he has the ability to transform his bodily atoms. He can heal his bodily cells and transform his brain-cells in cycles of seven years. Through intense unselfish meditation, he can and will become One with the Cosmic Mother. His purpose in life must remain clear: he seeks a connectedness with his Cosmic Mother. Having found her he then serves Her.

Prana - the Vibrating Life Force

Prana (Aum), as a vibrating pulsating individualized and Universal energy, must be experienced in meditation. The seeker now needs to practice, even harder, the processes of disconnecting from the five out-going senses and resting in the divine cave through *pratyahara* or withdrawal from the five senses and five organs of action.

This is done by first practicing the *Yoni Mudra* and the *Maha Mudra*. Both are *asanas* combined with *pranayama, pratyahara,* and *dharana* used to help the practitioner to progress further. These techniques are taught by *yogis* only.

Wisdom

The aspiring *yogi* wanting liberation transcends body consciousness and works from the level of awareness. He is partially liberated and functions through discrimination of the enlightening intellect, intuitive guidance is received while concentrating on his spiritual eye or *kutastha* opposite the *ajnaa* center.

The worldly man's mind and life activities are centered in the first three spinal centers or *chakras.* The seeker is advised to strive to keep his mind concentrated away from the senses of taste, touch, sight, smell, and hearing; rather, he should concentrate on the forehead, which is the seat of the spiritual eye and discrimination. It is this center of will, wisdom, and intelligence that empowers self-control.

The blissful soul who is perfecting himself in wisdom begins to know all things by intuition. He recognizes that his perceptions work through the instrument of senses, mind, and intellect. He knows that contact with objects occurs through the operation of the mind and the desire to indulge. Such sense desires have the capability to choke the discrimination born of Self-realization. These desires must be extracted from the subconscious and eradicated through the agents of spiritual perception, brought forth by meditation.

Any disturbance in the seeker's attunement with Cosmic Wisdom causes Nature's twentyfour components [five elements, five senses, five organs-of-action, five objects- of-senses, mind, intellect, ego, and *chitta*] for sensory perceptions, to dilute his awareness of consciousness in Oneness. The unenlightened seeker does not see his source; he only sees the elements that shroud the self. When the *sadhak* succeeds in freeing his awareness of body perceptions, he realizes that his lost and found wisdom is the only liberator of his mortality.

God does not speak to the average seeker, a beginner on the spiritual path. The only way a *sadhak* or seeker discovers the Will of God is by serving a true Master and becoming attuned to his guidance. By following the Master's instructions, the seeker becomes ripe for wisdom. Having risen from the identification of the first three mundane *chakras*, he has succeeded in controlling the senses.

The *sadhak's* devotion in the beginning is imperfect, conditional, and spasmodic. He practices external forms of devotion, all the while doubting and questioning the relevance of the teaching. In the later stages of evolution, the *sadhak* or seeker has unshakable and unconditional devotion to the Lord. He now becomes manifest through his devotion to the *guru*, respect for the words of all scriptures, control of the senses, and meditative practice.

> and *Adi Shankara* wrote (sage who lived fifteen hundred years ago and is the founder of the line of sages that produced my Master): "If you find peace in the presence of a *mahatma* [sage]; if you are inspired by his speeches; if he is able to clear your doubts; if he is free from greed, anger, and lust, if he is selfless and loving; with whom if you compare your own life you feel ashamed of your own weaknesses..you can take him [her] as your *guru*.."

Yoni-mudra or the Closing of the House

Each stage of the pranayamas begin with expiration or rechaka and end with inspiration or puraka. Inspirations made through the nose make a sibilant "sssss" sound and all expirations make the sound of "hhhhh"

Only one breathing technique may be done during a sitting or you may devote time to do them all in succession at the end of yoga meditation.

- Breathing is initiated by the diaphragm and the lower chest muscles. Air is filled from the bottom up towards the base of the neck (between the two collar bones).
- Ensure the asana keeps the spine erect by pulling the shoulder blades together and contracting the lower abdominal muscles **at all times during meditation.**
- Sit erect, neck and head straight in one line, with chin parallel to the ground and therefore head, slightly lifted.

In these preparatory stages, be aware of the sensations of breathing in the lungs while breathing normally through the nose. Keep the eyes closed and focused at the bhrumadhya in the east between the eyebrows.

1. Always start pranayama after expiration and end it with inspiration.

- Now follow the breathing into its four components:
- **inspiration - pause - expiration - pause.**
- Keep the eyes passively closed and receptive to the inner gaze of Infinity in the divine cave;
- Concentrate the ears to become alert and receptive to the inner hearing;
- First listen to the breath sounds and adjust by synchronizing the flow and tone of the breath;
- Do not inflate the abdomen while breathing: It is the chest that needs inflating by using the diaphragm which has been freed by contracting the lower abdominal muscles.
- By contracting the lower abdominal muscles, the contracting diaphragm descends and the contracting intercostal muscles lift the breast bone for inspiration and inspiratory pause (antara kumbhaka).

You are now connected to the "mains" of Stillness.

- During expiration, the diaphragm and intercostal muscles relax for expiration and expiratory pause (baahara kumbhaka).
- This completes one cycle of breathing: continue this for ten minutes until the whole body, and especially the limbs relax.
- This now is surrendering to the Lord. Exhale and pause silently. Now watch the movements of the breath; next, look at the Cosmic Vision in the divine cave with the tongue rolled back; listen to the Cosmic Sound and feel the silence!

You are now connected into the "mains" of Silence.

- Try to prolong both the inspiratory pause and the expiratory pause without exerting to cause discomfort.

2. Closing the openings of the body in the Yoni Mudra:

Remember always to have the eyes focused in the east with the tongue rolled back.

- Raise both hands to the face so that the elbows are at the same level as the shoulders. You may use a T-bar to rest your elbows on, instead.
- Gently press the thumbs on the tragus of the ears to shut them and to keep out all external sound.
- Close the eyes and bring the index fingers over the eyelids.
- Gently draw the upper lids down with the index finger.

Cover the lower half of the eye with the middle finger to keep out the light. Keep the eyes passive and receptive.

- Press them gently with the fingers.
- Place the middle finger on each side of the nostril and narrow the nostrils. Place the little finger under the nostril on the upper lip in order to feel the flow of the breath.
- Now watch the breathing.

- After inspiration and at pause, place slight pressure on the eyes, narrow the nostrils and close the ears. Look at the Cosmic Vision and listen to the inner sounds.
- With expiration and pause release the pressure.
- The seeker can hear the inner sound of Aum as the ears are closed by the thumbs. The pressure on the eyes allows one to see various colors of dazzling light or the sun, which one encounters during meditation.
- It is very difficult to maintain this mudra, with the arms abducted unless you have a T-bar such as the ones yogis carry with them. Wrapping a tight bandage over the ears and temples while doing pranayama in the yoni mudra is an acceptable alternative to this.
- At the end of Yoni Mudra, inhale and complete the exercise.

and the Master wrote about Knowledge as a pre-requisite to Meditation:

"Read what is in my discourses and become one with them. Then come with me into my world of Peace and Joy.."

Realization of the Self

Self-realization is difficult to attain because the average man's attention through the five senses is turned outwards towards the perception of objects rather than inwards towards the Self. Even with free will, man is habit-bound. He does not attempt to change his material habits into spiritual habits. Since each person is on his journey back to his own Source, sooner or later he must yield to the divine pull and enter the Cosmic Home.

As long as bad habits are not causing any disruptions in his life, man is not anxious to return to the Cosmic Home. When man is fiercely battered by the storms of cosmic delusion *or Maya*, only then does he commence an inner call for help. The response to this call is an inner pull of the Divine.

Only those who cling on to unfinished mortal desires have to reincarnate to play the delusions of Cosmic Nature, on the surface of life. Many sincere seekers desirous of returning home neither force themselves to seek the Cosmic Home through ever intensifying meditation nor do they persist in their search for His presence.

Some learned *yogis* have stated that a *sadhak* who continuously prays for communion with God for three days and three nights, or even twenty-four hours, will realize God. Even when advanced *yogis* are reborn, they do not automatically come under the sway of delusion when they are reborn. Having performed good actions in past lives, they have silenced the agitating effects of past *karmas* through self-discipline. Their hearts are free of the ripples of likes-and-dislikes; they are able to reflect and concentrate on the Self and find shelter in the Self.

In the new reincarnation, the *yogi* knows the secret of the *law of karma* and knows how to escape from the wheel of delusory living. By entering meditation, this *yogi* learns to perceive the presence of God in his physical, astral, and causal bodies. He knows how to unite his heart with the bliss of the soul; he retains this divine awareness even at the time of his death.

Even these *yogis* need to practice to become centered and grounded in the practice of meditation and reject the constantly troubled changes of the body, mind, and intellect. They must learn to be prepared for their mortal death when the soul, that is, ego consciousness, gradually retires with his astral and causal bodies into the astral planes of existence.

> When still in my early twenties, my father, an accountant by profession, allowed me to witness the severing of the 'umbilical cord' with the manifested Cosmic Mother. He called for me in the wee hours of the morning. On my arrival he informed me that he was leaving on a long journey and needed help to get ready. He warned me not to interfere with his body if he became unconscious.
>
> He visited the toilet and also had a bath. He emerged fully clothed and unable to stand. He coughed and turned quite blue. I was alarmed. I had still not been exposed to cardiogenic shock and my father knew I did not have the wisdom to understand what he was doing!
>
> I helped him sit up on the bed and he spoke to whoever was left at home that night. He bid my fortytwo year old mother good bye and asked everyone to leave his room. He called me last of all. I realized he was dying and he consoled me that he was only "...changing his coat...he would always be with me". He then ordered me to leave.
>
> I watched him sit erect in the asana of meditation and he placed his breath in the lap of the Cosmic Mother with a "Hari Aum'!

Ego and Death

As long as desire for physical life remains, the ego remains adamantly lodged in the brain and the spinal cord, or the divine cave. The body now enters a tug of war with physical death. If the body dies, the ego escapes through the astral body into the astral world until it is reawakened to his innate material desires recorded in his causal body. Surging for self-expression, the deluded soul seeks a proper home and environment for his next earthly journey as a limited mortal.

A *yogi* who has been trained in the technique of meditation has learned the ability to disconnect life-force and mind from the senses; he is able to withdraw his ego at will. He carries his life-force, mind, and ego upwards through the five *chakras* and unites with the bliss of the soul in the *chittamaya kosha* in the *ajnaa chakra*. Finally, he withdraws his soul and unites it with the Spirit in the *atmamaya kosha* in the seventh *chakra*. He makes a grand-exit into the Cosmic Soul and can decide for himself if he wishes to return to this world of the mortals.

Kapalabhati Pranayama or Kriya

"Kapala" stands for skull and "bhati" means light. In this pranayama, the inspiration is slow and the expiration vigorous. The pause after inspiration is four or more seconds and at the end of expiration the pause is short and negligible.

Kriya generates prana to invigorate the whole body and the divine cave. To practice kriya too long is like stoking an engine continuously: it can burn out the body because the breathing is so forceful.

In this pranayama, breathing is through the mouth. It cools the system with inspiration and warms it during expiration.

- Sit in an asana of your choice with eyes gazing at the cosmic vision in the divine cave, tongue rolled back and watching the breath.

  Now, with back straight, lower abdomen pulled towards the spine and lifted to the navel, bring the shoulders back until the scapulae meet with the chin parallel to the ground.

  Do basic pranayama for five to ten minutes using the 'Hum' saa..So'ham' technique, until the body and mind are still and the inner ear hears an inner silence with Aum in the backdrop.
- Become "spine conscious".

  Exhale deeply .

  Now inhale slowly through the mouth.

  Form a crow's beak with the lips and draw up cold air by inspiration by making a sucking sound of "haw".

  Draw the cool air from the base chakra to the back of the neck and bend it forwards from the ajnaa to the Kutastha or Christ center. Hold the inspiratory breath for four seconds.

  Now exhale down the spine feeling the warm air in the back of the throat . Make a hissing sound "hee" during expiration (by contracting throat muscles). Do not pause. This makes one full cycle. Restart inspiration as described.

  Continue this for 30 cycles, gradually increasing the number as able.
- Repeat this until concentration is centered in the divine cave (up to fourteen times twice daily).

  Magnetize the spine by sitting erect with both hands folded at the base of the head. Contract and relax the four parts of the back until the area become light and weightless.

  This exercise allows the seeker to enter the astral phase of the divine cave in the brain and spinal cord. Now watch the breath for ten minutes and listen to the inner cosmic sound. Ensure that your gaze is fixed at the Cosmic

Vision and the tongue is rolled back.

End the exercise with inspiration before opening your eyes.

Padma Asana or Asanas in Mahamudras

I . i. Again, sit erect on the floor. This time, sit with left heel against the anus and right foot stretched in front.

- First practice "stretching" by stretching down to hook the finger around the big right toe with the body bent forward and the two hands sliding down to the toe.
- Do this while focusing on the bhrumadhya in the divine cave between the eyebrows, with the tongue rolled back.
- Draw the right leg back into the folded position and repeat the same for the left leg.

ii. Next practice kriya pranayama with this asana:

- Start with expiration.
- Next inhale with the mouth open.
- Take in cool breath into the chest with an open mouth curled in an "O".
- Make a sucking sound "haw" during inspiration.
- Feel the coolness at the back of the throat .
- Pause at the end of inspiration for four seconds.
- Now, exhale a warm breath (felt at the back of the throat) with the teeth together.
- Make a slight hissing sound : "Hee..ee" during expiration, and do not pause. Quickly start to inspire again.
- Initially focus on the sound of the breath and feel the breath move between the navel and the throat chakras.

The end of expiration completes one cycle.

- Now transfer the attention to the spine and become conscious of the divine cave.

iii. Combine the two mudras by doing the kriya pranayama with the leg exercises.

- Start with the left leg first and then the right. Repeat up to six times each - twice daily: Tensing the lower abdominal muscles during the exercise releases the diaphragm and intercostal muscle for breathing.

This also improves the venous return from the lower half of the body.

iv. Sit with right foot tucked under the buttock and left foot extended. Begin by exhaling.

- While inhaling through the mouth make the "haw" sound. During inhalation slide the hands down the left lower leg and hook fingers around the big toe. Hold the breath there for four seconds.

- Now while exhaling, slide the hands back at the groin while making the sound "heee". Straighten the back with lower abdomen contracted towards the navel and pause.
- Now tuck in the left leg and repeat the same for the right leg. This makes one cycle.

For those unable to sit on the floor in the padma posture (lotus position):

- Mahamudra asanas are practiced by sitting on the floor with the legs extended in front or, alternatively may be done by sitting on a chair to do the exercises.

During these exercises, always remember to focus the gaze between the eyebrows in the east, with the tongue rolled back.

Energizing Exercises and Pratyahara

Just as air surrounds beings and water surrounds fish, beings are surrounded by cosmic energy - Aum. It is this Aum that enlivens the body from within and without.

- During meditation, the practitioner is asked to focus on the bhrumadhya in the east, between the eyebrows and listen to the cosmic sound of Aum through the right ear.
- Once centralized in the divine cave, he must invoke his Will to maximally contract and then relax each of the following twelve groups of muscles in an upward direction: toes and feet - calves - thighs - buttocks and perineum-lower, middle, and upper back - left and right abdomen - left and right chest - fists - forearms - upper arms - shoulders - sides of neck, face, and head.
- Repeat this three times, each time willing the that the muscles are energized with Aum radiating out of the divine cave to all parts of the body. Collapse the energy back into the divine cave during relaxation.

Next, contract each group of muscle until all the groups are now contracted:

- Contract all the muscles in total - the muscles should be vibrating at maximal contraction while willing the Aum into the body; continue contracting until you sense the vibrant energy of Aum in the whole of your being.
- Now relax the whole body together and become aware of the same Aum. Watch the breath and watch the changes in every cell of your body.
- Repeat three times.

This technique of pratyahara and energizing can be repeated for hours; it can be combined with pranayama; the attention should be to maintain silence within the divine cave. The inner gaze should be on the Cosmic Vision. The tongue should be rolled back. The hearing should only strive to hear the inner sound of Aum in the stillness of the divine cave. This together is dharana and dhyana.

Always remember the position of the eyes and the tongue and watch the breath. These yogic exercises are best taught by yogis.

The Physiological and Psychological Basis of the Mudras

The purpose of *pranayama* is to develop steadiness in the body, to keep the mind and emotions in balance and the intellect sober. When the practitioner observes the flow of breath being absorbed into his astral system, he notices that there is a transformation. Body, breath, mind, intellect, and the ego become one. The seeker loses his identity, and the knower (who watches or Consciousness) - the knowledge (who looks or Awareness), and the knowing (who acts and contacts with world-of-OET) become One.

Combining *pranayama* with *pratyahara* allows the seeker to become not only *prana* as life-force, but also *prana* as creative-energy or *Aum.* Prolonged practices lead the seeker into the silence and stillness of his divine cave, first resting in his astral plane and then in his causal plane.

Lost in this oneness, the practitioner is aware of a harmony which is, without doubt, special. He experiences acute awareness. The experience is subjective and personal. He alone can hear and is able to hear the sound of the breathing in his stillness. He alone can feel and enjoy the soundless silence of *Aum.* This is the quest of the Self.

The inspiration or *puraka* is the absorption of cosmic energy. The pause at the end of inspiration or *antara kumbhaka* is the union of the individual self ("Me") with the Self ("I"). Expiration or *rechaka* is the surrender of the individual energy. The pause at the end of expiration or *bahara kumbhaka* is the merging of the "I" with the Universal Self. This is *nirvikalpa samadhi.* Such a practitioner constantly breathes, lives and experiences *Tat Twam Asi* or That Thou Art.

From a practical level, *mudras, pranayama and pratyahara* improve the health of the practitioner, preventing diseases of the bone and slowing the heart and respiration to match the lowered basal metabolic rate. The whole process reduces the rate of cellular decay associated with aging.

Analysis on the Higher Mind or Chitta

Love is a universal currency and must be used freely. Man must learn to give and accept this gift from Mother Earth. Love can be allowed to enter your spiritual heart to remind the seeker that it is given freely. It empowers the mind and intellect and is recorded in the causal being as an image of a positive experience. Sorrow is the separation of Man and Creation. True love is a connectedness of the seeker with Creation.

What is this thing called "mind" which keeps us both prisoner and yet can experience such luminosity of the divine?

- It is like two selves, neither sharing the experiences of the other.
- We can neither walk away from the part that holds us hostage nor can we continue to live within the orbit of the Light.

What is this mind that demands to have everything explained, when there is really nothing to be explained, only experienced?

- Can the mind understand the knowing of the heart?
- If the mind has no form, then what is it that we experience?
- Are mind and consciousness the same thing?

If the brain is the physical seat of the mind, how does it function?

- What energy does it use to think?
- How does it transmit thought into the power of speech?

What is consciousness? Does it bridge the world of phenomenon with the world of the Absolute?

> and the Master said: "Reject everything about the Mind when looking for the Self, the Unborn Mind..."

One needs to possess the faculty of Love so that the Laws of Nature reveal themselves to the seeker. Their mighty powers allow the seeker to perceive the Oneness and Wholeness of the Universe. *Prakriti* refuses to reveal Her secrets, unless Her children love Her.

Wanderers along the Path of Spirituality are already in possession of images, of concepts, and of habitual separation from the Universe. Only the receptive mind has the ability to gaze and become inspired by the communication of the "Me" in his awareness with the "I" of my individuality and its connection with Creation (the Total "I").

Possession of the Intuitive Knowledge that all creatures, things, and beings are our "mothers" at some time or another in our previous lives, triggers an inner understanding. This empowerment will allow the seeker to feel, think, and expand into the vision of Oneness. The seeker realizes that images of his past lives embedded in his causal beingness is a perpetual dance in the Circle of Life.

Awareness and Consciousness

Mind is awareness, an expression of Consciousness with access only to limited consciousness. Consciousness, on the other hand, is unlimited in dimension.

- It is the substratum of awareness of the mind, and thus anything beyond the mind cannot be expressed.

In Eastern thought, the mind is the *sixth sense*. To discover and achieve its potential, it must be investigated thoroughly. Life is experienced through the five senses. The Mind interprets these experiences because it is empowered through the ability of creativity of *pranic energy*.

The mind interprets all experience within the limits of its past (conscious, subconscious and unconscious) and therefore will not expand into greater possibilities of superconsciousness.

- Emotional insecurity makes mind expansion impossible.
- The mind is unwilling to rise above its mental-emotional restrictions or lower astral planes of existence.

Each seeker therefore goes through his own private-hell when letting go of his mental and emotional security support systems, a pre-requisite necessary to go beyond the accepted limits of the mind - free of concepts and opinions.

The seeker experiences a rocky path, progressing from being a sleepwalker, then hypnotized conditioned being, and finally an aware person, receptive to the goal of Cosmic Consciousness.

Harnessing the Mind

The mind operates through the conscious (awake state of *tamas*), the subconscious (dream state of *rajas*) and the unconscious (deep sleep state of *sattva*) states of being. Each of these states has a qualitative mental characteristic, the *gunas* or qualities of matter.

To keep the mind *sattvic*, the mind must be cleared of all concepts. A pure mind has qualities of desirelessness, detachment, dispassion, and surrender. It becomes preoccupied with the happiness of others. In this way, the mind attains transparency.

Since the *rajasic* mind is connected to concepts, the possibilities of creation and destruction, a passion for activity, and a need for constant entertainment through indulgences, it must dedicate all passion and energy to *karma yoga* or Path of Action for a higher ideal.

The *tamasic* mind is preoccupied with instincts and thoughtless desires. Selfishness clouds understanding, and the mind is inaccessible. Devotion to a personal ideal is the path for such a person.

Unconscious Higher Mind or Chitta

Unconscious mind activity (images and ideas of previous births) crystallizes into the subconscious state as dreams. The unconscious mind (the *karanic* or causal mind) is also able to permeate into the conscious mind as habits, concepts, and opinions.

All things are created in the higher mind through the creation of concepts, which give the *chitta* (mind, intellect and ego) a framework to understand its own formulations within its own limits. When there is a decision made by a Collective Mind, it becomes the collective effort of many minds: It becomes a force of Collective Destiny. When values are clear, the mind gathers energy and will discriminate between self-gratification and the power that benefits others.

The Secretary of State had arranged a one day Seminar for the various ethnic groups of the city. The new immigrants were concerned about the necessity of a Cultural Identity. By the end of the day, it was apparent that the definition of 'culture' was different for each group present felt they may become victims of their shaky destinies. That evening, The master defined Culture and Collective Will:

"When a people live in the same geographic area for a long time, respecting and following common higher values of life and living, their life acquires a special fragrance of a unique aroma. This is the culture and collective destiny of the people.."

Intellect or the Desiring Mind

Intellectual thought is a refined capability of the logical mind. It expresses itself as concepts, interpretations, generalizations, thought associations, differentiation and distinguishing abilities, and the storing and retrieving of memory: all are the result of training given to the mind, through formal education.

Mind control is essential in order to restrain the energy *(Shakti)* and power *(Shiva)* of this faculty. Drifting minds are easily agitated. Learning to control the mind and direct it increases awareness and frees the seeker from mechanical thought and action.

The mind must be aware of the background noises of thoughts which emanate from persons, news, television and other distractions, leading to the loss of one's individuality. The mind can twist facts in memories to suit itself, just for the sake of such an individuality.

Exercises in Mind Power

Daily reflection will clarify the many areas in which the seeker has developed concepts and conditioning. Patanjali asserts that reconditioning is done through CMC (Concentration, Meditation, and Contemplation) at the *chitrini*, the point of three in one. (Please refer to Figure 16).

This occurs in the midbrain region where the astral thalamus is the seat of the *kutastha*. The *ajnaa chakra* is where the causal being resides as an astral being. The pineal gland and the pituitary gland is where the neurohormones and neurotransmitters are released for evolution of the physical, physiological, and the psychological bodies. (Please refer to Figure 12). This is achieved through the use of Will Power and the ability to focus, to give attention, to accept, and to let go of old concepts and conditioning.

At the start, new concepts are substituted for old ones, through the process of learning. Clouded thinking is now replaced by clear thinking (clairvoyance and clair audience are fall-out effects of such efforts).

Chitta

After the *sadhak* or seeker has received the instructions of the wisdom of *Sankhyan* philosophy, he must be shown the secret celestial route of meditation by which he can be led out of the prison of *karma.* Through meditation, when the ego is united to the soul and the soul to the Spirit, the ego loses its delusion of being a mortal whose actions are governed by the law of *karma.*

He has learned the knowledge of the 24 principles of Nature or *Prakriti* or Elders that play with the Spirit [five elements - mind - intellect - *chitta* - five senses - five organs of action - five objects of senses]. He realizes the truth of this theoretical knowledge when he reverses his steps, beginning with the grossest and linking himself with the origin of these twentyfour qualities.

He realizes that Nature or *Prakriti* or the Holy Spirit, is the basic creative power of Creation which expresses as *Mahat* or Cosmic Intelligence through:

- *Chitta* or the power of feeling which is the basic individualized intelligence in the ego, mind, and intellect complex;
- *Buddhi* or individual discriminative intellect or desiring thought;
- *Ahamkara* or ego or the "Me";
- *Manas* or the sensory mind;
- Five *gyanaindriyas* or organs of perception;
- Five *karmaindriyas* or organs of action;
- Five *tanmatras* or life forces or *pranas*; and
- Five *mahabhutas* or elements or the vibratory motions of matter expressing as solid, liquid, or gas.

Polarized by *manas* and *buddhi, chitta* triggers creation and becomes the root cause and substratum of the remaining 20 Evolutes of the individual and cosmic creation. The *desire for manifestation* is now acted upon by the three qualities of Nature of *sattva, rajas, and* tamas; from this arise the five organs of sense perception or *gyanindriyas*; the five organs of action or *karmaindriyas;* the five vibratory elements of space, air, fire, water, and earth; and the five physiological *pranas* or life-force empowering circulation, crystallization, assimilation, metabolism, and elimination.

> "And round about the throne were four and twenty seats; and upon the seats I saw four and twenty elders"..Revelation 4:4.

The *sadhak* dissolves the 24 principles in succession through the techniques of meditation described so far. He now merges his personalized awareness of feeling or *chitta* into the Awareness of *Aum* or the primordial cosmic vibratory *creative-force.* He finally enters into the Consciousness of *Aum,* the Spirit.

By graduated steps, the seeker converts all his awareness of matter into the consciousness of the Spirit. This is a realization attained through direct intuitive experience. He now knows for sure that all Matter is Spirit and Spirit is Matter; the Holy Spirit or *Aum* or Prakriti or Awareness and *Purusha* or God or Consciousness are One and inseparable. They together are *Shiva* and *Shakti.* The seeker frees himself of the delusory powers of *Maya* and begins to see the Universe as a dream of God.

The *sadhak* who knows the art of *yoga,* experiences the joy of meditation and will not immerse himself in new desires and new *karmas.* The Cosmic Energy of *Aum* as Will, finally destroys all tendencies, and sense-enslaved habits of past existences. He frees his Will and vibrates it in harmony with the Universal Collective Will.

Patanjali describes this state as *chitta vritti nirodha* or the cessation of modification in feelings. His perceptions are not through the excitable distortions of Nature; but rather arise from the calm perspective of pure soul-wisdom. He knows the afflictions of the excitable body, mind, and intellect are not that of the soul. He learns to control the instruments of excitability and can perceive the separateness of the soul and his matter envelopments, the *koshas.* (Please refer to Figure 4).'

Genesis of a Mortal

The first manifestation of the Spirit is Cosmic Light. God vibrates His Cosmic Consciousness and Intelligence as the Creative Cosmic Energy or Cosmic Light of Awareness. This Cosmic Light or Energy exists in man as the microcosmic sun in the physical thalamus or the spiritual eye, which becomes visible during meditation when the *sadhak's* awareness and the two currents of the physical eyes is concentrated between the two eyebrows in the *kutastha* opposite the *ajnaa* center. (Figure 8 and Figure 21)

All the intelligent creative power of the omnipresent Cosmic Energy is present in the spiritual eye. Through it, the soul descends into an embodiment of an individualized soul; it is also the route through which the soul ultimately ascends to Spirit. (Figure 9 and 11)

After the soul emerges from Cosmic Consciousness, it experiences a slightly lower vibratory state of Cosmic Light of Awareness; he then loses the awareness of being Spirit and becomes an individualized causal being encased in an astral body. This occurs within the *pituitary-pineal-ajnaa* complex.

The outwardly projecting power is imposed on the soul and the seeker has a "feeling" or awareness that he experiences his existence. This feeling triggers thoughts and thinking by the intellect. When this feeling is distorted by delusion, the ego evolves into existence and "Me" is created. Intelligence manifests as thought, ego, and discrimination.

Afflicted by delusion, intelligence gives rise to the *blind sensory mind*. The mind coordinates with the seeker's sensory mind and the *will* for *activation of the senses* and organs of action. The *desiring intellect* thinks the seeker desires through contact with the world of objects and imagines the object of his desire is real. It is the mind that is responsible for all human endeavors; the Cosmic Energy manifests as the life-force in the astral and physical body which is directly under the vagaries of the mind; in the causal plane, Cosmic Consciousness and Energy manifests as intuition. (Please refer to Figure 10).

Self-hypnosis

Self-hypnosis may be achieved without going into a trance state. It can be continuous. This is different from being hypnotized and being under the will of another person. The seeker can self-induce hypnosis and use it as a tool under certain circumstances for self-development. Auto-suggestion by mentally or audibly talking to oneself is a form of self-hypnosis.

The *asanas* or postures, *pranayama* or breath-regulating exercises, and *pratyahara* or withdrawal from the senses through *dharana* or concentration, use the power of subtle suggestion to constantly remind the seeker of his *yogic* aspirations.

Life itself is a constant flow of suggestions and influences for the purpose of desired changes. Certain colors and their association with specific qualities are also forms of self-hypnosis. They create desires and have associations with their own self-hypnotic effects.

What we see with our eyes and hear through our ears exert a particularly powerful suggestive influence on the mind. Millions can be manipulated by those who know how to exercise the power of suggestion.

This kind of *exploitation of others* create *karmic* debts. All teachers (with stronger or more powerful minds) are warned that they will some day have to account for everything said and done to influence the minds of the weak, the untrained, or the simply ignorant.

Trance

Trance, which is a state of sleepiness by suggestion, is a condition sought out by "mediums" to use the body as apparatus to function for a purpose. This state is not available to recall, because it lacks the presence of a conscious awareness.

Predictions

Predictions must be made within the limits of space and time. They can be made when the mind is in a state of deep reflection (astral plane of being) for a long period of time.

At a general level, predictions have a powerful suggestive-influence, bordering on hypnosis, and can therefore create the fulfillment of the prediction.

Seekers are warned not to aspire for such powers. Absence of foresight and irresponsible attitudes can have disastrous influences (mental and emotional) on the party being influenced. This becomes an act associated with a *karmic* debt in the future.

Many sincere seekers can suddenly turn in the opposite direction from their spiritual goal because of disappointments. They can be heard making cynical remarks and resorting to the dangerous manipulation of others for their own needs. These are egoistic desires for the control of others and must be guarded against.

The objective of the work done so far is to achieve self-mastery over the lower forces. Meditation techniques can be used to overcome any obstacle; but without vigilance one can be drawn into its supernatural powers.

The seeker is therefore warned that one's most powerful faculty is that of *discrimination and a keen awareness: be sure you know what you want to invite into the house of the mind. Always invoke the Divine Light and keep the mind focused on the Light, within the kavach or protective shield. With each pranayama, expand the awareness into the Collective Consciousness.*

Understand the awesome power of the mind, which as the vehicle of expression of the Self is, therefore, very precious. *Consciousness, subconsciousness and unconsciousness result from active life force or prana.*

Care must be exercised when working with the mind. Apply what is learned. The Power of Creativity is Neutral. It must be applied slowly, courageously and through dehypnotizing oneself. *A constant reminder is made by the invocation of awareness of the Divine Light.*

Psychic manifestations may side-track the seeker. It is best to control the power manifesting as psychic phenomenon by creating a *kavach* or protective shell.

Manifestations of a spiritual experience have the power to transform the seeker. They create an acute awareness of the Holy Spirit or *Devi's* presence which is Her promise in Her gesture of *varada*.

Examining Samadhi or Oneness

When a practitioner enters the state of *samadhi* in meditation, he experiences a sense of oneness between the concentrating mind (object) and the subject (Self). This union is very different from that experienced during concentration or *dharana* and meditation or *dhyana*.

The ultimate union of the individualized mind with the Self is a vivid realization that the everything is in the Self and the Self is in all. It is a state of Universal Consciousness experienced in *samadhi* (oneness).

The continuous practice of meditation in *dharana* (concentration) and *dhyana* (meditation) takes the mind (object) deeper and deeper into the astral planes. The practitioner experiences the concentrating mind (object) gradually becoming integrated with the subject (Self) in a partial union.

When subject (Self) and object (mind) become synchronized and synonymously experience Universal Consciousness, this unity remains sustained and supported at its base by the subject, the Self. The subject (Self) and the object (mind) cannot remain differentiated: the mind must become the Self (subject) by leaving behind the mind (object).

In the realms of the higher astral planes, the Supreme Self or God or *Brahman* provides the higher dimension and a special realm where the subject (Self) and object (mind) merge with the Supreme Self or Being. Here, individual "beingness" vertically merges with the higher Beingness. With it there is an ascending-transformation within the divine cave and beyond. In this higher astral plane, there is no differentiation between the practitioner and the other "beings" that have ascended to this plane, because none have any individuality or group distinctiveness.

> During his first stay with our family some twentyseven years ago we were discussing the ecstasy of Oneness and the Master related a fascinating story of his own experience in *samadhi*. My understanding at the time was immature, but it remained a target the arrow of my spiritual journey would take and is taking.
>
> My Master had studied at the feet of another mystic-yogi, *Swami Tapovan Maharaj* who lived near the mouth of the *Ganges in Gangotri*. For many years, the young seeker served and watched his Master guide seekers who visited him. The young renunciate who was later to become *Swami Chinmayananda*, one day experienced the ecstasy described in scriptural texts and falteringly expressed by *Swami Tapovan*.
>
> The young renunciate felt an intense disgust with his physical manifestation and disappeared in one of the many caves in the Himalayan foothills near *Gangotri*. Here he fasted without food for many days until the body began to shed, starting from the surface and progressing inwards. *Swami Tapovan*

had only forty days to find his young *sishya* (student) and I had the audacity to ask why!

And the Master replied: "... Your physiology must have taught you that during the first forty days of fasting the surface of the body or fat and muscles are broken down for 'energy' to sustain the body. After forty days, the central vital organs get 'eaten' up: this is the point of no return and physical death must soon follow".

It was close to forty days when the young renunciate was found and he required expert resuscitation for many weeks. He was nurtured back to health by his own Master, *Swami Tapovan Maharaj* and the monks in the mountain. I have often wondered if our Master suffered severe damages to his heart and pancreas at that time!

Experiencing "Beingness"

Individualized "beingness" is the association of a person's physical-physiological-psychological (BMI) bodies with the causal body. That brings us to a question: does God in His "Beingness" also have a body? The answer to this is "yes". The Cosmos is His Body, which is also made up of physical, mental, and causal bodies.

Once this "beingness" ceases and the body is abandoned, its unique identity is not lost. The object's unique identity (mind) is suspended and the subject (Self), which is the source of all beings, emerges and manifests in the mind (object) as the subject (Self) in a state of oneness.

The Supreme Self assumes His various forms through the individual mind as the experiencing "Self-Supreme Self" union in *samadhi*. This state does not free him of his past *karmas* (causal body). Therefore, experiencing Universal Awareness in the higher astral dimension is still not the highest spiritual achievement.

"Beingness" exists in the physical, astral, and causal dimensions. "Beingness", at each level, is distinct, but also comes together to make up a single person, collectively matching with the person's *karmas*. However, an individual cannot attain and become Universal Consciousness unless he is able to transcend his particular *karmas*.

Universal Awareness in the Astral Plane of Mind-Intellect

The partial union that occurs in the astral plane is a type of *samadhi* which has transcended the material world but has enveloped the astral and causal dimension. Here, the spiritual being can sustain the mind (object) and becomes one with the other minds (objects) in the astral dimension. However, the object is still separate from the subject (Self).

> We were discussing experiences in meditation when one of my daughters shocked me with this statement: "The Master took me into the domains where I can see myself sitting [physical body] in meditation from above [as astral being]."

This type of separation from the atomic body or matter and into life-energy or 'lifetrons' is an expansion into an astral being. Union with the Total Astral Being in the astral dimension is associated with strong emotions of pleasure and comfort. The mind-intellect feels comfort in this realization of Universal Awareness.

Of note is that some psychics have the ability to enter other astral beings in the astral plane. "Unions" such as this may be characterized by "acquisition" of the other astral body. If the spirit is agreeable, the union is cheerful and agreeable.

If the astral being is antagonistic, the practitioner becomes uneasy and depressed. If the union is with an emotional astral being, the practitioner experiences strong "feelings".

This type of interaction with another astral being can take place in the astral plane as the "combined-beingness" of the practitioner with one who has become disembodied at physical death.

Oneness in Causal Dimension - Vasana or Ideational

When the practitioner transcends the astral world, he achieves oneness in the *karana* or causal dimension. He experiences a sublime oneness which is beyond the simple emotion of feeling-good, but is tainted with the desire for its prolongation.

Before entering *samadhi* or oneness, the practitioner undergoes frightening experiences. With the template of his previous lives now in total ruin, he, the ego feels both insecure and anxious.

The mystery of life begins with a basic life-force and the desire to live. Life-force blossoms as energy and travels through life as creative expression. Through *sadhana* the seeker has directed this creative energy to become transformed and identifiable as spiritual force. It is this return journey, the force of which will carry the seeker to final enlightenment. He has passed through different levels of awareness in his spiritual journey. The final spiritual unfolding is fraught with negativity, self-doubt, and even fear.

This bewilderment experienced by this new can be alarming: he feels lost and insecure. At this stage, the practitioner MUST have the faith to invoke the *Guru* or God who will carry him across this difficult threshold. The energy of his spiritualized life-force will move him towards persons and situations which will attract the seeker to what is best in and for him.. The seeker is urged to appreciate each opportunity and live each moment to the best of his ability. He will reach his desired destination if the desire is perfection: this desire for selfperfection can be a hard taskmaster!

Many practitioners give up meditating at this stage and dabble in supernormal abilities like those of psychics in the physical world. *Yogis* who are Masters at leading the ardent seeker across these difficult thresholds are always alert to their existence, wherever they might be. Call for the Lord of your heart or your own beloved Teacher and he/she will take you home.

> and the Master wrote:
>
> "The ancient masters of our country were such mighty stalwarts who stood amidst life's storms as firm as the great Himalayas. Their emotions and sentiments made their hearts bleed for the suffering of humanity, but their heads were above the clouds in the ever peaceful realm of the high levels.."

Encountering Frightful Images in Causal Dimension

Before the practitioner enters *samadhi,* the ego ("Me") must be shattered and discarded. In this instance, the practitioner or his "beingness" faces its own death. Without the death of the "Me", the seeker cannot transcend the causal or *karanic* dimension.

The practitioner must depend on his *Guru:* this faith will carry him into the spiritual dimension of his being. While transcending the causal dimension, he will be confronted with demonic obstructions to his progress. The seeker must have implicit faith in the abilities of his or her teacher. The seeker will be taken to safe shores.

> and the Master wrote: "The secret might of faith is that power in the human mind to hold on to what he intellectually believes, but has not come to experience in life. Faith and devotion to the guru are necessary in order to ease the student's path and level down the slopes en route his pilgrimage. Faith is a very powerful secret source of energy in the human bosom".

The obstructions come from beings trapped in their own individual *karmic* beingness in the causal dimension. It is inevitable that the practitioner will encounter these beings causing images of terror. At this stage, the mercy of the Higher Self must be called upon.

A Japanese mystic wrote the following as a cure for phenomenon and frightening images encountered during deep meditation:

Call your *guru* for help.

Instead of raising the current of *energy* up and down the divine cave, raise the current of awareness from the base *chakra* to the *agnaa chakra* at the base of the brain and then forward to the *bhrumadhya* between the eyebrows.

Now instead of descending down the divine cave, carry the current down <u>in</u>

front of the body and back up through the tail to the crown in a complete ellipse.

Repeat this until the phenomenon and fear resolves.

Causal "Beingness"

At this level of causal or *karanic*-beingness, the practitioner has attained oneness at the *karana* dimension, but there is still distinction. Here the psychological characteristics are:

- Meditating consciousness has been purged of the conscious and subconscious mind (memories of the inferior mind);
- The greater conscious mind is clear and untroubled by wandering-thoughts because the unconscious mind (causal) has also nearly been purged;
- This higher consciousness of the unconscious mind (causal) remains as his base beingness, even though the shell of the ego has been fractured and the inferior mind is rendered powerless.

The higher awareness in the *chittamaya kosha* or sixth sheath of Awareness, flushes out the inferior awareness in the *anandamaya kosha* or fifth sheath of *karana*, but neither are as yet destroyed. The experience is so powerful that the practitioner falls into a trance and is now under the influence of an infinitely greater awareness. The trance experience cannot be recalled.

The meditating causal being gradually replaces the lower mind or inferior awareness with the higher mind of higher awareness. Progress is judged by the practitioner's growing ability to recall the trance experience. The trance will gradually disappear; and the seeker will understand the nature of his previous lives. He will also have insight into the path of his own spiritual efforts. He will know what needs to be done to get to his destination.

This level of awareness is a superconscious state which is beyond the conscious [awake], subconscious [dream], and unconscious [deep-sleep] states of beingness. This awakened-causal-state of being is in fact an acute state of awareness which is experienced at the *kutastha* between the eyebrows. At first it seems like a trance and then as a clear self-understanding through pre-cognition or clairvoyance of present and past lives.

Phenomena in Astral and Causal Dimensions

When the practitioner's astral being merges with the Universal Life-Force *in the astral dimension*, he experiences acute Awareness at the center of Will in the *kutastha chaitanya* of Universal Intelligence behind and between the eyebrows.

When the practitioner's causal being residing in the *ajnaa* center merges with the *kutastha*: the seeker experiences a sublime state of super awareness of existence, knowledge, and bliss. Once the practitioner becomes adept at this depth of meditation, he has the ability to leave his physical dimension and enter the astral planes of the Universe. He is able to *travel the astral realms* through the phenomenon of astral projection. The body is light and exists as 'lifetrons' or energy, rather than atoms of matter.

Levitation of the energized-physical body will occur because it has become transformed and is one with all the spiritual centers or *chakras* in the divine cave. The seeker who transcends his causal-beingness is able to enter the domains of the seventh or *sahasrahara chakra* beyond the causal dimension. He experiences Universal Consciousness or superconsciousness.

When the practitioner has reached this stage of meditation, he *gains control of his physical being.* He can levitate, walk on water, disappear and transport himself to other distant sites, even perform psychic-surgeries without actually cutting the flesh, and repair defects in the physical body of his ailing *sishya* or student, from an astral dimension.

Different types of **psychic healing** can be performed from different dimensions:

- from an astral dimension;
- from an intermediate dimension between astral and causal dimension; and
- from a causal dimension.

At the astral dimension, healing occurs through the transference of life-energy by concentrating on the afflicted area. This phenomenon is called *materialization.*

Even while in meditation, the practitioner has the ability to gain control over things in the physical dimension in proportion to his spiritual progress. When he is able to enter the causal dimension, he can create things or make them disappear. He can control and regulate the life-force energy.

P.C. Sarkar, a famous magician of India initiated the disappearance of the Taj Mahal for a few minutes in front of a few hundred of people around the famous monument. The act was not mass-hypnosis.

Psychological Differences in Astral and Causal Dimensions

A practitioner who has reached these levels of meditation can enter the state of *samadhi* or union and can then have power to control the functions of the body and effect changes in the external world. Only *yogis* who are aligned with the Laws of Nature or the Cosmic Mother, have the ability to transform the world, for the benefit of Man!

While motionless, the *yogi* is aware of the meridian flow of kinetic or ki-energy through the *nadis or* meridians. He is able to arrest respiration and the heart at will. Knowledge of this is the basis of understanding networks of energy meridians in the body. This knowledge is the underlying principle in the study of acupuncture, *ayurveda, hatha yoga, and reiki.*

Some skillful acupuncturists have a keen intuitive understanding of the flow and obstacles in ki-energy within the channels or *nadis*. They also have the power to control the flow of such ki-energy by using pressure in their fingertips, to enter meridians of persons under their medical care.

The practitioner not only can identify these powers in himself, but is able to recognize the aura of each *chakra* awakened in another person. He is now able to develop enough self-control not only to project ki-energy on another, but is able to restrain it in himself.

A *yogi* who enters *samadhi* in an astral-dimension can arrest his respiration and slow the heart rate. The psychic who enters *samadhi* in the causal-dimension is able to arrest the activity of the heart. The majority of psychics are able to enter the lower astral-dimension only.

Psychics in Samadhi

The ability to enter *samadhi* in either the astral or causal dimension is associated with considerable improvement in the psychic's own physical well-being. He has gained awareness of his body and control over its physiological and psychological functions.

However, his *karmas* draw him back into life, determine his state of health while he lives, and finally ushers him out. Since life is a process of fulfilling a predetermined sequence of *karmas*, their consequences can be eased but never escaped. Those who evade the *karmic* effect only postpone it until a later life.

The most beneficial course is to cultivate a spiritual life and enter *samadhi* to minimize the extent of physical suffering. Unhealthy *karmas* will have to be endured as disease and sickness in this or later lives.

Psychic healing does not attempt to remedy *karma-caused disease*; it only assists the inherent restorative powers of the patient's own body.

Masters and evolved beings have the ability to protect their *shishyas* in this world and or even from the astral world. Many of his *shishyas* have felt the Master's presence and influence in their times of need. This fact is felt and expressed the world over by many in a common echo!!!

Man's Possessions

Man's possessions consist not only of the material objects he acquires and gathers around himself, but also the sum total of all his illusions of Nature with which he has identified himself as ego: these include his body identifications, his sensuousness towards objects of pleasure, his feelings, his sensory inclinations, his habits, and desires of past lives.

Unless realization of the Self becomes established as part of soul consciousness, man cannot renounce his attachments to his inner, as well as outer possessions. He will remain enslaved by the *karmic effects* arising from the activities they engender.

Wherever man goes, his egoistic *karma* accompanies him in all his pursuits. When man attains inner non-attachment through meditation, he becomes a true renunciant; he performs actions with mental discipline, free of expectations.

> and the Master said:
>
> "Man is part of that vibratory activity and integral part of the Cosmic Plan projected out of the Cosmic Self. Man must evolve back into the Cosmic Self, through activity in harmony with the Cosmic Plan inherent in Nature.."
>
> and he also wrote: "...God dedicated selfless actions performed in a spirit of devotion and self-surrender exhaust the existing *vasanas* and do not create, of their own accord, any more fresh tragic impressions, which in their turn would order fresh fields of activity.."

Self Discipline

Self discipline includes speaking the truth, calmness, sweetness of speech even under provocation, honesty, and self-restraint: these characteristics are aspired by followers of all religions. Sanctimonious beings who lose sight of God realization as their goal and destination, also lose their way while traveling the path of spiritualism and especially meditation. Those who intelligently practice austerity, motivated by devotion to the Self, find their self discipline helpful for uniting with the Cosmic Spirit.

> and the Masters said:
>
> "Religion is not for the unworthy, the unintelligent, and the abnormal. Religion is only for the most level-headed and balanced people ... people who are sound spiritually, psychologically, and physically. Cowards cannot progress in spiritual life. Spiritual life is meant for the person who enjoys good health, who is alert in mind and intellect, and who has a deep 'craving of the soul'. Only such a thirsty, fully blossomed human being, who has lived life fully, can come to *vairagya* or dispassion..."

Seekers who follow the eightfold path of *Raja Yoga* neutralize the agitation of the *chitta* or feelings. These individuals are able to see an undistorted reflection of the soul. They not only practice *yama* restraint *and niyama* adherence to restraints, but they can control body postures through *asanas* and make it respond to their will by sitting for long hours of meditation and *samadhi.*

The practitioner next learns to control and regulate breath through *pranayama.* His mind disconnects from body awareness by switching off the life-currents to the senses, which now connects with awareness in the spinal cord and brain in the divine cave.

This interiorization is *pratyahara* or the withdrawal of the mind and life-force from the objects of senses, senses, organs of action, and the physiological *pranas* [*pranaya, apanaya, vyanaya, samanaya and udanaya*]. The inner spiritual journey is towards the astral and causal divine cave or spinal cord and brain.

Having mastered the body, mind, and life-force, and after learning interiorization, the seeker devotes long hours concentrating on the soul through concentration or *dharana,* meditation or *dhyana,* and ecstasy of Oneness or *samadhi.* He learns to meet with the Spirit of *Aum* which he listens to through the inner ear. He learns to expand this feeling of *Aum* into the expanse of the vibrating *Aum* beyond his physical and astral bodies and into the Universe.

The seeker attains oneness with *Aum* vibrating in the Universe and the ecstasy is an awareness sensed at the *Kutastha Chaitanya.* At first the seeker encounters the fusion in the Krishna-Christ Center between and behind the eyebrows. Later, he experiences himself beyond himself and in the Universe. This exercise dissolves all likes-and-dislikes and desires that interfere with intuitive feelings or *chitta.* The calm *yogi* unites the soul with Spirit.

> And the Master writes:
>
> "The indifference to religion of the apparently educated man of today is not so much due to the futility or hollowness of the Science of Religion as such, but his own incapacity to understand the text-books of Religion in the world. This is true not only of the Hindus but men of every faith..."

Summary of Universal Philosophy

Manifest Creation is the Dream of God whose first manifestation is LOVE. When unmanifest, the Infinite created the first vibration: the great divider or *Maya.* She, accompanied by Her three *gunas,* danced the dance of delusion. She gave Immortal Man the illusion that he was mortal. This dizzy Love-dance made the Indivisible into the divided, the One into the many, the Inseparable into the separable, and the Infinite to the finite!

This *Maya* is Love and the seed of visible creation. The Universal Idea of a Causal Creation contains the blueprint of both the physical and astral creation. The Tree of *Maya* is born of Love. Love brings energy [positive] and electrical sparks [negative] together to create sub-atomic particles [neutrons, protons, electrons]. Love brings the atoms closer in an act of Love to create molecules and then cells, and finally a man's body. Every movement of closeness is an act of love and a grosser but invisible manifestation of Creation.

Out of this Invisible Love arise the Invisible Word [AUM or Amen], Time, Space, and Size. The conscious atom has a mind [negative polarity reaching for objects of desire] and wisdom [positive polarity reaching for the source of creation]. When magnetized, the polarities merge to become the Ego. The Ego desires and the 35 causal essences of creation are manifest (the 19 ideas of the astral creation and 16 matter principles of physical creation). Physical Creation is visible. The Astral and Causal Creations are invisible, but vaster.

Ordinary love or *sneha* is attachment to a person, people, or thing. When separated from the object of attachment, there is restlessness and pain. There is a sense of duality. When the object of love ceases to satisfy, the seeker discards or hates it and moves on to new attachments. This is not Love! This type of love is in contrast to God's love or *prema*, from which the body, mind, and intellect originate. The closeness and oneness of this type of love cannot be fathomed by the mind or intellect; it is beyond our understanding.

To contact *Prema;*

1. Sit in a position of your own choice with back and head in a straight line, chin parallel to the ground. Roll the tongue back and concentrate your gaze in the Cosmic space between the eyebrows. Watch the feel of the breath.
2. Place the interlocked palms of your hands on the medulla at the base of the skull. Touch and feel this area of the head. Merge in this sensation at the back of the head.
3. Pray for true love. Over time, the seeker merges with the energy of love alone. He is freed of the sense of duality and attachments. He is suffused by a unique continuous energy. The world becomes his home. He works for the welfare of the Universe. His thoughts are preoccupied with doing his duty to both friend and foe. He has the intuitive knowledge that the body, mind, and intellect (BMI) is the residence of delusion (Maya). It is the plane where the law of cause-and-effect is manifest.
4. *In deep meditation, when the seeker becomes unconscious of his body, he enters the domains of changelessness and true love. He sees the seven centers of Consciousness.*

Conclusion

The Causal Being carries within its memory all the images, desires, habits, concepts and likes-dislikes of past lives and corrections made in the present life. These images speak constantly. The seeker may or may not listen to this inner guide. The intuitive mind hears the commands and the psychological:physiological body, listens. The seeker discovers that his body, thoughts, life, and his world images, are of a heightened awareness of the Ultimate Truth. Now what you see of this world, is a reflection of your inner integration. This realization empowers the seeker with expansion, and self-connectedness.

SECTION SEVEN

Topics in Section Seven

Self-Mastery Removes Blindness of Creation

Unknown to us everything and everyone is endowed with Infinite Power. Once Man becomes One with the Cosmic Mother his Mind blindness disappears through the innate power of Intuition.

Intuition has the ability to search both his heart and soul. The search takes Man to Wisdom. Here in the Christ-*Krishna* Centre, in the Centre of Universal Intelligence, Man acquires an innate Wisdom which is a product of his own self-effort.

The Spiritual Journey is far from complete. The traveler must continue to experience his own Changelessness. He will eventually see the seven spiritual centres as seven candles within the Altar of God. He will see a Collective Vision through an inner perception.

He will realise that his own Personal Vision was a downward and outward perception of Mother Nature. The Spiritual Journey has been a powerful upward journey of increasing self-discovery. Bon Voyage.

Sahasrahara Chakra

Preamble

To unleash the Power of Light and Energy within yourself is to create the future every seeker desires for himself. Man feels trapped when he feels he is a pawn in Nature's game. Meditation is a spiritual tool of profound relevance in the Journey of Self-Understanding. The seeker makes choices and brings to his life, a complete balance. The mind emits positive emotions of love and goodwill. Thoughts and speech affirm that the seeker is attuned to the Cosmic Vision. He enhances his life quality by reaffirming the imagepower of the Cosmic Mother, working on his foundation causal beingness. The seeker is able to put aside his mundane thoughts and enters the deeper mysteries of the Mind of God.

Sahasrahara or Seventh Chakra
The Crown Chakra

The crown *chakra* is sometimes called the thousand-petaled lotus or, also the secret *chakra.* Although ALL *chakras* are considered secret, this is the most secret.

In the divine cave and at the brow is a **reflection** of the *kutastha chaitanya* or the Christ-*Krishna* Centre, which normally resides within the *ajnaa chakra* in the medulla. The sixth *chakra*, threads through all of the mundane-beingness of "Me" in the five lower centres and unites them with the autonomic astral channels or *nadis (Ida, Pingala and Chitrini).* This confluence of channels occurs in close proximity to the "I" in the *Brahmanadi* in the centre of the brain. This is the secret residence of the evolving *chitta* or mind-intellect-ego complex. Here seeker's Awareness senses the closeness to Consciousness.

> "He that dwelleth in the secret place of the Most High [Awareness in *kutashta*] shall abide under the shadow of the Almighty [Consciousness in *sahasrahara*]." ..Psalms 91:1.

Suspended here, in the *ajnaa centre* is his causal beingness. The practitioner of meditation already has the knowledge of and has experienced the pleasures of his physical-beingness. He understands emotions and the mind in the lower astral-beingness, through knowledge gained so far. He also understands the higher astral-beingness of images and intellectualism.

The practitioner has reached a bursting-point. Despite the near complete union in the causal dimension during meditation, the mind is still full of mundane thoughts and is in danger of re-entering the mundane world.

To comprehend and pass into the *sahasrahara* or seventh *chakra* requires an ability to dispassionately view any scene of sensuality and depravity. Total equanimity is the only way to enter this domain of superconsciousness beyond, the causal dimension.

When the Life-Force of the astral body pierces all the *chakras,* it ascends to the seventh *chakra* through the *brahmanadi* to enlighten the astral causal brain. Here, in *samadhi*, the Self is experienced in oneness with the Supreme Self and in the Self everywhere.

The mind and intellect are transcended and now become instruments of the Self, the "I" instead of the ego. The "Me" awareness experiences its own consciousness. It is an unattached awareness, free of consciousness-of! He experiences Awareness-Consciousness or combined *Purusha-Prakriti or Shiva-Shakti.* He first experiences Collective Consciousness within the central nervous system or divine cave. He realizes there is an actualization of a risen Energy released and vibrating on the top of his head. He hears, sees, feels, the Word. It is the call of 'many waters'! It IS *Aum.*

The *sadhak* or seeker becomes a total feeling or *chitta* of harmony which is characterized by peace, quietude, and joy. It is a spontaneous experience where although the seed had been planted by him, the expansion and growth of the tree is beyond his control. Thereafter, Mother Nature continues to work on Her own, unlocking all hindrances on the Path of the seeker.

This center contains subtle seats of all the previous centers. This is the place where Energy of Awareness unites with the Light of Consciousness. Once unified, its powers of Universal Consciousness are unlimited. The Life Force Energy threads all the *chakras* like a rosary, threading through the central channel *(brahmanadi)* with the perennial source of the Light of Consciousness.

Once the connection is established, the transcendental experience of identification with the Universal Spirit becomes a synthesis of the integrated whole, felt as a joy born of spontaneity free of reactivity, impulsiveness, notions, speculation, and imagination. It has no form and no ego. It has no cause for being. There is no need for activity.

Life-Force Energy opens the brain to unknown dimensions. *Maya* or delusions of ignorance of his identity, no longer holds Her sway on the practitioner's daily living. The brain becomes a computer of Collective Consciousness, capable of directing Nature's Universal Law. The seeker enters effortlessly into the domains of subtle communication through the vibrations of *Aum.*

In this state, the seeker is awakened to a level of awareness despite the roaring of active life. The *Devi of* Life-Force Energy retains Her power until absorbed into the Supreme *Brahman.* The screens of the five matter sheaths now drop off, one by one. Starting from the skin to the soul they are: *annamaya* or the food sheath; *pranamaya* or the physiological sheath; *manomaya* or the psychological sheath; *vignanamaya* or the intellectual sheath; and *anandamaya* or bliss or the causal sheath.

Even at this stage, the journey is not complete. The *chitta* or mind-intellect-ego complex has to be erased, and all vestiges of individualistic personality transcended. The seeker enters into the *chittamaya kosha* of soul-awareness and, by the grace of God and *Guru,* he enters into the *atmamaya kosha* of Self-consciousness in the crown *chakra.*

With the help of the human form, the *Atman* or soul enters the Self and secures union with the Universal Self. Here there is no objective ("Me") or subjective ("I") mind; all fancies and ideas are destroyed in the fire of the beginningless, limitless Supreme Spirit. Here lies the primary seed of the Universe, the very source of bliss, the ultimate goal of Divine Love which unfolds and delights into waves of *Sat Chit Anand* or Truth-Knowledge-Bliss which truly Exists!

Synchronization of Concentrating Efforts

Progress in *Dharana* or Concentration allows brain activity to become synchronized in proportion to the depth of the effort in meditation. With this, the stimulation of the neoencephalon or cerebral hemispheres is gradually lessened. In the meantime, the activity in the paleoencephalon (brain stem, hypothalamus, limbic system) is heightened. (Please refer to 21).

The brainstem at the Mouth of God is thought to be the centre of the unconscious or causal mind. Therefore when the *dharana* synchronizes the mind at this level, suppressed ideas and images surface into consciousness as images, to disturb the practitioner's efforts.

Many months of disturbances hound the practitioner. Steady effort at *dharana* will eventually weaken the conscious mind until the unconscious mind is completely purged.

The effect of wandering thoughts and images can be lessened by starting the *Humm'saa Soo'ham* Technique of breathing. The *Kechari Mudra* or rolling the tongue back to touch the uvula or palate roof while doing *pranayama* and *pratyahara* is another method to stop thoughts from disturbing the practitioner.

The disruptive effects of wandering thoughts and images should be disregarded for their content and attention re-focused. They are "forgotten physical, mental and psychological experiences." They must be purged for they have the propensity to cause psychosomatic disease processes. Many of these diseases begin by affecting the autonomic nervous system. Then it influences the blood chemistry and finally disrupts the bodily functions themselves.

Dharana or efforts at concentration are the means through which all the accumulated debris of the past is gradually eliminated. Cleansing takes time. Once the process is complete and the subconscious and unconscious minds have been freed of past experiences, all imbalances disappear.

The *Kechari Mudra* or rolling tongue back also helps the mind and the body to achieve a state of balance. Once this is achieved, the practitioner is able to contemplate or practice *dhyana.* He experiences momentary oneness between "I" as *Aum* and *"Tat"* or "That" at the Christ Centre or *Kutastha Chaitanya* of Universal Will and Intelligence.

Although the union is brief, the experience will leave the practitioner with a feeling of intense bliss. This is what needs to be achieved and realized as a first step to emancipation. Efforts at deeper and deeper meditation take the practitioner to union of longer duration's. There is a gradual transcendence of ordinary awareness with body and the nervous system's activities with the environment of materialism. The ego becomes progressively fractured. The practitioner experiences a great presence of a powerful consciousness.

This meditative-state is the means by which an individual as *chitta* or mind-intellect-ego complex leaves his *chitta* behind and escapes the physical limitations of the body and its contacts. Through intense long meditation, the seeker in bliss enters his enlightened *chitta-state.* His efforts are relentless until he enters the *chit* or Self. This is the only way to rise into the superconscious- state and its vast potential.

As the efforts deepen into successes, breathing becomes gradually slower and each breath is unconsciously held longer at the end of inhalation as well as exhalation. At this stage of progress, the practitioner may become aware of disturbances from astral dimensions. These are contacts with beings who have both reached the same level of spiritual evolution and with whom the seeker shares a strong affinity. When confronted by such a situation, invoke the name of the Lord or the *Guru*, with faith, for protection and deliverance. The *Mrityunjaya Mantra* is powerfully effective.

Once the practitioner acquires the ability to rise above the physical restraints of his body, he will become aware of his astral mind and body. He realizes this is a distinct body, all its own. The practitioner now develops a "third person view" of his physical body, astral body and "I".

In deep meditation, he may "look down" on his own motionless physical body from an elevated position, as if effortlessly hovering in the air. He may be able to see through the back of the head and through solid walls and closed windows. The experience may last a few seconds and should not breed fright in the practitioner. The phenomenon is called astral projection of the senses which have become supersensitive and function beyond their physical capabilities. These out-of-body experiences can be fatiguing and the practitioner must rest to restore himself, in the beginning.

The practitioner who is able to rouse the Life-Force/Energy up the spine through the five lower *chakras* will hear astral sounds of the element the spiritual center represents. The practitioner's body has undergone transformation and the vibrations of his density is consistent with his identification at each *chakra*. The particular sound heard is the level at which his energy has been raised:

- *Muladhara* awakening produce sounds of birds chirping or bees buzzing;
- *Svadhisthana* awakening produce sounds of tinkling bells;
- *Manipura* awakening triggers ringing sounds;
- *Anahaata* awakening produce mellow flute sounds;
- *Vishuddha* awakening drums the uniform reverberation of *Aum.*

These inner sounds should be listened to calmly and without alarm while the mind becomes synchronized into a tranquil state of both stillness and silence. Continued meditation allows these sounds to fade away.

Occasionally, the practitioner may feel a *sense of expansion and growing to fill the room.* This sense of extension is an indication that the practitioner is ready to free himself from the bondage of the flesh. He is ready to embrace the astral dimension or even to experience the dimension that transcends even the astral worlds.

At this stage of development, the practitioner watches his breath. His *respiration stops for longer periods and may even stop altogether* for periods of three to five minutes. During these periods, the mind becomes completely transparent. If the practitioner concentrates at any of the *chakras*, he will experience them radiating their own specific radiance of unique brilliance. He will not lose touch with his physical body but will experience being charged with divine energy and power of perfect peace and serenity.

These *experiences last only minutes* but, in most cases after the meditative period, the practitioner feels a sense of pervasive vitality, joy, and lucidity of the mind which lasts the whole day.

Although the *experience of ecstasy is achievable, some have experienced the opposite.* The practitioner may undergo a terrifying experience of being alone at the edge of a deep dark chasm or may feel his existence is coming to an end.

When visited by such experiences, invoke the name of the Lord or *Guru* or recite the *Mrityunjaya Mantra. The Spirit will Never abandon the meditator who is willing to live through his karma in order to kill the ego.* If the meditator wishes to enter the astral or causal dimension of beingness, the Spirit will fill the seeker with pure white light. This *state of spiritual illumination* can last for days of trance.

Under repeated exposure of awakening into superconsciousness, *the practitioner will be blessed with visitations from his Ideal.* He experiences oneness of all things in himself. He is now free and serene.

To reach the ultimate state of samadhi, the *Tat* or That at the *ajnaa chakra* must be awakened to the *Sat* or Truth at the *sahasrahara chakra*. Meditation efforts therefore *are efforts at raising Aum or Life-Force or Prakriti, to Tat at the Will Centre of Universal Intelligence in the Kutastha. Then it is the uniting of Aum with the Tat. Finally, it is the uniting the both Aum and Tat with Sat. All religions of the world agree That-You-Are or Aum-Tat-Sat.*

The Spiritual Eye or Third Eye

The spiritual eye is the single eye of intuition and omnipresent perception at the *Kutastha Chaitanya* or Christ Center of Universal Intelligence. It is seen with your inner gaze while focusing at the brow in the divine cave, between the eyebrows.

> "The light of the body is the eye: if therefore thine eye be single, thy whole body shall be full of light." ..Mathew 6:22.

A deeply meditating practitioner "sees" the eye as a ring of golden light of *Aum,* surrounding an inner sphere of blue light of *Tat.* In its center is a five pointed white glowing star of *Sat.*

The golden glow epitomizes the vibratory realm of creation or Cosmic Nature or the Holy Spirit of She the *Devi.* The blue sphere represents the *Kutashtha Chaitanya* of Universal Intelligence or Christ-Krishna Consciousness or the Son. The five pointed white star is the vibrationless Spirit beyond creation or *Brahman* or God the Father.

The spiritual eye is the gateway into the ultimate state of divine consciousness in *samadhi.* As he enters the spiritual eye the practitioner experiences superconsciousness in *samadhi.* It is an ethereal joy of soul-Spirit realization of oneness of *Aum* with the *Aum* of Cosmic Intelligence in all Creation.

> "No man cometh unto the Father, but by me [the son or Christ Cosnsciousness}." John 14.6.

Through the central star in the spiritual eye (opposite the *ajnaa chakra*) in the forehead, the *yogi* sails his Awareness into Omnipresence of Cosmic Consciousness, while hearing *Aum* and merging with the divine sound of many waters. It appears as vibrations of Light and Energy that constitute Creation.

> and the Master wrote:
>
> "Happy New Year. Salutations.
>
> "So happy to see you and the grandchild. You look rested, peaceful, and cheerful within.
>
> The Spirit has ***started*** working in you."

That too after twenty years of teaching and hammering at my ego!

Summary Instructions on Meditation

Do not be satisfied with the theory of meditation. Practice and apply its lessons. Divide the body into twelve parts and recharge [contract and relax] the parts, three times each, starting with the feet, calves, thighs, buttocks, four parts of the back, abdomen, chest, hands, forearms, upper arms, shoulders, head and neck.

Roll the tongue to stretch the hypoglossal and glassopharyngeal nerves; this opens the mouth of the divine cave for maximal entry of the life-force or *prana,* through the medulla. Turn the gaze to the *bhrumadhya* between the eyebrows and look at the Cosmic Vision in its Infinite expanse. Visualize the altar of God in the brain and spinal cord. Become aware of effortless breathing. All of these four movements have the quality of Existence or *Sat.* It is the power of intuitiveness (a sixth sense) that recognizes *Sat* as an inner current.

Ego expresses through an outward flowing current. When man practices meditation techniques, his awareness resides within the divine cave. He then receives direct advice from Him because he has focused and diverted all his currents (spinal and cranial nerves) towards the altar of God in the Divine Cave.

Existence or *Sat* can assume countless names and forms but can be classified only into three forms: Energy or *shakti,* Manifest Joy or *ananda,* and the Omniscient Feeling of Consciousness or *chit.* Combined, they are *sat-chit-anand* or the visible creation.

In meditation, the seeker's awareness moves inwards, and he feels he is made of the substance called energy or *shakti.* He feels his own inner bliss or *ananda.* His consciousness acknowledges his existence or *sat* in his word, time, space and size. At first, his awareness is shadowed by his desires manifesting as *vasanas* gifted with a will or *chetana,* and a desire for enjoyment or *bhoga.* Meditation takes the seeker deeper into himself through the power of listening. He admits here in his own silence that he is the changeless infinite *sat-chit-anand.*

The seeker's listening becomes gradually more channeled. He accepts all outer as well as inner sounds without judgment. He watches the silent periods between sounds and directs both the sounds and the silent periods into the divine cave. He gathers all the sounds and the silences at the *ajnaa chakra* and watches them being transformed into love, peace, and joy. The seeker acknowledges the presence of God. God manifests as silence, power, vigor, wisdom, love, patience, stability, and a powerful creativity. The seeker realizes his immortality as he witnesses his own transformation. He is now "twice born".

He acknowledges his own Truth and Immortality. He confirms that all change is a dream delusion of divisiveness. His thirst for God causes a reversal of the flow of the cerebrospinal fluid in the brain and spinal cord. He now knows that every desire is possible if he remains undistracted and single-pointed in his quest for God. He begins to realize that every atom in creation has life and every activity is through the power of God, whether within the atom or outside it.

Understanding this inner expansion allows the meditator to rise above all sense of duality. He is exposed to circumstances and situations that give him the opportunity to develop immortal friendships with every name and form.

He feels and acknowledges that his own body is the Kingdom of God, where he meets the Changeless Reality behind his own changing mortality. His cells begin to transform even more from head to toe. There is lesser and lesser distance between himself and God and eventually no sense of separation from the Infinite.

His meditative efforts give him the wisdom of the Image of God, His dream image. He realizes that he cannot meet God without loving His Image, the manifested Universe. This personal experience gives him a loving understanding of God. He finds the common thread binding all names and forms and he sings the glory of God for a Collective Good.

Man's search for his own immortality is possible through the science of meditation. Life has to be synthesized by reducing the distance between matter and energy. Separation from the inner core of his being (Seat of Brahma, the Creator) has to be reached through a gradual inner journey. The meditator has to enter through the door of his own will and desire at the *kutastha* between the eyebrows. The deeper he concentrates, the deeper he enters the seven centers in the brain and spinal cord. He develops even-mindedness, patience, and humility. His inner vision is freed of the sense of duality.

He transcends physical concentration, matures through astral concentration, and sees the 'star in the east'. He is now able to enter and interact with the forces of the causal world. He watches for all types of changes without any expectations. This acceptance of life's changes reduces the distance between outgoing energy or *apana* and ingoing energy or *prana*. The past, present, and future become connected with Timeless Eternity. The meditator finds his immortality within himself! He now has the wisdom to accept everything as it should be. The world is perfect according to divine plan.

The meditator now places God in his brain and spinal cord where the mystical neurons dance to the tune of the Infinite Creation. Here there is really no field of violence. Identifying with the forces of his astral being, he sublimates all sense of ego and duality. His personality changes. He is transformed from a limited to limitless being!

The meditator realizes that his human body was designed for his own evolution through the thought or idea of will. Without a spiritual training, it would ordinarily take man one million years to evolve naturally. However, once the seeker has committed to finding God and his own immortality through meditation, it will merely take one lifetime. Meditation begins with physical transformation, during which time the personality changes. The next step is a merging with the astral energy.

The last effort in meditation is to synthesize energy with thought which convert to the Light of Awareness as *chitta* (enlightened mind-intellect-ego complex). The seeker now leads a God-centered life by harmonizing all polarities of differences. He experiences true love, free of pain and pleasure, duality, concepts, habits, and desires.

His intuitiveness develops in proportion to the duration of his meditative efforts. Once he discovers his immortality through intuition, he sees the power of God within himself. Virtues and evil tendencies both undergo transformation within the spinal cord at the six lower centres. This is the battlefield of *Kurukshetra* referred to by *Krishna* in the *Bhagavad Gita*. When both virtue *[five pandavas* represented by the first five *chakras]* and vice *[one hundred kauravas]* are erased, the meditator enters the field of *dharmakshetra* located between the *kutastha* [Christ-Krishna Center between and behind the eyebrows] and the seventh center or *sahasrahara chakra* located in an area that is tenfinger wide.

Controlling the senses involves feeling all twelve parts of the body until every cell is transformed. Sensation to these parts is withdrawn and placed within the altar of God in the divine cave. The inner physician heals all cells. Attention is especially given to the first two astral centers [coccygeal or *muladhara* and sacral or *svadhisthana chakras]*. Aging begins when these two centers are not attended to. With aging, man discovers that his body below the waist undergoes progressive decay. The lower limbs feel heavier, less agile, and unstable. He develops diseases of organs in the pelvic and lower abdominal cavities.

Having reached this state, he now turns to finetuning the five senses. He begins with the sense of touch. Normally, feeling the outer word of objects triggers physical nerve impulses in nerve tracts and fibers. The seeker is asked to remain even-minded to all grades of touch whether hot or cold, soft or hard, or in pain or pleasure. This practice helps develop will-power over desire and lust.

Next, he feels the inner touch of his own energy-filled astral being. He watches his own breath and its movement inside the body. He moves this awareness of his breathing into the divine cave. He is in contact with the awareness of the touch of breathing. His mental powers gain strength, and his personality acquires magnetism. While feeling the touch of his breath, care must be taken that his gaze is at the Cosmic Vision and that the tongue is always rolled back.

The meditator concludes that if creation is the condensation of divine consciousness, then name and form are inseparable from the space they occupy and the space that surrounds them. The universe therefore is space without boundaries. Everything and everyone occupies this Infinite space. Enter this into the divine cave and visualize the Universe in the expanse of the Cosmic Vision in the *bhrumadhya* between the eyebrows.

Taste sensation is also a manifestation of God's love. Eating involves feeling or touching food, seeing food, and tasting food through taste sensations. Focusing awareness on the act of eating leads to a refined awareness of taste. Man is asked to stop eating as soon as there is a change or non-enjoyment in the taste faculty. This prevents overeating and accumulating unnecessary impurities.

A diet conducive to meditation is suggested. Man is a fruit-eating animal whose diet should be composed of whole grains, nuts, fruits, and vegetables. Sight and smell of such foods create a delight in his chosen meal. Eating foods that are incompatible to the herbaceous man results in assimilation and accumulation of toxic molecules within cells. These are capable of causing symptoms of ill-health, including cancer and allergies.

Perfect health is the result of the synthesis of the body with the intellect. Only a perfectly synthesized being has the supercharged sensitivity to assimilate the essence and fragrance of food, fruits, and the flowers in creation. These are also assimilated into the bodily cells to create a perfect body capable of serving humanity.

The impact of the type of food eaten and the service capability of the meditator is of great importance. If there is a sense of peace, comfort, self-satisfaction, and perfect health, the meditator maximizes his service through the act of love and understanding.

This understanding is intuitive. He acknowledges the presence of the soul or *chit.* In all his inter-actions, whether in meditation, working, or awake, his gaze is fixed at all times at the *kutastha or bhrumadhya* between the eyebrows. When preoccupied with this awareness, the seeker becomes freed of anger or *krodh* and jealousy or *matsarya.*

An evolved seeker who wishes changes in dubious environments and difficult persons should focus in the area of *dharmakshetra.* This is a ten finger width area of the brain between the *bhrumadhya* at the Christ-Krishna Center (center of sixth or *ajnaa chakra)* and the *sahasrahara* or seventh center. During meditation, religious and moral thoughts can be beamed out from here to humanity as well as to individuals.

During physical exertion, avoid wasting out-going energy. Instead, focus into the brain and spinal cord while working and divert the energy back into the divine cave. This allows man to remain balanced between the forces of his out-going and in-going life-forces. There is then no physical tiredness. His performance also remains efficient.

Before and after consumption of food or expulsion of bodily wastes (defecation and urination), pull in the abdomen and the perineum for a few minutes.

Since senses only perceive mortality and therefore change, train all the senses to see changelessness in the sky until all concepts of duality disappear. Feel the touch of air in the space in this infinitude of space as well. See the waves of water rising and falling in the expanse of space, air, and ocean. Hear the outer and inner sounds and merge them with the eternal expansive sound of eternity. Protect the sense of smell and taste. Loss of these result in the loss of bone-density and physical weakness felt below the waist, as in the aging process.

Expose the body to the sun, and especially at the medulla. Feel the Light enter your very being through every pore in the body until you are able to experience light in every atom and cell of the body.

Water consumption should be controlled by thirst which is usually felt 90 minutes after eating a meal. Warm water is recommended for those with tendencies for acidity and flatulence. Do not eat unless hungry for at least six hours after the last meal. Meditate four hours after the last meal.

Meditate regularly and experience the changeless state of bodilessness, formlessness, and infinitude.

Once the meditator acknowledges and finetunes all sense transformation, he knows he is on the path to self-evolution. He accepts all change as necessary. They are blessings from God. The mind must be watched. Intellectual reasoning must be made without judgments.

Pranayama or controlled breathing is used to expand the aura of *prana* or life-force in the medullary area. The larger the area, the better and more abundant is the source of energy for the divine cave. Rolling the tongue back opens the mouth in the medulla even wider. Increased cerebrospinal fluid flow charges the neurones to store more *prana* within them and in all cells of the body. When there is life-force expansion in the total body, physical breathing stops.

Everything and everyone in Creation has this Infinite Power, but they do not know how to become one with it. Meditation removes the blindness of the mind and senses. The mind, synthesized with wisdom, creates the power of intuition. The meditator's devotion allows him to see and hear the seven astral chiming stars in his divine cave. The heart center experiences intense love. There is connectedness between the cells of the body and the astral centers.

Over time and intense meditation, he experiences changelessness and God-consciousness. He realizes he and creation are controlled by prophets and *guru* through the *ajnaa chakra.* He develops a collective vision where there is no difference in the body, the people and Nations of the world. The Universe is as it should be: a changeless reality. Man's life is designed to search for his own Immortality.

Conclusion

We started as a seed of causal beingness-that is the first step of manifestation. The ideas in this state inspire life to take birth. We may be unaware of it, but within the seed lies the *whole plan* of a perfect unfoldment.

Embedded in the plan are memories of past hopes, dreams, fears, concerns and talents. Every cell that is within the seeker's body summons him to reach for the Sun: the path reveals itself as the seeker walks.

The territories the seeker travels eventually lead him through planetary fields, where celestial influences direct his energy towards higher spiritual information which is released by guiding forces already known to the Self.

At this level, all the desires, beliefs, wishes, feelings, thoughts, memories, longings and expectations of the seeker become windows to the Cosmic Self. Once this Unknown is glimpsed, the seeker finds the doorway to the Infinite.

SUMMARY GUIDELINES TO SUCCESSFUL MEDITATION

1. *Before undertaking meditation, the practitioner must first ask for guidance in his quest for spiritual growth.*
2. *Create a cave or shield guarding oneself from all interference.*
3. *Choose the place and posture (whether seated on a chair or in lotus pose) for your regular meditation.*
4. *Ensure that the back is taught and straight; head and neck thrown back a little; the shoulders pulled back together; with hands at the abdomen thigh junction; abdomen below the navel pulled in; now enter the divine cave in the brain and spinal cord through the east between the eyebrows by gazing at the divine cave of brain and spinal cord. Here become One with Awareness.*
5. *Close your eyes and focus your inner gaze and 'look' at the Cosmic Vision at the kutastha.*
6. *Start pranayama using the Ham "saa So" ham technique to regulate breathing. Watch the regularity of breathing by feeling the cold and warmth of the ingoing and out-going breaths in the back of the throat.*
   Start after expiring. Feel the movement of air through the nostrils.
   Synchronize inspiration - pause - expiration - pause. Once the process is smooth, rest in the pauses as long as possible.
7. *Energize the twelve groups of body by contracting [until they quiver] and relaxing [feet, calves, thighs, four parts of back, abdomen, chest, hands, forearms, upper arms, shoulders, neck, and head]. Look at the withdrawal and re-infusion of the life-force - AUM, in and out of the body parts. Do this with gaze at kutastha and tongue rolled back, and back arched back taught and straight.*

Continue this until the body parts become weightless and withdrawn into the divine cave. This is withdrawal of the senses into the divine cave or pratyahara.

Now listen to the inner sound more and more attentively.

Enter deeper and deeper into the Cosmic Vision at the kutastha.

Watch the breath coursing in and out through the nostrils for a long time, doing all of the above as well.

8. *Transfer your attention to the spine of the divine cave and continue the pranayama-pratyahara.*

   Magnetize the spine by first folding the hands at the base of the head and arching the whole back into the hands. In sequence, arch back to the left, then right, then back, and forward.

   Connect with the astral centres of the divine cave by first physically contracting these sites until you enter the astral centre in the cave. Rest your arms and watch the breath coursing through the nostrils. Repeat this for each chakra.

   The rest cycles include: rolling your tongue and eyes backwards, looking at the divine vision of Infinity, watching the breath through the nostrils, listening to the inner sounds of AUM, and remaining withdrawn and within the cave.
9. *Drop your arms in the lap and concentrate on the sound Aum (or Amen or Amin or Hum), listening only through the right ear with the inner ear; this is listening to the inner sound and then the Cosmic Sound*
10. *Hold the eyes up [above the senses] and back into your inner gaze at the kutastha. Allow the "spiritual eye" or "third eye" to materialize over many attempts until it becomes clear at the Kutastha (site of will and universal Intelligence) or the Christ Centre, between the eyebrows. Now bring "Aum" to the Kutastha.*
11. *Practice the Kapaalabhati or Kriya Pranayama by breathing through the mouth. This has to be taught by an experienced Master of Kriya Yoga.*

    Next inspire starting at the base chakra and raise a cool breath up the six chakras and forward to the brow and pause.

    Here get centralized at the kutastha Centre of "Tat".

    Inspiration is done by making the sound: "Haww" through the open mouth. Expiration is the descent of warm breath felt at the back of the throat, from the throat to the base chakra while making the sound "heee".

    Continue until centralized and end with an inspiration.

    Continue until the divine cave becomes radiant.
12. *Once the body has been stilled, you have now entered your silence. Turn the gaze to your inner vision and your ear to your inner listening and listen to the pranava or Aum in your own inner being for as long as you can. Now become body conscious.*

13. Do Energizing Exercises before starting meditation or at the end of it while still in contact with Aum. Convert the body into Aum alone.
14. There is still enough energy to project to one you want to heal or help

This is the seeker's ultimate centre of power. From this point on, only love, the light of Consciousness and the Spiritual Energy, passes through the seeker to create ongoing awakening on his path of perfect balance and beauty. This progressive awakening is an awareness that many celestial forces are at work, helping the seeker from all the higher planes of existence.

The seeker has learnt to walk with Mother Nature and to abide by Her laws. He knows Her ways benefit Her Plan for the Universe. He now takes part in the transformation, because he and the Mother are One. The separation is finally resolved. All polarities disappear, and his life on earth becomes a conscious creative working relationship with the Divine Mother.

His personal desires for name, fame, wealth, and possessions have been transcended. He acts in the present for the moment. He is completely aware that the present is the future. His life is balanced. His life and death are one in this very life! His ultimate understanding is that he lives and transforms in Her Infinity until there is perfect understanding and unison between the experiencer-experience-experiencing.

This text is based upon both the *Sankhyan* Philosophy taught by the Master and the *Patanjali Yoga Sutras*. When I first completed writing this text, I had reservations about its content, as the latter had seldom been addressed in the study of meditation, and I wondered how readers would receive this synthesis. Imagine my delight when I found that the Master, too, had commented and written on *Patanjali*.

In December 1999, as I was putting the finishing touches on this document, *Swamini Sharadapriyananda* sensed my continuing anguish and reassured me with the following words:

> "Remember these are two different means of approaching the Supreme. One, through the head and the other through the heart. When you use the head it is *Jnana*. When you use the heart it is *Bhakti*. Both paths are recognised by the Masters. There is no conflict between your movement between devotion to the *Guru* and the path of *yoga* that you are interested in. What matters is that you reach the Goal. By what means, who cares?

Aum Tat Sat

Acknowledgements

- Swami Tejomayananada of Chinmaya Mission Worldwide, for the use of the voluminous material written and commented on by Swami Chinmayananda.

- "The Bhagavad Gita" by Paramahansa Yogananda of Self Realisation Fellowship.
- "Human Physiology" by Tony Nader, International President of Maharishi Ayurveda Universities.
- "Steps Towards Self Realisation" by Swami Yogi Satyam of Prayag Yoga Anusandhan Sansthan of Allahabad.
- B.K.S. Iyengar - Author of 'Light on Pranayama' and 'Light on the Yoga Sutras of Patanjali' who personally wrote back allowing me to use statements made in his writings.

ADDENDUM FOR SPECIAL INTERESTS

Addendum

The Universe is Transcribed in the Brain and Spinal Cord

Preamble

Unknown to the modern man, the Spirituality of India is to love and work with each other. The modern man judges the land of my forefathers as a stagnant undeveloped and backward area of the world. As one of Indian origin, I salute Africa for breast-feeding me. I bless Eire for teaching me to serve mankind, in both selfish and unselfish ways. I honour Canada for allowing me the luxury of studying the Science of Spirituality under a Master, *Swami Chinmayananda*. She, my Canada, is a young country and her people are just learning to have a Vision for this vast and beautiful land.

I prostrate to India, the Land of my forefathers, where the people's lives are designed to Search for their own Immortality through the Power of Love. In this Power, there is no decay nor division. There is only a Power to Transform everything and everyone. Love accepts no divisiveness among people or Nations. May the Spirituality of India Unite all Nations of the World.

**Physiology of the Physical, Astral and Causal Bodies

Introduction

Through the ages, since Time took its birth from a Moment in Eternity, Man has asked the same questions: What is the essence of human nature? What is his real potential? Are disease and suffering his lot? Can man perfect himself? Can humanity live perfectly and in harmony with its environment? Can society achieve perfection?

**This section is both philosophical and of medical interest. It may be ignored by those not interested in it.

Human Physiology is the material expression of Mother Nature or *Prakriti.* The Laws of Mother Nature are obeyed implicitly also by the human body. The same laws that govern the Universe, are built into the construction of Man. These facts are articulated in the *Vedas* since time immemorial. It seems as if there is the same mind-boggling potential for a higher evolution, through transformation, in the human physiology as there is in the Universe.

Man has the ability to enter new knowledge into a practitioner's silent intervals of meditation and transform his causal being template in the divine cave of the brain and spinal cord. This then allows for the release of altered but more evolved neurotransmitters and neurohormones from the master organs of the body: the hypothalamus and the pituitary glands. The observed result of this gradual evolution and transformation of Man as a result of the release of these bodily hormones and transmitters, is a healing and changing of all functions of all systems of the body. This is possible through their influence on the life-force or *prana* along their specific *nadis* or channels..

The rules are implicit and within the strict boundaries of accepted principles called *chhandas* or prosody *[maharishi yogi*]. There is a capability of a higher quality in all bodily functions. This capability allows man to aim for a perfected state at all levels of his body coverings or *shariras* and sheaths or *koshas*.

Meditation can physically, mentally, and physiologically transform the body. Starting at the atomic level of every cell, meditation allows for a progressive transformation over time during which a seeker practices deeper and more intense meditation. The physical body undergoes change by first altering the energy structure of the astral body that nourishes it. The changes are permanent and forever recorded in the DNA molecule in the seeker's causal template.

If children are taught the *yoga* of meditation and are exposed to the study of *Vedic* literature at an early age, this information enters their silent intervals of stillness and silence. The result is a transformation and growth in a growing child's neurons.

The neuron is the most evolved of all cells in creation. This is especially true for the human neuron. When a child's neurons are exposed to divine and soul elevating environments, he gradually evolves into a perfected being. This child who will in time become an adult, becomes capable of perfect action and speech, according to the natural Laws of *Prakriti* or Cosmic Mother.

All matter in the body and the Universe or *Prakriti* is endowed with *Awareness.* Everything from electron, proton, neutron, atom, to every molecule, is alive. It is endowed with life in varying grades of evolution. Mother Nature or *Prakriti* draws Her powers from the Spirit or *Purusha* whose characteristic is *Consciousness.* It is Consciousness or Light that is inseparable from Her Energy or Awareness. They are inseparable and function as One like the Sun and Its rays of Energy!

Purusha is the eternal observer who witnesses-and-watches all changes taking place in Mother Nature as well as in the individual meditating brain-body. Since He is the repository of all available Universal and Cosmic Knowledge, He is a *rishi* and the experiencer of consciousness; He does not take part in any action.

Prakriti or bodily matter is awareness. Changes made in the template of the causal being are recorded here as observation. The causal being looks and supervises all the changes being entered into Her [Nature's] causal template. These changes are requested by the meditating seeker who aligns his desired wishes with those of the Cosmic Mother.

Because all wants are placed at the feet of the Cosmic Mother or a similar ideal [idol worship through prayer], She is therefore called the *devata,* the personal icon. If prayers are granted (through intense single-pointed meditation), permanent changes are recorded in the causal being and there is a transformation triggered in every cell of the body. The result of this afferent meditative input into the causal template is a transformed or altered observing or interaction with the world of objects, emotions, and thoughts (OET).

Permanent changes made in the causal template of the brain now stimulate a transformed set of orders for the masterglands of the body. They are now direct the hormone and autonomic glands [pituitary-hypothalamus] to alter the quality of the transmitters being released. The result is a changed or transformed stimulation of all the target organs they control in the autonomic system as well as the endocrine system.

Because the dynamism of the end-organs is altered within the strict command of the transmitters, they are said to have a *chhandas* quality or are products released in accordance of specified strict principles.

All subsequent observing, feeling, hearing, seeing, tasting, touching through the instruments of perception and organs of action is in alignment with the soul-aspiring meditator. This is the basis of evolution and neuronal transformation! In meditation, the observer, the observation, and the observing become aligned in perfect harmony.

Any observation by the ideal *devata* or causal icon is a wish granted through the master glands in the brain. The strictly principled changes are permanent, silent, and unmanifest in Man's causal beingness.

From these two sets of neurons (causal [thalamus] and master neuro-endocrine glands [hypothalamus and pituitary] of the body), all manifestations are possible. All the Laws of Nature reside in these silent centres of the brain. In fact, the whole DNA structure of the entire universe resides in this silence. It is here that creative intelligence of Mother Nature resides. It is here where the whole possible manifestation collapses into an unmanifest potential.

Here, Awareness resides as existence or *sat* in the stillness of the divine cave. It is in the silence of the divine cave that all possible knowledge or *chit* resides as Consciousness. In this silence and stillness within the divine cave, the evolved man has transformed himself into bliss or *anand.* He thereafter functions from a higher level of *seeing, experiencing, and knowing* of Mother Nature. He knows he IS *sat-chit-anand.*

All possible Knowledge resides within the *observer* who is the *rishi or* seer. He has the Cosmic Intelligence and Consciousness to direct *awareness* in the *chitta* [mind-intellect-ego complex] to become dynamically transformed with all new knowledge possibilities. The causal template is moldable and therefore records all new *observations.* The ideal *or devata* changes according to the desires of the being.

This special quality of *dynamic transformation* in Man and in the Universe is described in the six *vedangas* or auxiliaries to the four *vedas.* Here, special teachings are given to students of life and living for self-evolution, self-transformation, and regular self-reevaluation. The processes being taught are the same as those taught in *raja yoga* of *Patanjali.* An individual's receptive causal template learns and records what he desires and then makes the necessary changes in the DNA molecule.

The human physiology, therefore, encompasses all possibilities, provided the bodies or *shariras* and sheaths or *koshas* are cared for, in accordance with the Laws of Nature. The highest form of human dignity is seen in a person who possesses a complete mastery over all the Laws of Humanity and can project all in one single awareness. He knows there is order in Creation and that there is only One Knowledge which is the substratum and basic knowledge of all life. He knows that every life evolves stepwise to a higher order through transformation.

In light of this realization, it is understandable that *hurting the environment* or the human physiology through *indulgence* violates the laws of nature and the very fabric of life. Natural Laws are implicit, immortal, invincible, self-sustaining, self-referring, and impossible to dominate. Disturbances in the natural makeup of the human body, therefore, results in pain, disease, and suffering.

All actions and thoughts that are in accordance with the Laws of Nature, are projected as a pure Awareness in the causal body. Matter is Aware and lies within the cusp of the Spirit or Consciousness. When the seen [matter or *prakriti*] and the seer [spirit or *purusha*] are aligned with seeing [action], there is no suffering or pain. Life flows in the fullness of contentment because there is complete alignment in the human physiology.

To make such a state a continuous possibility, man must live within the one Knowledge and its mighty Self-Organizing Power. Man's fluctuating mind must be transcended through meditation to reach an exalted awareness. When this happens, every state of his awareness (conscious, subconscious, and unconscious) is supported and sustained by unalloyed Awareness-Consciousness or superconsciousness.

Over *time,* the transformation in the physical and astral planes permeates back into the conscious awake state as a sustainable self-referral. Man now moves from individual awareness to Cosmic *Awareness* and eventually into a unified field of One Wholeness of the Self in the Total Universe.

To ensure there is permanent physiological and psychological transformation, *time* is an important factor. All processes unfold over time. Reading and listening to *vedic* or scriptural literature or true preceptors of the Truth and intense meditation enhance and accelerate this transformation over time.

Bal Vihar and Yuva Kendra

Schools for Children and Youth

Every growing child should be exposed to Scriptural Literature, which carries within it a complete system of rehabilitation. When a child learns to listen, sing, and speak the subtle and profound knowledge of this literature, perfection is created in his or her human physiology, starting in the causal template. His life gradually becomes characterized by a physical and mental perfection. He then has the ability to attain the highest dignity of life by physiologically transforming his, thought, speech and action into one stream of perfect alignment.

This learning should start as early as is possible and practical, to ensure that the messages of truth and idealism are entered into the silent periods of their growth. With proper nourishment, guidance, structure, and cultivation, the un-evolved impulses brought from previous lives are transformed into evolutionary expressions of perfection.

Diet plays an important aspect of being able to move into different states of awareness. The healthier the body [healthy eating habits] is, the easier it is for the future seeker's psyche to free itself from his physical anchoring and concerns. This awareness of diet determines the child's future health also. Good diet habits must be inculcated early in the life of the child and youth.

The child is given seed *mantras* at specific ages in his life. At first, he is taught to meditate on the *mantras* as he gazes at the sunrise and sunset. His concentration is usually quiet and thoughtless; there is a progressive awakening of the seed. Parents must make sure that the child or youth has spent the previous day eating and resting sufficiently for this feeling of perfect quietude.

If the parents are knowledgeable, the child will be willing to abide by the rules of eating, playing, studying, and sleeping. The child learns that he is now happy to abide by the rules. He has enjoyed the joy of his own silence. He now has learnt to reproduce the experience of perfect warmth, harmony, and energisation by abiding by the rules.

The growing child and youth is able to make healthy choices for a healthy physical body. He eats what has been prepared for him in love. He imbibes these vibrations of loving and caring parents, teachers, and elders. The regenerative efforts are subtle.

These regenerative and transforming energies are entered through neuronal connections at synapses in the child's nerve fibers. They are highly influenced by and further sensitized by Nature's stimuli. Depending on the type of stimuli to which they are exposed, certain connections become established in the brain very early in life. These connections are part of a new transforming in a child's individuality.

Each sensory and emotional experience leaves traces in the neuronal physiology of the synapse space, where the incoming or afferent stimulus is transformed into an outgoing or efferent action in the nerve reflex arc. Repeated exposure to the same love experience leads to a neuronal transformation which eventually becomes permanently recorded within the child's causal template, as a good habit or tendency. Conversely, lack of stimuli prevent connections from forming and the development of the child is hindered.

Timely exposure to the most appropriate stimuli in the proper sequence will ensure development of a physiology capable of achieving its full potential - a mastery over the Laws of *Prakriti* [Mother Nature]. As the child grows, so does his sense of responsibility towards all his actions. As a youth and young adult, he gains mastery over responsible action and understands the *karmic* law of cause and effect. He has the ability to enjoy the qualities and splendour of *maya* [Universe in all Her Qualities] and Her beauty. Parents teach him the reason for his likes and dislikes or *raaga dvesha.* He is taught to overcome this tendency by harmonising the pulls of opposite polarities in Nature. Such gradual mastery leads the young adult towards a life aiming at near-perfection.

Transformation and Evolution of Man and Nature

Through proper training in meditation, it is completely within our reach to speak spontaneously and act in accordance with the natural laws. The 'instinctive' ability to make no mistakes in thought, speech, or action is the orderly evolutionary direction, and it is available to man in his own physical anatomy and physiology.

By studying the dynamics of the silent spaces at interneuronal junctions, one can appreciate that there are silent intervals which occur during the conduction of an impulse. The stimulating impulse can be sounds of syllables, verses, and *mantras* already in the *Vedic* [scriptural] literature. A serious student of neurophysiology and psychology can learn the *mechanics of transformation* of any state, situation, or condition.

Maharishi Mahesh Yogi calls these spaces 'gaps'. He claims that intercellular spaces between cells in the body, are similar to the gaps between *mantric* sound. These are silent areas where new informational inputs induce changes and transformation in the cells around. Since the neuron is the most evolved of all cells in the body, the effect of such activity in and around the neuron leads to the highest achievement possible in a transforming man who is meditating.

Just as a presynaptic impulse collapses into the silent gap and another transformed expression emerges at the post-synaptic end, so too it is for the evolving neuron. If the space is perfectly aligned and balanced, the emerging expression is perfectly in tune with the expected sequence of expressions. The new syllable or impulse will undergo the same process of collapse, and a third expression will emerge.

For every collapse, a new state arises. In neurophysiological terms, the impulse collapses into the *silence* of the next space. The emerging impulse depends upon the *quality* of the presynaptic impulse and on the inner dynamics of the intercellular and synaptic space. This is the basis of neuronal transformation and evolution in man.

The dynamics that ensure a proper sequential flow of one state to another therefore depend upon the *mechanism of transformation* within the space. What is collapsing within the space? How does this collapse take place? Is the space perfectly balanced? Is the space in its simplest state? Is the space noisy (fluctuating) or silent? All these factors determine the purity of the next stage of progression. The intended result can be perfect only when the state of pure *silence* is realized as perfect.

The *self-correcting mechanisms* available within the structural dynamics of *Prakriti's* Laws of Nature always put everything back on the *highway of evolution*, so that the Laws of Nature can continue to delight in an undisturbed flow of Her expressions. Look at how a Perfect Knowledge in *Spiritual* literature of all religions continues to rejoice man and creation with their perfect, flawless sequence of thought, sounds, syllables, and verses.

The state of balance of the spaces where the impulse must collapse need not express itself in overt action. The dynamic nothingness can impart its *quality* into the space in the synapse of the nerves, as well as, in the causal neurons of the medullary or *ajnaa chakra*.

Here in the divine cave, the *silent witness* in the cortical or *sahasrahara chakra,* just 'watches' all the incoming and the outgoing impulse as 'experiencer' or *rishi* who is already endowed with all the possible Knowledge in the Universe. Awareness agrees to all the changes the mortal desires. She is the icon and therefore the *devata who* 'looks on' and in *silence* holds in Her *memory* all the changes being made in Her mortal causal being in the spiritual thalamus [planetary Sun within the brain].

The memory of this new knowledge is aligned with the memory of Total Nature. This memory in the DNA molecule of the thalamic neuron maintains and ensures that there is *order in creation* - the Unmanifest Causal Body of the Universe. This is the secret of transformation in an individual mortal and also in the Universe, in one single act. This is the Path of Evolution through *sadhana of meditation.* Ultimately individualized *dhyana-samadhi* takes the seeker to Oneness with Mother Nature..

All human behaviour, speech, and action follow this flawless system of collapse and emergence of all inputs into the afferent systems of the nervous system. What emerges depends on what was collapsed and upon the purity and balance of the silent, self-referring gap between thoughts, decisions, words, and actions. This is a display of the indomitable power of the natural laws of *Shakti or Prakriti* [Cosmic Mother], which maintains order in the whole universe. Nothing is ever wasted. Nothing is ever lost. Through the perfect mechanics of *transformation,* everything unfolds with great precision.

Mastery over the natural Laws of Nature is available to each one of us where its *source lies,* in the silence of the intercellular and synaptic space - in *atyantabhava,* the self-referral *pure awareness.* Acting from this level means acting while established in silence and stillness of the body, mind, intellect, and ego or *chitta.*

Acting while established in the silence, in the Yoga of Meditation, is action in non-action. It gives real freedom from any boundaries imposed by partial and non self-referring impulses, including desires that cannot find fulfillment. These unfulfilled desires or *vasanas* collapse and emerge out-of-tune with the Cosmic Symphony, leading to Stress in the Fabric-of-Creation.

Desires or *vasanas* are what brings the mortal to a rebirth of manifestation. Mother Nature will offer all possibilities for these to be fulfilled. If the mortal aligns his action in accordance with Her *dharma* [virtuous and righteous actions enjoined by all scriptures of the world], there is harmony. It is unrighteous actions for indulgences that create stresses in Her creation, both, in the microcosm and the macrocosm!

In meditation, the desire for oneness with the Divine Mother is available to all seekers. One need not become a monk nor does he have to give up caring for his kith and kin while seeking his own immortality. Many seekers wait until old age to enter spiritual life. They are of the opinion that a spiritual life demands a rejection of all worldly pleasures, desires, and family responsibilities.

The Master was challenged by a Western seeker about his right to enjoy the world and its bounties. The Master first defined *vasanas* as desires for pleasure. He then explained that even a meditating monk can enjoy the gifts of life, if the attitude is refined with a perfect understanding.

"... *Vasanas* express themselves as **desires** for indulgences. These become thoughts, which express as gross actions in the outer world..." repeated the Master for the umpteenth time during the *Yagna,* pointing suggestively towards the famous *'BMI Chart.'*

A newcomer to the talks at a *yagna* [lecture in philosophy] found this a bitter pill to swallow and he expressed his dissatisfaction to the Master at a *satsang* or meeting with the wise. He felt the *Swami* was feeding him with seeds of 'Eastern Passivity.' To the Occidental Westerner who since childhood is trained in becoming a 'dynamic, aggressive materialistic Victor,' this was unacceptable. He felt he was being given a philosophy of 'Inaction'.

The Master continued:

"... *Vyasa's* [author of *Bhagavad Geeta* and transcriber of the *Vedas]* son, *Sukadeva* was himself a great mystic who believed unswervingly in the *path of 'non-action'* [meditation] *as the state of 'perfection'* or *samsiddhi. Sukadeva* was ordered by his father *Vyasa* to go to King *Janaka* for 'further training' [in worldly actions]. Obediently, he took leave of his father and hiked towards *Janaka's* palace.

"King *Janaka,* was a 'realized' soul. He had a daughter and therefore could not abdicate his throne despite his wish to spend his time in meditation. He therefore continued to serve his Kingdom as a righteous King should. This was part of his *dharma* or duty.

King *Janaka* was notified that *Vyasa'a* son, *Sukadeva* was on his way towards his Kingdom.

"On arriving at the gates of the palace in the centre of the city, *Sukadeva* parked himself and awaited further instructions from his *'guru' Janaka.* The king decided to ignore *Sukadeva* who remained calmly at the gate, on the sidewalk, without food or shelter, wrapped in his meditation upon the Lord.

"After many days, King *Janaka* decided to invite *Sukadeva* to the palace and received him with pomp and reverence befitting the young sage. He was bathed and clothed by maidens. The King's Ministers arrived and invited *Sukadeva* to be present at the King's Court for a gala evening performance.

"*Sukadeva* was brought into *Janaka's* Court that evening. After the usual traditional prostration, King *Janaka* gave *Sukadeva* a beautiful silver vessel filled to the brim with oil, and ordered him to hold it without spilling even a drop of it.

"He then ordered the evening performance to begin. It was a spectacular performance of music and exquisite dancing. At the end of the performance, King *Janaka* turned to *Sukadeva* and with royal indifference asked him how he had enjoyed the performance.

"*Sukadeva* replied: 'My attention was so totally aimed at not spilling the oil in the vessel which you had ordered me to hold, that I was oblivious to the show.'

"The King condescendingly admitted that when one is so fully absorbed in such a drab function as observing the 'oil,' he could not have been aware of the world of music and dance.

"How can one, 'actively' merged in the supreme Bliss of the Self, ever become distracted by the world-play outside? *Sukadeva* had learnt what he had come to learn. It was time for him to leave.."

Our Western friend was now even more confused than before:

'Why does the *Swami* contradict himself', he commented.

> Days later, the *Swami* added
>
> "..Act you must. Therefore, do your duty or *dharma* according to your own *svadharma* or according to your own beliefs or desires or *vasanas* or tendencies."
>
> The Westerner remained confused. Then came the final advice
>
> "..Act in a spirit of sacrifice for the benefit of the community, in accordance with your duty, without anxiety and desire for the 'fruits of action'. Your inner alliance should remain a perfect meditation."

The Westerner smiled back knowingly. The penny had dropped!

A*tyantabhava* or non-existence of a state, is always available inside the seeker and also in *Prakriti* [Universe]. It allows space for possible changes and manifestation to take place. An adept seeker learns to master the mechanics of what is the most appropriate impulse required for transformation to take place in the memory of the seeker who is already connected to *Prakriti* [Mother Nature].

The secret of meditation is to sit where the *atyantabhava* or self-referring awareness is, and become a master of all transformations, thus guiding his own destiny. This is the Secret of Creation, the Secret of the Creator, and the Secret of attaining Oneness with Her . No struggle, no strain, no pain is ever necessary!

The secret to the fulfillment of all desires is to act while established in the self-referring state of the silent space or gap of pure awareness - in the *atyantabhava* of complete non-existence. One can achieve anything, be anything, create gardens out of mud, move mountains, and shake the cosmic structure, when actively resting [meditating] in this stillness and silence!

It is in this same silent still mechanics of transformation that the understanding of immortality lies. The whole dynamic of change and evolution happens through transformation. No impulse of the self-referring absolute ever dies. Every thought, particle, and galaxy is transformed. It never dies, it only becomes something else. The first law of thermodynamics also points to this reality: all transformation occurs in the silent unbound pure level of extreme non-existence which is immortal in its self-referring nature.

Every fluctuation in thought (*vritti)* is always with reference to itself. It is the real Self of everything. Each impulse of knowledge, each impulse of the Natural Laws of *Prakriti,* or indomitable *Shakti,* is a vibration or *pranava Aum* that supports the universe with Her Creative Universal Intelligence. Every one of these impulses finds its course in creation, collapse, and re-emergence. Consequently, the ever-changing field of relativities, cause-and-effect, and changing qualities, is itself immortal.

There are two values of immortality in *Prakriti or Shakti*: one is its own level of self-referral in pure silence; the other is in the field of dynamism. Here, although fully awake in both the states (observer-observation), in the field of dynamism (observing) there are no boundaries. There is only enjoyment of every new possibility, gain, and an ever-changing new experience. As each impulse collapses, from it emerges a new experience, delighting Man in *Prakriti's* play-and-recreation or Her *lila*!

Having discovered this secret, all that Man has to do is to strive for oneness with the Universe in both Her silence and also in Her dynamism. It is never too late to start, wherever we are at:

> and the Master said:
>
> "The present alone is the time when we can work and achieve, gain and gather, give and serve. In the past we can 'now' do nothing! In the future, we can 'now' accomplish nothing. In the dead moments of the past and the unborn moments of the future we can never act. These living dynamic present moments are the only fields to be hammered at, wherein are all the glories of life, all the gains in existence..."

A *sadhak* or seeker, who awakens into this reality, experiences the never-ending bliss of creation, its play, and its ever serene, peaceful fully awake, unbounded limitless Self. The seeker emerges as the totality of everything, the glory and joy of creation, liberated from the cycles of change, discovering immortality and the unlimited dignity of life. He rejoices in the glory of the Cosmic Administrator.

Modern Science Recorded in Ancient Vedas

Vedic Literature is the age-old literature of India which has been preserved in a large collection of books by *rishis* of yore (seers of truth) in the four *Vedas*. Some of this literature is still "oral" and is preserved from generation to generation in old *vedic* families.

However, we owe our greatest appreciation to sage *Vyasa* who compiled the material in the *vedas* and other *vedic* literature, over 5000 years ago. Some 2000 years ago, *Patanjali,* another *vedic* scholar, focused on man's central nervous system as the miniature template of the Universe, from where all orderliness of nature emerges.

The Laws of Nature *whisper* constantly to themselves. They describe all Natural Laws to themselves and record all potentials through a system of self-referral in Cosmic Intelligence. The whisper intonates itself in a series of synchronized **hums** of varying frequencies and vibrations: those able to "hear" these whispers realise that the whole universe is a Vibrating Infinity, from atom particles to galaxies.

The Laws of Nature refer to every law known and unknown, and include physics, chemistry, biology, anatomy, physiology, and biophysics, including the laws governing every individual life. Thus, *there is order in the infinite diversity in nature.* The sound value of the underlying hum in diversity means that it requires nothing outside itself to justify the existence of the entire universe. It is self-sufficient by virtue of its self-referral and its ability to transform in accordance with the Laws of Nature.

Knowledge has an amazing self-organizing power. The more precise this knowledge is, the greater is its organizing power. Pure Knowledge of the Infinite is consequently transcendent and unmanifest and combines the power of Pure Awareness and Consciousness into Itself. In it are contained all the possible interactions of the Laws of Manifestation in one unified field of experience. The universe is born of relationships of its own components, a system of dynamics which structures its diversity. These dynamics are self-interacting and therefore have a self-sufficient, self-sustaining, and self-referring quality, independent of anything outside itself.

It follows, therefore, that the Manifest Universe or Intelligent Awareness is created in and is an expression of that Unmanifest Conscious Intelligence or *mahat.* When man lives in accordance with the laws of nature that govern his anatomical, physiological, psychological, and intellectual processes, ill-health and irrational behavior do not arise. Man is able to fulfill every aspiration or desire to the fullest through the support of the Eternal Mother of Creation and Her Laws of Nature. She is the Cosmic Homemaker.

When a *group of people collectively understand and adopt this spiritual life-style*, they can create a coherent *collective awareness* eliminating stress in the fabric of creation. There is a palpable raising of the standard and quality of living. Society progresses towards a healthy life-style free of disease, stress, crime, and anti-social behavior.

This profound insight, that there is absolute order prevailing in the universe, leads one to the conclusion that the self-referring abilities of the unmanifest intelligence gives the objectified manifest universe its own self-referring quality, despite multiplicity and diversity. There is a connectedness between the unmanifest intelligence and the manifest intellect. It is this connectedness which gives an eternal order to creation and evolution.

The listening and reading of scriptural material from childhood, allows for a sequential evolution of the developing central nervous system which resides in the divine cave. Perfect nurturing of a child's neuronal physiology eventually becomes a habit and concept. The growing child who is exposed to the Laws-of-Righteousness or *dharma,* matures into perfected sequence of progressive awareness. This is also the basis of progressive gains made by seekers during *sadhana* of meditation.

Meditation is the ability to transcend the mundane mind and its mental activity. When the physical, psychological, mental, and intellectual sheaths are *stilled,* the individual's awareness settles quietly in its own restful alert awareness - in *silence.* Here, the individual who now rests in his own stillness and silence, transforms within the boundaries of his own self-referring state of consciousness.

Over time, all past stresses are erased. There is a new transformed creativity, capable of orderliness, dynamism, and exalted creativity, which inspires and upholds all thought, speech, and action. *What is exciting about this transformation is that the laws of nature uphold and sanction every desire of this transformed central nervous system.*

The human physiology as *chitta* (mind, intellect and ego) residing in the *ajnaa* centre has the ability to be aware of itself, in structure, thought, and action. The human physiology also has the ability to know and experience itself as the enlightened *chitta* or pure awareness or Universal Intelligence in the centre-of-will between and behind the eyebrows in the spiritual eye reflecting within the physical thalamus [microcosmic Sun in the brain's planetary system].

Once this perception in awareness has become manifest in the understanding of Man, he has the ability to change the settings of the control systems of the body, mind, intellect, and ego. All changes are recorded in the memory of the *devata or* ideal [microcosmic Sun or thalamus] who has the ability to stimulate the master glands within the brain and spinal cord. The master glands controlling the autonomic nervous system and the endocrine glands now release altered neurotransmitters and neurohormones which transform every cell in all the sheaths of the mortal.

The transmitters are strictly structured and follow strict principles of change, in accordance with the amount of transformation that has taken place in the silence periods of meditation. The transmitters have a *chhandas* quality and the manifested actions are in accordance with the inputs made into the silent gaps of the afferent nervous system.

When the observer *(rishi),* observation *(devata),* and observing (under *chhandas*-like controls) is synchronized into a harmonious experience *(samhita),* an exalted Oneness with the Whole is realised.

Human Cell and Intercellular Space

The human cell differs in size and structure depending upon its function in the body. Between cells, there are spaces or gaps containing fluids and molecules, permitting communication between like and unlike cells in the body. The *central nervous system* within the divine cave acts as the master clerk with the ability to organize and coordinate the activities required to integrate perfectly all the bodily functions.

The *basic cell* of the nervous system is the neuron. The neuronal cell body contains all the information (DNA) required for the neuron to function as the combined observer, observation, and observing *(or samhita)*. The *rishi* or observer is the eternal witness who merely 'watches' without becoming involved with the changes occurring in the awareness of the neurons of the *devata* in the thalamus. All silent observations in the *devata* are registered in the causal body for posterity. (Please refer to Figure 20).

The postsynaptic efferent impulse is a transformed message influencing the release of altered neurotransmitters and neurohormones from the hypothalamic-pituitary axis. The effect of this 'altered' state is the evolution of the cell which acquires a principled or *chhandas* quality capable of eliciting appropriate motor and verbal responses when man makes contact with the world of objects. (Please refer to the Chart: 'Transformation through Meditation' before the Introduction to Vedanta).

**Nerve Tracts and Peripheral Nerves

Collections of neuronal processes with identical functions travel together as *nerve tracts* within the spinal cord and as nerves outside the cranium and spinal column. Within the brain, they gather as *fasciculi,* also called *white matter* of the brain. Collections of neuronal cells with similar functions are nuclear aggregates *of gray matter* within the brain and the spinal cord. Transmission of messages between neurons occur at synapses in *synaptic spaces* or gaps. The experience and experiencing may be motor, sensory, and autonomic.

**The Brain and Spinal Cord

The nervous system consists of pairs of cerebral hemispheres, the midbrain, the pons, the cerebellum, the medulla, and the spinal cord. Each has the ability to function through a whole range of man's experiences.

The cerebral hemisphere is divided into four lobes: frontal, parietal, temporal, and occipital. The surface is highly convoluted into *gyri (folds) and sulci (grooves) that have neurons or gray matter which are a few millimeters thick and are histologically very distinct from each other. The gyri of *all the four lobes are interconnected* by association fibers. The two sides of the brain are connected through the corpus callosum and the anterior commissure. (Please refer to Figure 20)

These four lobes become *integrated* by sinking down through the six layers of neurons of the cerebral cortex, where the experience is of a unified awareness in the deeper parts of the brain. This is the neocortex or the neoencephelon wherefrom the waker functions as a *conscious* mortal.

*There are 196 gyri or surface convolutions covering the brain. Some have matched these to the 196 statements made by Patanjali, the author of Patanjali Yoga Sutras.
**Please omit if not interested in medical sciences

Deeper to this lies the mesocortex or *subconscious* dream brain. Deeper still lies the limbic cortex which encircles the whole brainstem and the subcortical structures of awareness. This is the *unconscious* deep sleep area of the brain which experiences bliss and existence. This is the level of the thalamus or centre of will. This is where *all emotional and motivational transformations take place.* The changes are recorded in the causal centre *[ajnaa chakra]* in the diencephalon in the apex of the medulla.

The subcortical structures of the cerebral hemispheres are the deeplying basal ganglia. From this level of control, *human physiology plans and executes the complex motor functions involved in planning, higher cognition, and the execution of strategies.* The basal ganglion has connections with other motor functions, and the limbic cortex. With these connections, the brain is *involved in cognition, memory, orientation in space, behavioral patterns, and motivation.*

The diencephalon (basal ganglia) lies within the cerebral cortex and the midbrain. It is composed of the thalamus and the hypothalamus. The *thalamus* is the sensory information centre *transmitting emotion and awareness to the cerebral cortex.* It can be likened to a door between the outer world and the inner world within the cerebral hemispheres.

The *hypothalamus* plays a major role in the autonomic *bodily homeostasis.* It receives inputs from the limbic system and *expands by transforming* the stimulus *through a feedback system,* thus regulating motivation and the autonomic nervous system. It is here that life-force vibrates and beams in its Light [Consciousness] and Energy [Awareness] as *prana* [AUM] through the medulla. This individual connection permeates into the various sheaths and bodies of the mortal. As long as there is life in a mortal, the mains at the medulla always remain connected to the unseen Cosmic Life-force.

The cerebellum wraps the whole midbrain, the pons, and the medulla. It *integrates* all information from motor and sensory inputs originating in the cerebral *cortex.* Through the spinal cord it preserves the balance of the body despite the forces of gravity, through the inner vestibular nerve system.

The brainstem or diencephelon is composed of the *reticular formation, the midbrain, pons, and the medulla.* Also embedded here are the nuclei of the *cranial nerves.* This area is concerned with *sleep-wake cycles and biological rhythms* of the body. It is of interest that the twelve cranial nerves emerge below the level of the *kutastha* between the eyebrows. The gaze into the Cosmic Vision is beyond and above the level of the individualistic mind and senses.

The spinal cord or myeloencephalon consists of collections of motor and sensory tracts capable of activating organs of *perception*, organs of *action and of behaviour.*

Perfect *integration of all functions* of the different components is possible through feedback loops existing within the system itself. To ensure 'instinctive' control and balance, the efferent response is *multiplied by maintaining continuous contact with the source* of impulse.

For neurophysiological information to be relayed, an *afferent stimulus* must be *processed through eight* synapses. The progressive transformation of this stimulus takes place in the spaces or gaps at synapses. It stands to reason that the integrity of the eight factors of the synapses must also be perfect.

Each, the eight factors elaborate a particular 'processing.' During *sadhana* or spiritual effort, there is a gradual transformation of the quality of neurotransmitters and neurohormones being elaborated from the hypothalamic-pituitary axis. The effect is a gradual transformation of 'eight matter factors' in the seeker's seven psychic centres or *chakras* residing within the divine cave.

These eight factors are products of Nature or *Prakriti* - they are:

- Ego or *ahamkar,* which *re*sides in the medulla.
- Intellect or *buddhi* which has the discriminating quality capable of clearing channels for onward conduction. It resides on the hemispheric surface and is connected to deeper structures of the brain.
- Mind or *manas*, which is capable of emotion and thoughts. It is represented by the limbic complex. The thalamus [centre of willed transformation] and the causal template in the *ajnaa chakra* are capable of influencing the qualities of *transmitters being* stimulated for release by the pituitary-hypothalamic axis. These neurohormones and neurotransmitters make their influence felt through the autonomic nervous system and the endocrine glands.
- Space or *akasha,* which exists within synaptic spaces or gaps in the autonomic nervous system channels is for the purpose of specific effects of neurotransmitters and neurohormones; it resides in the psychic *vishuddha chakra* or cervical plexus.
- Air or *vayu* which exists within the gap spaces for exchange of gases; it is represented by the *anhaata chakra* or thoracic plexus.
- Fire or *agni*, which exists within the gaps for the transmission of impulses through a feedback system of electrons and electrolytes; it is represented by the *manipura chakra* or lumbar plexus.
- Water or *jala* which exists within the gaps for ionic constitutions and osmolar values; it is represented by the *svadhisthana chakra* or sacral plexus.
- Earth or *prithvi*, which gives structure to boundaries between gaps along cell membranes; It is represented by the *muladhara chakra* or coccygeal plexus.

These eight factors combine, integrate, and *modulate into the DNA molecule* of the neurons of the brain and spinal cord residing in the divine cave. It has recorded within it all the rhythms, cycles, structures, and laws of nature and also of the human physiology.

The basic unit of DNA is a codon with sixtyfour possible permutations which determine the type of transformation possible in the structure and function of the neuronal cell. Depending upon the structure of the neuron, it has a *memory bank* of every exposure and action endured through its millions of incarnations. The full memory of the present existence for elaboration of any studied action or perception resides on the surface layers of the cerebral cortex.

Feedback Systems of the Nervous System

Sensory Nervous Systems

During *wakeful existence*, man experiences his environment through specialised *sensory channels* which sustain a qualitative wakefulness. All five sensory modalities are represented, giving man his observer or *rishi* status who merely 'watches'.

The perceptual (special senses) and sensory equipment allow him to organize, balance, and decode all incoming stimuli and record them as observations in his *devata status*. The *devata* merely 'looks' at the transformations taking place within the individual. It reacts by making the required desired adjustments. This is where the psychic 'third eye' *or Kutastha* resides in the divine cave and is intimately connected with the causal being in the *ajnaa* centre. It records all inputs, whether for self-improvement or for indulgences!

> Eshaa braahmi sthiti partha nainaam praapya vimuhyati. Bhagavad Geeta II.72
>
> This is the Brahman-state, O Son of Pritha [Arjun]. Having attained this, none is deluded. Once established in thereign [in enlightenment], even at the end of life, one attains [every desire including] Oneness with Brahman.

All bodily functions are fulfilled through processing systems, parts of which are experienced and others which are not. Inputs such as eating, drinking, breathing are experienced as *offerings of sacrifice or yagna* to the body. These are metabolized *in the fire of physiological digestion, psychological emotions or feverish thoughts,* all depending upon the *intent of the sacrifice*.

If the inputs are for *indulgences,* these are metabolized in ways that cause injury to bodily functions. This is the result of 'inputs' causing the release of appropriate (harmful to the body or otherwise) and specific neurotransmitters and neurohormones from the master organs in the brain. The specific agents released are then capable of a changed efferent stimulation. The experiencing in the body is in strict accordance with the afferent desires and inputs.

This is the basis of altered actions and relationships with the world of objects after sincere *sadhana* desiring oneness with the Cosmic Mother. All of the eight factors of Nature of the Man must undergo permanent changes. According to sages, it takes at least eight years of sincere concerted effort to make visible changes in the habits, concepts, and likes and dislikes of the seeker.

Sensory and Autonomic Nervous Systems

Two categories of processing systems exist: *Shukla* (white) and *Krishna* (black). Somatic or white inputs (sensory) are open to awareness; the autonomic or visceral or black inputs (sympathetic or *pingala* and parasympathetic or *ida*) are not.

The *Shukla* or somatic inputs are consciously experienced on the body surface through fifteen modalities of perception: sound, sight, taste, smell, cold, heat, sharp pain, burning pain, light touch, sense of air movement, pressure, vibration, proprioception (limb position), joint capsular sense, and the sense of balance. The last three correspond to sense with reference to a mid-point of the body.

The *Krishna* or autonomic inputs are channeled through the autonomic ganglia of the cranial nerves and the sympathetic-parasympathetic systems. They are all controlled by the hypothalamus or the master autonomic ganglion. This gland lies below the thalamus, and is close to the pituitary gland. It is under control of emotions and also the conscious brain.

Four aspects of these the visceral-autonomic systems are recognized. They include inhibitory and excitatory modalities of each of the sympathetic and the parasympathetic nervous systems. These release neurotransmitters. The pituitary gland is part of this system. It is the master gland for hormonal secretions of the body. It releases neurohormones.

Together they respond to the thalamic ability to make changes in the DNA codon of neurons in the thalamus. The thalamus makes changes in response to afferent inputs. The changed message is then communicated to the hypothalamus for changed neurotransmitters and to the pituitary gland for changed neurohormones

Somatic or *Shukla* sense modalities, are also channelled and controlled by the thalamus in the basal ganglia of the brain. The thalamus corresponds to *Surya* or the Sun. It is a midline structure in the depths of the brain. In addition to controlling the hypothalamus and the pituitary gland, it controls all *sense modalities* of the body. (Please refer to Figure 20).

The *Bhagavad Geeta* refers to these physiological, anatomical areas of the nervous system and also confirms there is an established astral connection of the physical body. It is the spiritual northern path back to the Self or the southern path towards unfulfilled desires.

> *agnir jyotir ahah shuklah shanmaasaa uttarayanam*
>
> *tatra prayaataa gachch-chanti brahma brahma vido hanaah Bhagavad Gita VIII. 24*
>
> Fire, light, day, the bright half of the month (full moon), and the year: departing by this path [northern path in meditation and at the time of physical death], men who know brahman go to brahman [do not reincarnate].

The *visceral-autonomic nervous system* is channelled and controlled by the *hypothalamus* which is associated with *Chandra,* the moon. As previously stated, the hypothalamus lies below the thalamus and controls the autonomic nervous system through the release of neurohormones. It also orchestrates the parasympathetic channels through the moon-channels or the *ida*. The moon channels unconsciously cater to man's *indulgences* and process the inputs in accordance with the *intent* of man. In conjunction with the thalamus, it reciprocates in the control of the sympathetic or sun-channels or the *pingala.* (Please refer to Figure 21)

> dhumo ratris tathaa krishnah shanmaasaa dakshinaayanam
>
> tatra chaandramasam jyotir yogi praapya nivartate Bhagavad Gita VIII.25
>
> Smoke, night, the dark half of the month, and the year: departing by this path [southern path of sensory desires], the yogi gains the light of the moon and returns [reincarnates].

Awareness "Looks"

The *reticular activating system* in the brainstem controls the *waking and sleep cycles* of man. During sleep, all sensory inputs are prevented from reaching the wakefulness centre of awareness. The process of waking up involves the integrating of all sensory inputs into the thalamus and eventually the cortex of the brain where all <u>watching</u> takes place.

The thalamus <u>looks</u> at all the sensory inputs in the causal template of the *ajnaa* and instigates appropriate responsiveness in the five senses. It induces wakefulness and triggers appropriate actions with the world of objects. In deepening meditation, *pratyahara* secures a withdrawal from all sensory inputs while fully aware [that he is pure energy] within the reticular activating system. This awareness induces a transformation within every cell in the whole body. The changes are <u>felt</u> as light energy or *prana* in every part of the body [during an inward journey]. The body is now felt without the grossness and density of matter [as while on an outward journey] .

> *shukla krishne gati hyete jagatah shaashvate mate Bhagavad Gita VIII.26*
>
> These two, *shukla* [incoming northern] *and krishna* [outgoing southern] are held to be the world's eternal paths [of evolution].

The other brain stem nuclei form part of the reticular activating system and control the waking, dreaming, and sleeping cycles of man. While in this pure aware state of meditation, man is in his *chitta* state (mind-intellect-ego) and is under the control of the thalamus, the sun or *surya*. The ancient seers of all faiths call this the spiritual eye. It is the *Krishna* or Christ Centre of Universal Intelligence which must be entered to reach the doorsteps of Awareness and eventually, Consciousness. It is the gateway to your connectedness with the Cosmic Mother.

In the *chitta* state in meditation, the seeker gets a sense of relief from his imprisonment in his body which has been preoccupied with his senses, thoughts, and desires. The veils are lifted and blindness of past births, which were once invisible, become manifest in his understanding. He has intuitively understood where he is and where he is heading to.

Action through Motor and Skeletal Systems

The musculoskeletal systems of the body give man their shape and moving capabilities. It also has the ability to cover all the inner physiological systems of the body. The body is capable of shrinking and expanding and moving from major joint levels. The purpose is to *establish individualistic harmony with his environment, through mobility and adjustments.*

The vertebral column has the shape of *Arjuna's* [*Krishna's* student] bow. When held taut and firm, it upholds all of the physiological systems of man's body. It remains undisturbed and unchanged while upholding all transformations that course through its *tunnel,* experienced as a 'blue' passage in death experiences. It is invincible despite the assault of diversity of change in the environment. It is geared towards maintaining an evolutionary balance and perfect order within the universe. The cavity of the brain and the spinal cord is the 'divine cave', the altar of God.

The spinal cord houses the five *chakras or* centres of psychic energy in the *plexuses* of the spinal cord. Here, the entire human physiology sits in silence and dynamism. Old molecules of DNA are constantly being destroyed and new ones produced, recording every change in the inputs being made by man within the thalamus.

Their structure and function have a quality of invincibility which obey all the laws of *karma* and *gunas* and of *relativities.* This profound influence is left "on record" as habits and change; they eventually make their effect felt in all the bodily enzymes, their biochemistry and in the immune systems. *Here lie the blueprints of a healthy or a diseased bodily state* in the present and future bodies to come.

The Body's Pacemakers

Bodily pacemakers are an integral part of the feedback mechanisms of the human physiology which is orchestrated from different levels in the midline by the human nervous system. They include the cardiac plexus or *anahaata chakra* where mystical rhythmic sounds are heard by *yogis.* The thalamus controls all sensory inputs into the brain. The hypothalamus controls the type of neurotransmitters being released. The pituitary gland determines the types of neurohormones that must be released. The limbic system enjoys the effects of these changes. The remaining basal ganglia determine the health of man's physical structures and their coordination. The medullary centre of *ego* brings in the life-force or *prana* and breathes life into all the physiological functions of the body. The cortex of the cerebral hemispheres are centres of memory, intellect, and social-behavioural norms. (Please refer to Figure 20).

Anhaata Chakra or Cardiac Plexus

Seven sympathetic ganglia on each side of the spinal cord modulate the *rhythms of the heart.* These are connected to four thoracic parasympathetic segments (vagal) enervation. The integrating quality of the two autonomic systems is responsible for the cycles and rhythms of its physiology which controls cardiac rhythm, circadian rhythms, metabolism and hormonal secretions, and its relationship with the rhythms of nature.

The integration of the autonomic nervous system with the heart centre is through the faculty of thoughtless love for the Cosmic Mother. It is one of the halves yearning a connectedness with the second or other half: Love.

Hypothalamus

The hypothalamus synthesizes releasing-factors to *activate the pituitary gland*, the *neurohypophysis* and the *autonomic nervous system*. Its control therefore, has an expanding quality on the endocrine, biochemical, and physiological responses: together they bring about a new state of balance in the bodily functions.

The hypothalamus produce long sequences of aminoacid strings which can be cut at various strategic points to become specific messengers with specific influences on the physiology of the bodily functions. The changes are easily done and are in response to the changes demanded by the mortal. The changes are made in the thalamus first.

Hypophysis or Pituitary

The pituitary gland maintains a connectedness with the neurohypophysis/ hypothalamus and the autonomic nervous system (sympathetic and parasympathetic). It is activated by the hypothalamus and the limbic systems. Responses are expanded by multiplication through a feedback system which maintains homeostatic balance in the organs it influences. Through a self-referral system, it controls at least eleven hormones of the body, not to mention the neurohormones and neurotransmitters released by the two sides of the autonomic nervous system.

The feedback loops of the *hypothalamic pituitary axis* and the *sensory-motor systems* have a self-adjusting quality capable of measuring needs and feeds components of balance. The range of transformation anticipated is part of the adjustment and resetting mechanism. The role is played by neurotransmitters, neurohormones, and hormones. This ensures proper functioning in all the organ systems of the body, including the circadian rhythm.

Transmitters have the ability to activate cell *membrane receptors* and allow for transformation at all the *eight end-organ levels* (gastrointestinal, haematological-immunological, pulmonary, neurological, cardiovascular, musculoskeletal, endocrine and dermatological). Specific transmitters open doors at specific receptor responsive sites to allow for biochemical transformation.

The psychic centre of the *ajnaa chakra* resides in the base of the brain opposite the pineal-pituitary bodies, the hypothalamus, and the thalamic areas of the brain. It is the causal centre of the unenelightened *chitta* [mind-intellect-ego complex].

Limbic System

The limbic system is divided into four components and make connections with the lobes of the cerebral cortex. It has the ability to *transform* a specific stimulus into an *adaptive* expression of a global experience. The response takes into account the *emotional needs* of the individual, also taking into account the *inner and outer requirements* of the person. The limbic system's role of transforming a value into an expanded expression allows for adaptive *adjustments in overall balance and homeostasis.*

This is the psychic area where the thalamus *(prakriti)* allows itself to be hammered at the *kutastha* itself, without itself changing. The sole purpose of this evolving awareness through the processes of *sadhana* is to secure a connectedness with the Cosmic Mother. The limbic system responds to the demands made at the thalamus. (Please refer to Figure 20 & 21).

and the Master wrote:

"...*Kuta* means anvil. Everything that comes in contact with the anvil changes, but the anvil itself never undergoes any change. When pure consciousness is being perceived in an undifferentiated manner in the intelligence of all beings from *Brahma* the Creator, down to an ant or *brahmadi pipeelika paryantam*, then it is called *kutastha...*"

Basal Ganglia

The basal ganglia occupies the centre of the brain. It is likened to the planetary configuration around the sun. The thalamus is the sun or *surya,* around which *all motor and sensory activity is centred.* It is the "king" of the basal ganglia and interconnects with all the other nuclei through the corona radiata. This is the psychic centre of the causal being. (Please refer to Figure 21).

The hypothalamus (moon) also lies in the centre of the brain under the thalamus. It deals with feed-back functions relating to *emotions, behaviour, bodily temperature, reproduction, and hormonal cycles and frequencies*. The hypothalamus represents the moon or *chandra* of the solar galaxy in the brain.

The putamen or *shani (saturn)* is the farthest satellite from the thalamus. It functions as a centre *receiving inputs which must be retransmitted* to other parts of the basal ganglia. Its major concerns are motor activity and it has the ability to limit or obstruct inputs. Diseases of the putamen are related to chorea, loss of bodily tone, dementia and premature death.

Aligning with the putamen, but deeper to it is the globus pallidus which is the *guru* (jupiter) or instructor *capable of a high order of instructions to action*. It is responsible for planning and execution of *complex actions*. Its functions are related to the limbic system. It ensures inner balance taking into account the natural laws of action.

Deep to the globus pallidus is the substantia nigra or *mangala* (mars). It activates and inhibits the putamen and the caudate nucleus. It is involved with *precision of movement* and maintenance of *steadiness* while performing voluntary movements. Diseases of this centre are characterized by tremors, inability to initiate movement, and rigidity of tone. The person is afflicted with a sense of insecurity, fear, and lack of initiative.

The amygdala's function is related to the tail of the caudate nucleus or *ketu*. It is the *emotional centre for fear*. It is also connected to the red nucleus, which is related to *mangala* (mars) as well. Its hallmark is *emotional courage, precision, and sharpness*. Pars compacta is part of this complex of nuclei.

Pars reticula *or shukra (venus)* is the counterpart of pars compacta. It connects with the limbic system and has limited control over action. Its main characteristics are *instinctive and sexual behaviour, and emotions*.

The subthalamic nucleus *or buddha (mercury)* lies just below the thalamus. It has the *discriminating quality of the intellect*. It receives inputs from the thalamus and the other nuclei surrounding the thalamus. Its outputs are moderated by the influence of the inputs.

The caudate nucleus is a large C-shaped collection of cells, with the head *or rahu* (*ascending lunar node)* connected to the putamen (*shani) or Saturn;* the body of the caudate nucleus encircles the thalamus *(surya) or sun;* the tail *or ketu* (*descending lunar node)* connects with the amygdala *or mangala (mars)* in the temporal lobe. Here it is the *seat of emotions, learning, and memory*.

The head of the caudate nucleus *or rahu* is involved with *saccadic eye movements, memory, and the ability to change in behaviour patterns*. When this area is diseased, the affliction is of irritability, absent-mindedness, depression, fidgeting, clumsiness, recurrent sudden falls, disturbances of speech, and facial expressions. Eventually, the individual loses all cognitive functions and reasoning capabilities. Similar disorders transpire from disease of the putamen *(shani)* with which it is connected.

The tail of the caudate nucleus *(ketu)* lies within the temporal lobe, close to the amygdala *(mangala) or mars*. It is closely connected to *learning and emotions*. Diseases of this area are characterized by feelings of unreality, visual and auditory hallucinations, depersonalization, fear, anger, delusions and paranoia. Irritative lesions of the tail of the caudate, manifest as intense emotions, ardent religious zeal, extreme moral opinions, and lack of humor. Destructive lesions of this area present with inability to understand or express emotions. Panic attacks and anxiety disorders are afflictions of this area of the brain.

The deep subcortical nuclei of the brain are likened to the nine planets *(nava-grahas)* of the universe revolving around the sun *(surya)*. The twelve cranial nerves in the brainstem contribute their individualism to the emotional and intellectual make up of the individual. Their association with the nuclei of the brain give them a *bhava* or mental attitude or purity of disposition. They are connected to the four elements: air, water, fire, and earth..

Brainstem Nuclei

A constellation of neurons exists in the brainstem which are connected with the hypothalamus (moon). The cell groups have a variety of functions and therefore are specific with special neurotransmitters. Their connections with the thalamus, hypothalamus, basal ganglia, cortex, brainstem, spinal cord nuclei and other structures of the central nervous system renders them subject to the intrinsic rhythms of its own individualism.

At the time of birth, a newborn is *exposed to a new set of conditions* created *first* by a *new environment* away from the mother and *second* by the *phase of lunar activity on the hypothalamus.* From the moment of birth, the *lunar and planetary cyclically influences* the *hypothalamus and its connections in the brainstem.* The body is influenced by Nature's orderly progression of cycles into day and night, months and seasons, and annual cycles of planetary influences etc,.

These constellation of neurons in the brainstem are monoamine transmitters and are involved with activation processes in the brain relating to:

- Connections with the cortical nuclei and the cranial nuclei *(12 bhavas)*;
- Levels of awareness while awake, dreaming, or sleeping;
- Behavioural patterns of arousal;
- Regulation of reflexes;
- Coordination with autonomic functions;

- Responses to pain and stress;
- Maintaining constancy of the internal milieu through breathing, feeding and temperature regulation;
- Connecting internal cycles with the cycles of the planets in nature.

Cortical Nuclei

The twelve cortical areas of the brain are connected to twelve *bhavas* or attitudes, one specific for a cortical area on the right or left side of the brain. Some cortical areas exist only on the right or the left side; others are interconnected on both sides. Taken in the context of totality, they regulate the individual's *physiological responses to life, whether social, family, or otherwise.*

The twelve *bhavas* or attitudes that are connected to twelve cortical areas of the cerebral cortical areas include:

- Head's *bhava* (*tanu*) depicts the person's innate nature as regards appearance, body and self-image, ego, intellect, personality, response to grief, and orientation to birthplace and position.
  This attitude is connected to the right and left occipital-temporal areas of the cerebral cortex, which regulates appearance, facial recognition, memory, self-image, personality, and language.
- Facial *bhava*, especially of the right eye *(dhana)* depicts the person's learning, and facial expressions through visual identification and his ability to attract wealth of precious stones and metals, and materialism that is pleasing to the eye's sense of sight.
  This innate attitude is connected to the right occipital lobe which is responsible for vision, visual identification of face, and facial expressions of others.
- The *bhava* of combined throat, neck, shoulders, arms, and hands *(sahaja)* depicts vitality, valor, courage, travel, and sensuality.
  It is represented in the right parietal lobe: their perception of space and the sense of touch leads to integration into a somatic sensation and perception of their body in space, especially while connected to courage and valor.
- The nose, heart, lungs and chest *(bandhu)* convey confidence, maternal happiness, beliefs, comforts, and love for homeland.
  They are represented in the right limbic cortex for the perception of emotional and instinctive pleasures recorded in the hypothalamus by a mother's nurturing.
- The abdomen *(putra)* allows for learning, intelligence, knowledge, success in the fields of education, liaisons, partners, children, and natural inclinations.
  The right frontal cortex allows motor control of actions in accordance with inclination of the mind, knowledge, and learning.
- Hips, umbilicus, and the intestines *(ari)* are aggressive *bhavas* towards opponents, competition, enemies, adversity, obstacles, worries, anxieties, voices but is able to deal with intelligent speech, through consultation.

They are represented in the right prefrontal cortex which is the seat of intuitive thinking felt, as deep gut-feelings. This area of the cortex regulates mood, motivation, and is the focus of mental diseases caused by worries, conflicts, oppositions, and anxieties.

- Abdomen below the umbilical level *(yuvati)* relates to life, power, desires, marriage, travel, business, trade, and partnerships.
  This area or *bhava* is represented in the right and left temporal cortex; it is connected to the autonomic control of all organs above and below the navel and bladder. Desires for indulgences, pleasure of sensory gratification, and impressions of memories of these are recorded here as future inclinations.
- Excretory and reproductive organs *(randhra)* have the *bhava* of vulnerability, transformations, recall of past and future events, research into material and mystical topics, violence, and aggression.
  The left prefrontal cortex controls *bhavas* of occult and mystical interests, aggression, mood regulation, research, and prognostications through analytic and discriminative intellect. Discrimination of desire associated interests of the reproductive organs are modulated here.
- The *bhavas* of the thighs *(dharma)* are important in destiny and fortunes of the individual; righteous conduct, religion, philosophy, higher learning without pains, affluence are all the result of paternal nurturing.
  The left frontal cortical area represent the thigh. Actions are dependent upon the inclinations of the mind as nurtured by paternal influences.
- The knees *(karma)* support activity, occupation, status, honor, position, respect, vocation, profession, name, and fame in public life.
  The left limbic cortex and the thalamus which matures under paternal nurturing determine personality and vocation.
- Calves and ankles *(laabha)* render *bhavas* of income, gains, fulfillment of hopes and aspirations, not to mention greed.
  The left parietal cortex integrates all sensory inputs of physical comforts, sensory fulfillment and lead to income and materialistic prosperity.
- The feet and the left eye *(vyaya)* function in the fields of investments, foreign travels, expenses, financial losses, falls and sin.

The left occipital lobe records visual discrimination when exposed to visual attractions and temptations.

The connections of the cortex with the twelve *bhavas* are the result of the influence of nurturing by parents and environment on the DNA molecule. It has the capability of receiving information necessary for the creation and maintenance of a new structure and function to align with the environmental needs.

The two helices of the DNA molecule are exact mirror images of each other. One of the strands is the template and the other is the coding strand. The coding strand is the "silent witness" *(Purusha)* who only "watches" as *saakshi* and does not take part in the formation of the m-RNA; it only ensures that the memory of the value is intact.

The second helix functions as a "catalyst" *(Prakriti)* for transformation and eventual expression of the information available on the strand, but does not itself change. This strand only "looks" in awareness.

Between them they orchestrate all change in the person during meditation. Depending upon the changes secured, Man's actions in the world of beings, objects, and environment are a mirror image of what has been aligned by the observer-observation-observing complex.

and the Master wrote:

"A *saakshi* or witness is a person [in common parlance] who has seen an incident but has not got involved with it. In philosophical parlance, it is He who is the cogniser of the manifestation [into names and forms] and disappearance [merging into unmanifest state] of the knower, knowledge and the knowable, but Himself is devoid of manifestation and disappearance. He is self-luminous [because of His being unmodified and unaffected by the above two states] and is called the *saakshi* or the witness [who 'watches'].

"It can be said to be the connecting link among the three states: Waking, Dreaming, and Deep-sleep. The actionless bird in the *Mundakopanishad* as well as the Sun who illumines everything, represents *saakshi*..."

Thalamus the Centre of Will

The thalamus is the center for logic or *nyaaya* with the capability of distinguishing and deciding. It *relays* sensory and motor inputs to appropriate areas of the cerebral cortex. It also transmits motor information from the basal ganglia and the cerebellum to the motor cortex of the cerebrum in the frontal lobe. It is involved with both the sympathetic and parasympathetic reactions of the autonomic nervous system, and is involved in the maintenance of arousal and awareness.

The thalamus and its satellite nuclei *receive inputs* from all these areas, maintaining a to-and-fro connection between all the nuclear centers, thereby regulating overall neuronal health and excitability both in sleep and arousal.

The thalamus is the *center of will power*, capable of integrating *intellect* with discrimination and decision-making. This translates itself in every action, behaviour, perception, and motivation. Its ability to analyze perception requires logic and justice: only then can there be a decision to initiate a particular action. Therefore, the thalamus and its connections have the ability to comprehend the specific, as well as the whole.

Thalamic perceptions may become inhibited, excited, or remain neutral. The reaction is from a *point of consideration in awareness* which is the *chitta* or the mind-intellect-ego complex [in the *ajnaa*]. The point of consideration corresponds with specific values, whether they be extraneous, specific, relative, or a changing values. The reaction is a holistic response to all the factors discussed, whether this is inwardly directed or is more desire motivated.

If the response is *holistic,* it has taken the Laws of Nature into account and uses the neurotransmitters and neurohormones to make the necessary changes in the contents of the divine cave, that is: the nuclei of the brain, brain stem, and the spinal cord centers are transformed and acquire a specific or *chhandas* quality.

If the response is *inwardly directed*, awareness and intellect have been involved and the transformation is an observation by the causal body or *devata* whose quality is that of the unenlightened *chitta* (mind-intellect-ego). If the response is *transcendental,* mind and intellect have been eliminated and only awareness as *enlightened chitta* is experienced as a unified whole in a pure awareness. The observer of the responses has a *rishi* quality of *chit*. The experience is that of an uninvolved witnessing consciousness.

Perception by the thalamus, by virtue of its connections with other parts of the brain, covers sixteen modalities of logic. The thalamus integrates all the information to execute a valid response.

Perception through logic *(tarka)*, is a *faculty of the intellect which is patterned in accordance with the structure of natural laws.* This means is that the structure of thought and the structure of matter are the same.

Logic, therefore is a progression of thought through the processes of being reasonable and rational, according to common sense and evolutionary laws. Logic is evolutionary because it has the ability to change behaviour, cognition, and re-orientated memory. It is dependent upon a widespread connectedness with a variety of information centers in the brain, taking into account the situation, the object, and the concepts.

The processing of a final **perception** of any one individual therefore requires three things: *seer,* the *seen,* and the inner act of *seeing* unified as one whole from the point of view of a unified knowledge.

- The **seer** has a *rishi* quality of the transcendental, capable of being an inner observer or consciousness or *saakshi*. The **seeing** has endured transformation. The changes have a quality of strict transformation or *chhandas* quality. It takes into account the known principles of an external physical object. All subsequent experiencing is outwardly directed act of observing while acting with the world of objects.
- The **seen** or the linking of the seer and the seeing is the holistic response of the thalamus which has a *devata* quality of silent observation or awareness.
- The combined **experience** of the seer (subject), seen (silent link or object) and seeing is **knowledge**. Together they unite into a single field of perception or *samhita.*

Knowledge is perceived as different in different states of awareness-consciousness. These differences depend upon whether awareness is:
through matter as unenlightened *chitta* (mind-intellect-ego);

through pure awareness as enlightened individual *chitta* (causal) *;* or refined through pure universal intelligence as *chitta* (or pure *prakriti*) or through pure consciousness as *chit* (or pure *purusha*).

Patanjali defines seven states of awareness-consciousness: waking, dreaming, sleeping, transcending [sheaths], pure individualised awareness [causal], universal awareness or *dvaita* [thalamic as *chitta*], and unity awareness-consciousness or *advaita* as *chit:*

The thalamus or spiritual eye or kutashtha chaitanya or Krishna-Christ Centre is the door between awareness and consciousness. It holds within its bowers the power of will, wisdom, love, and desire to serve for its own sake of connectedness with the Cosmic Mother.

- The unenlightened *awake state* is a perception through all the five matter sheaths of the body: *annamaya kosha* (food sheath), *pranamaya kosha* (physiological or energy sheath), *manomaya kosha* (psychological sheath), *gyanamaya kosha* (intellectual sheath), *and anandamaya kosha* (bliss sheath). [Please review Figure 7].

  Perception at the thalamus (door) is coloured by the condition of the bodily sheaths. There is light outside it [in the world of perception of objects, emotions and thoughts - OET] but not inside the House of Awareness (thalamus). This is the Conscious or awake state.
- The *dreaming state* is perception of stored impressions, giving one an illusory reality. The light is not lit outside and there is darkness inside the house-of-awareness. Awareness is therefore processing stored thoughts from the Subconscious mind. This is the dream state of "Meness".
- The *sleeping state* has no perception at all. There is no light anywhere and the gates of the thalamus are closed. This is the restful Unconscious state of deep sleep of "Me & I -ness".

  When the individual practices the *yoga of meditation*, he is able to progressively enter this bliss-sheath as well as the remaining three deeper halls of this "house of the unconscious state". They can be entered through the door of the thalamus.
- The *transcendental state* of perception is without the body and mind, meaning that there are no physical sensations nor thoughts. There is light inside the House of Awareness (thalamus) but not outside it. The intellect and the ego perceive without any given specific value.
  There is awareness of perception of pure knowledge of "I-ness", the subject of the search during *sadhana*. The meditator has entered the halls of the unenlightened *chittamaya kosha.*
- The *individualistic awareness state* is a perception of *two values which leads the seeker towards enlightenment*. There is awareness that there are separate values: one inside which is non-changing as Self or "I"; and another which is outside which is constantly changing as "Me". One is permanent; the other is

not. The light of pure awareness shines equally both in the inside and on the outside - ***unenlightened chitta.***

- In the *state of universal-awareness* or *dvaita* state, there is a *clearer perception of the outside world of the waking state.* This refined perception is free of doubts, hesitations, and apprehensions. When the light is shining equally both inside and outside, the exalted perception is that the outside matter is a perfect dynamic expression of the inner silent spirit. Intelligence perceives the separate values in their combined pristine glory. This is a higher state of universal consciousness - ***enlightened chitta*** *state of pure awareness.*
- In the final *state of unity-consciousness* or *advaita* state, the inner awareness becomes consciousness and sees a unified field inside and outside. Individual awareness is constant in thought, word, and deed. The outer matter layers never again overshadow awareness. There is both stillness of matter (object or seeing) and silence in awareness (observation or seen): the experience of the whole is pure consciousness (observer or seer) - a ***chit*** *state is of combined awareness and consciousness.* The object and subject become one in a single enlightened vision.

Cerebellum

The cerebellum receives input from other brain structures concerned with the programming and execution of movements. It monitors and integrates peripheral information received from the spinal cord and the descending tracts. This *internal feedback* confirms the type of external feedback that is necessary for an action to occur. The type of action to be performed has to be confirmed and *aligned with* the *central information* in terms of the goal underlying the action.

The cerebellum, therefore, *sees the goal, specifies the performance, and fulfills the actual motor response.* It has the ability to give *specific value to each wave of the ocean.* These specific values of a thought or action must include:

- *dravya* or substance;
- *guna* or quality or property;
- *karma* or action;
- *saamaanya* or common factor;
- *vishesha* or specific factor; or
- *samavaaya* or aggregated value.

The integration of all the specifics are concentrated in the depths of the deep cerebellar nuclei (dentate, fastigial and interpositus). The cerebellum integrates the body's position in space, by timing movement and its direction, its relationship with the individual's awareness as regards his position and mental intention.

Yoga through Association Nerve Fibbers of the Cortex

Yoga of Meditation has the unifying quality of self-referring awareness. Despite the diversity of thoughts and physical psychological afflictions, meditation has the ability to cover all differences in spite of the bombardment of millions of inputs.

This integration is a function of the **association fibers of the cortex**. The fibers are axons of neurons located in the cortical gray matter, woven into a weave of a fine mesh. Bundles of U-shaped fibers connect gyri of the brain surface. Longer association fibers connect the right to the left brain through the anterior commissure and the corpus callosum. Some *yogis* say there are 196 association fibers to match the 196 aphorisms of the *Yoga Sutras of Patanjali.*

The *right* brain has a *general synthetic* quality to it while the *left* brain is more *specifically analytic.* The grand theme of nature is to connect specificity with generality to create a wholeness of totality. What this means is that everything is interrelated and everything is connected to the whole.

The cerebral cortex of the adult brain is divided into *six anatomical layers of cells* in the four lobes (frontal, temporal, parietal, and occipital) of each side of the brain. This is where all diversity of expression is represented. With meditation, the practitioner progressively enters the deepest layers of the brain where motor and sensory inputs are extinguished into each other.

The first layer of the cerebral cortex *receives inputs* from all the other layers, but sends *no projections.* The full potential of the brain emerges when the whole sustains the experience of pure awareness in all aspects of thoughts, perception, and action - a unity in diversity.

- The cell structure allows for a gradual withdrawal of all stirring for the sake of a transcendental self-referral which takes the practitioner into self-sufficiency, autonomy, and independence while in a field of increased inner-directedness.
- The second layer of neurons stills all unwanted noise and information from entering awareness. Deeper levels of meditation give the seeker a greater sense of intimacy and empathy for the whole. The seeker senses an **all-pervading wholeness.** The integration has a quality of complete **stillness.**
- The third layer is connected to the nerve bundles and cortico-cortical fiber and commissures. Widespread integration and processing within this self-referring ability gives it a **quality of omnipresence.**
- The fourth layer connects with the thalamus in an unmanifested state of a **sensory experience.** Once the seeker enters the thalamic level, there is a **silencing** of all sensory inputs and *increased emotional stability,* friendliness, loyalty, tolerance, respect for others, and compassion. This is a state of universal awareness of the unenlightened *chitta.*
- The fifth layer of neurons contain the pyramidal cells of the **motor system**. The experience is an unfolding of awareness with reference to a known quality. With the acquisition of an increased intrinsic spirituality, the integrated personality becomes more aware of his **own relationship with God's omnipresence.** This is a deeper enlighteneing awareness of the *chitta.*

This open-mindedness allows the seeker to see diversity in the context of a whole. He realizes he can combine the unmanifest parts into the manifesting whole. With increased mental and physical well-being, he finds a greater sense of social responsibility. This is a process of an unfolding persona into a state of increased creativity wherein the seeker may connect with *siddhic* experiences.

- The sixth layer of the cortex also contains pyramidal cells which send axons back to the thalamus and remains in balance with it, dissolving all unwanted inputs. Here lies the holistic integrated activity of the nervous system. The final stage of **dissolution allows a deep state of rest,** free of the physical and physiological functioning of the body. This is the state of "Unity-Awareness with Consciousness" of *chit.*

Oxygen consumption and carbon dioxide elimination are decreased and the tidal volume is reduced. There is a lowered respiratory rate and periodic breath suspension. The heart rate drops to basal levels; and all biochemical, metabolic and hormonal functions are suspended to hibernation levels.

Memory and Automated Reflexes

Memory or ***smriti*** exists in all structures within the DNA of every cell, but especially in the neurons of the gray matter of the hippocampus of the brain, the brainstem, and the spinal cord. This *perfect automation* is the result of a *perfect memory* at every neuronal level. This is further entrenched by the fact that a full range of possible connections have been established through the nervous system.

Memory is represented in all memory systems and reflex-arcs, which allow for rapid perception and action without the need for a lengthy processing and analysis. An automatic reaction occurs, governed by complete knowledge (in memory) of what is the appropriate motor, mental, or emotional response to any given situation. The response is always appropriate to the situation and can even consist of complex adjustments of social and traditional behaviour in the presence of changing circumstances or environmental demands.

Memory has the structure of intellect in that it displays the total potential of the observer or seer or *rishi,* whether at an individual potential value or at a universal potential value. With reference to memory of a cosmic potential, the individual's potential has an *absolute value that is capable of and ensures a spontaneous right action based upon the holistic value* of the individual's spontaneous adequacy. Simultaneously, the individual's spontaneous response computes in all the laws of nature into itself.

The interconnecting fibers of the reflex arc are silent gaps possessing the ability to see the response that is required. They have a *devata* quality, by virtue of the fact that the intellect *displays a total potential of the processes of*

observation. Taken from an individualized potential to a cosmic potential, the intellect has an ancient, eternal quality of awareness. The total potential of the individual's process of observation is found in the "great intermediate net" of the brain which monitors all inputs and outputs of the central nervous system.

It provides a correct response on the basis of intended action, individual needs, environmental demands; and actual response. The "great intermediate net" of almost 400,000 neurons correspond with the 400,000 neurons in the spinal cord. The neurons of the "great intermediate net" include all the neurons and their fibers *within* the nervous system.

The motor response is **seeing** and therefore, is mediated through an observed integrated value with known quality**:** all based upon established values. The spinal cord, which is the most ancient part of the central nervous system, gives expression to all automated channels. "Seeing" also has a structure of the intellect in terms of its ability to display the total potential of the blossoming of **human experience.**

It illustrates an individual potential of human experience and the ability to assimilate all the laws of nature in his every thought and action. Physiologically, this is represented by neuronal fibers which activate the musculoskeletal system controlling action and speech.

Descending and Ascending Tracts of the Central Nervous System

The *descending tracts* of the central nervous systems have a *chhandas* or specific quality, structured for speech and action. All of the eighteen descending bundles are motor tracts and structure expression of behavior, action, and speech.

The *fasciculi propria* are divided into six sets of *spiral-spinal fibers* which are short crossed and uncrossed, ascending and descending fiber systems, beginning and ending within the spinal cord. *All groups at various levels are within the same level of the spinal cord.* They are interconnected with their own intrinsic value within the spinal pathway. The fasciculi propria are effective "whirlpools" of activity, interconnecting and stirring structures for material expression.

The stirring quality of the spiral-spinal nerve fibers has a *devata* value of the **seen or observation**. The self-referring awareness inherent in them illustrates the underlying mechanics of processing and transforming through living examples of material expression.

The *ascending tracts* of the central nervous system bring every possible sensory experience to awareness. These sensory pathways channel individual expression to the higher cortical centers where they are perceived in a holistic value. The ascending pathway includes sight and sound, and act as channels that make every experience accessible to the cortex, in one symphony of experience.

For a seeker established in pure awareness (***chitta***), there is the opportunity to expand over time, into the experience of pure consciousness or soul (***chit***). Every experience starts to be perceived in terms of unbounded, infinite, and transcendental self-referring soul.

The use of sensory ascending tract of the central nervous system is the ultimate purpose of every experience in Meditation. Repeated exposure towards localized point values (points of concentration) leads to the gradual expression of these values as expression on one's own soul. The seeker acknowledges in sequence:

This awareness is Self:	***Pragnyanam brahman***
That also is my own Self:	***Tat twam asi***
All of this is my Self:	***Ayam atma brahma***

The use of the ascending channels leads to the most refined and ultimate of all experiences, where all point values are understood simultaneously in terms of the oneness of life:

This soul and cosmic soul are one:	***Aham braham asmi***

The four *mahavakyas* or great-sentences quoted above, are discussed and elaborated in the 14 main *upanishads.* There are about 300 *upanishads* in the four *vedas* which describe the transcendental experience of awareness and eventually consciousness, through a process of meditation described by *Patanjali in the Yoga Sutras.*

Mahavakyas are four *upanishadic* declarations, expressing the highest *Vedantic* truths about the identity of the individual soul and the Supreme Soul. Each is found in one of the four *Vedas.* The first *mahavakya* is found in the *Aitreya Upanishad* in the *Rig Veda.* The second *mahavakya* is in the *Brhadaranyaka Upanishad* in *Yajur Veda.* The third *mahavakya* is recorded in the *Chandogya Upanishad* in *Sama Veda.* The last of the four *mahavakyas* is discussed in the mighty *Mandukya Upanishad* of the *Atharva Veda.*

Conclusion

Every religion has strict warnings against acts that violate the personal space and awareness of other beings. Even while on spiritual paths, many seekers continue these violations against each other. *Yama and niyama* is about rules of conduct seekers must adhere to. *Kama* or passion and lust, *krodha* or anger, *lobha* or greed, *moha* or infatuation, *mada* or pride, *matsarya* or envy, and *ahamkar* or ego are referred to as the 'Seven Sins' in many other faiths.

- Lust or passion is wanting without regard to the wants of another. It stems from lack of respect for another and eventually for oneself.
- Greed is the urge of taking without giving back to persons or Mother Nature: it breeds death of generosity and world cooperation.
- Gluttony is over-consumption of Nature's gifts, whether this be of food, or Nature's resources; they cannot be taken without thought of leaving some for future generations.
- Arrogance and pride is the feeling that I alone deserve the gifts of the Earth.
- Envy is the secret desire for what others possess and you do not. This negativity creates death of self-growth and motivation in life.
- Idleness and sloth is considered a virtue by the working man who is employed. He refuses to work but demands more for his personal needs. He kills his personal responsibility and his will to survive with such powerlessness!
- Avarice is a combination of killing out of spite, hate, greed, gluttony, lust, and envy. Here man projects his desire to kill the shadow of his own failings.

These are poisons that need weeding. These tendencies are habits acquired through many previous lives. Transcending these tendencies is imperative for the sake of balance in one's own life. Only then can there be a balanced culture and world society.

The balance is between giving and receiving, planting and harvesting, taking from the Earth and giving back to Her. The balance is between oneself and others. It is about inner values and outer expressions. It is also about feasting and fasting, silence and speaking, freedom and self-respect, creative work and inspirational silence, time to seek God and time to allow God to manifest within.

In the Circle of Life, fulfillment of the body, mind, intellect and *vasanic* or causal desires gives man his creative urge to live and to strive in this life. The rules are clear. The interaction of man's desire must be in accordance with the Laws of Nature. Violation against any of the matter envelopment spells death and disease in that sheath during his lifetime. These are carried as burdens into future lives.

Aum Tat Sat

GLOSSARY

Glossary

A

Aabhaasa	Reflection
Aabhaasam	Effect
Aabhaasavaada	Doctrine holding that creation is reflection of Reality
Aabhaati	Shines or illumines
Aachaara	Right conduct, conduct or practice
Aadarsha	Ideal
Aadesha	Divine command from within
Aadhaara	Support and basis
Aadhibhautika	Elemental
Aadhidaivika	Pertaining to the heaven
Aadhyatmika	Pertaining to the Soul
Aaditya	Sun - a class of celestial beings
Aagama	The Veda as proof
Aahara	Food as an object of senses
Aahuti	Oblation offered in fire sacrifice
Aajna chakra	Seat of the mind in the sixth lotus of the yogis behind the eyebrows
Aakaanksha	Desire all round
Aakasha	Ether
Aalochana	Deep thinking or reflection
Aananda	Bliss
Aanandamaya kosha	Karana-sharira or blissful sheath or seed body which contains all potentialities
Aaradhana	Respectable worship
Aasana	Posture or seat
Aashrama	Hermitage or order of life of which there are four, namely., Brahmacharya or studentship, Grahastha or household-life, Vaanaprasta or forest-dwelling, and Sanyaasa or monastic life
Aatma	The Self
Atmabhava	Feeling that all is the Self
Atmabodha	Knowledge of the Self
Atmadrishti	Vision of seeing everything as the Self
Atmanishta	Established in the Self

Aavarana	Veil of ignorance
Aavaranashakti	Veiling power of maya
Abhava	Meditating upon Self as zero or without quality
Abhavana	Non-thought
Abheda	Non-difference
Abhedaahamkara	Ego that identifies itself with Brahman
Abhedabhava	Sense of non-separateness
Abhedabhakti	Highest devotion culminating in oneness
Abhedabuddhi	Intellect that beholds unity
Abheda chaitanya	Constant thought of identity of soul with Brahman
Abheda jnana	Knowledge of identity of individual with Absolute
Abhaya	Freedom from fear
Abhinivesha	Instinctive clinging to life
Abhiman	Egoism
Abhivyakta	Manifested
Abhyaasa	Constant practice
Achala	Immovable
Achintya	Unthinkable
Achetana	Unconscious
Achintya shakti	Inscrutable power
Achyuta	Unchanging or indestructible
Aadhaara	Support
Adi Shankara	Philosopher who lived 1500 years ago
Adi Shesha	Primeval serpent who supports the world on its head
Adharma	Contrary to right
Adbhuta	Wonderful
Adhibhuta	Elemental forms of matter
Advaita	Monism or non-duality
Ahamkaara	Ego the "Me" and "I"
Adhimatra	Degree of vairagya from sources of pain
Adhisthana	Background or underlying essence or substratum
Adhyatma shastra	Spiritual science
Adrshta	Unseen principle
Adrishtam	Unperceived
Adryshya	That which cannot be perceived
Ahimsaa	Non-violence
Ahuti	Offering an oblation at a solemn rite (usually into fire)
Ajnaa chakra	Seat of command and will between the eyebrows

Agni	Fire
Aghaada	Unfathomable
Agandha	Odorless
Agati	Stability
Aguna	Without quality
Aham	I or ego
Aham atma	I am soul or atma
Aham brahma asmi	I am God or Brahman
Aham etat na	I am not this
Aham eva sarvah	I alone am all
Aham Idam	I [and] this
Ahakara	Ego or self-conceit or self-arrogating principle of 'I am-ness'; three types: Rajasic : Dynamic egoism with passion and pride Sattvic: Egoism within sense of goodness and virtue Tamasic: Egoism expressed in ignorance and inertia
Ahamkarta	I am the doer
Ahamvritti	Self-arrogating thought
Ahimsa	Non-injury in thought, word, or deed
Aishvarya	Spiritual wealth
Ajaha lakshana	Amplified or added meaning
Ajapa-gayatri	Ham soham mantra
Ajati vada	Theory of non-evolution
Aja	Unborn
Ajnana	Ignorance
Akaara	First letter fundamental to sound or first letter of alphabet
Akarma	Inaction
Akarta	Non-doer
Akaasha	Fifth element or sky or space
Akhanda	Continuous or Indivisible
Akhandakara	Of indivisible nature
Akhandaananda	Unbroken bliss
Akhandabrahmacharya	Unbroken celibacy
Akhandamauna	Unbroken silence
Akhandasamadhi	Unbroken meditation in oneness
Akshaya	Undecaying or everlasting
Alakshana	Without distinctive marks
Alinga	Without mark
Amalam	Free of impurities of Maya
Amara	Immortal or deathless

Amatra	Having no sign
Amrita	Nectar
Anabhidya	Non-coveting of other's goods; not brooding over injuries received from others
Anaadi	Beginningless
Anaadikaala	Eternity or beginningless time
Anaahata chakra	Heart plexus or fourth lotus of the yogis where mystic sounds are heard opposite the heart
Anandamaya kosha	Sheath of joy enveloping the soul
Anna	Food
Annamaya kosha	Gross and outermost food sheath enveloping soul
Antahkarana	Seat of thought or conscience
Ananta	Infinite rendless
Antara	Internal
Antaradhvani	Internal mystical sound heard by mystics
Anantadrishti	Unlimited vision
Ananyata	Single-pointed
Aneka	Not one but many
Anga	Step or a limb
Antara kumbhaka	Suspension of breath after full inspiration
Antaratma	Innermost spirit in beings
Ap	Water
Apaana	Lower abdominal control of bodily excretions
Arjuna	Mighty bowman of the Pandava princes
Artha	Wealth as one of man's pursuits
Ashtanga Yoga	Eight-fold path of Raja Yoga of Patanjali
Anima	Subtlety or reducing mass and density at will
Anitya	Impermanent
Anistha	Not Lord but subjected to or impotent
Annam	Matter or food
Annamaya-kosha	Food sheath or gross physical body
Anugraha	Grace
Anukampaa	Sympathy
Anumana	Inference as a means of proof of knowledge
Anupalabdhi	One of eight proofs of knowledge of the existence of non-existence
Anuparmaana	Atomic in size
Anuraaga	Intense love for God
Anusandhaana	Investigation into nature of Brahman
Anushaya	Residue of karma which forces the soul to take a rebirth
Anusmarana	Constant remembrance of Brahman
Anutva	Smallness or subtlety

Anyat	Another
Anyatha	Separateness or state of being otherwise
Anonya	Mutual
Anonyaabhaava	Mutual non-existence
Anonyaadhyasa	Mutual superimposition
Apah	Water
Apamaana	Disrespect or disgrace
Apaana	Nerve current which governs abdominal region which has its center in the anus
Aparaa	Other or relative
Aparaadha	Fault or mistake
Aparaprakriti	Lower cosmic energy through which God projects all forms in Nature, gross and subtle
Apara-vidya	Intellectual knowledge or lower knowledge of the vedas
Aparigraha	Freedom from covetousness or non-receiving of gifts connective of luxury: one of the primary disciplines of yama
Aparinaami	Changeless
Aparokshaanubhava	Essence of intuitive perception and direct realization
Apavaada	Exception; negation; rejection; refuting a wrong belief: as rope believed to be snake or superimposing the real elements with a view of names and forms
Apavaadayukti	Using logic in apavaada
Apavarga	Liberation or moksha or final emancipation from bondage of embodiment Other three being dharma, artha, and kama
Aprameya	Immeasurable
Apraana	Without prana or life-force
Apunya	Non-meritorious or sinful
Apurna	Imperfect or incomplete
Apurva	Unseen; the hidden power of karma which brings fruits in the future
Archana	Offerings of flowers at times of puja or worship
Archiraadimarga	Northern path taken by the soul after death through which yogis depart in uttarayana into the world of Brahman
Ardhaangini	Partner in life
Arghya	water offering
Artha	Object of desire or wealth
Arupa	Formless
Asana	Posture; third stage of Yoga

Asat	Unreal
Asmita	Ego
Asthi	Bone
Ashabdam	Without sound while referring to Brahman
Asad-aavarana	Shakti which screens the existence of Brahman which is removed by aparoksha gyana
Asambhavana	Spiritual doubt
Asanga	Non-attachment
Asangabhavana	attitude of the mind of non-attachment
Ashanti	Absence of peace of mind
Asat	That which is not or non-being or existence of reality
Asiddha	Not perfected
Asmat	Pertaining to me or us
Asmi	I am or I exist
Asmita	Egoism or I-ness
Asmriti	Forgetfulness
Asparsha	Touchless or name of Brahman
Ashtanga Yoga	Mantra with eight letters:Aum Namo Narayana
Ashtanga Yoga	Raja Yoga of Patanjali: Yoga with eight limbs
Astetya	Non-stealing or one of the five items of yama in ashtanaga yoga
Asthi	Bone
Asthira	Wavering or unsteady
Asthula	Without grossness
Ashubha	Inauspicious
Ashudha	Not pure
Ashudha Maya	Maya preponderating with rajas
Ashudha sankalpa	Impure resolve
Asura	Evil tendency in man
Asuya	Envy
Ashvata-vrksha	Sacred peepul tree
Atarkya	That which cannot be reasoned out
Atigraha	Object of sense
Atindriya	Beyond reach of the senses
Atithi	Guest
Atyanta	Too much or to the extreme
Avadhuta	Ascetic who has renounced the world
Atma	Supreme Soul
Atharva veda	Deals with magical formulae, tantras and esoteric knowledge
Aum	Like the Latin "Omne" of omniscience
Avastha	Condition of mind

Avidya	Ignorance
Avidyanivrtti	Removal of Ignorance or moksha
Avikari	Immutable Brahman
Avinashi	Indestructible
Avirodha	Without contradiction
Avyakta	Unmanifest or indivisible when the three gunas are in a state of equilibrium
Avyaktadrshti	View from standpoint of the Infinite Whole
Avyaapti	Exclusion of part of a thing defined
Avyaya	Unchangeable or undiminishing
Ayama	Restraint
Ayurveda	Science of Health
Ayukta	He who has no concentration

B

Baahya	External
Baahya kumbhaka	Pause at end of expiration
Bandha	To close
Bhaagatyaagalakshana	Expression to define Upanishadic Statements that if the literal *appearance* is removed, the identity is revealed
Bhagavad Gita	Song of the Divine
Bhagavan	Lord Narayana or Vishnu of the Trinity
Bhaagvata	Adorer of Bhagavan
Bhagvatam	Puranic scriptural text about Vishnu
Bhakti	Worship in adoration
Bhautika	Material or elemental or composed of physical matter
Bhaavana	Feeling of devotion and unity
Bhaava	Attitude expressing relationship with God
Bhaya	Fear
Bheda	Difference or splitting
Bhoga	Worldly pleasures
Bhiksha	Alms
Bhikshu	Monk
Bhokta	Subjective experience of enjoyment
Bhram	Delusion or illusion
Bhrashta	Fallen from the way of yoga
Bhrumadhyadrishti	Gaze at the space between eyebrows
Bhraanti	Erroneous knowledge or vision
Bhrumadhya	Gaze in between eyebrows
Bhuh	Earthplane: the first of three worlds
Bhuvah	Ether: the second of three worlds
Bij	Seed

Brahmamuhurta	Ninety minutes before sunrise
Bija mantra	Mystic syllable uttered mentally in meditation
Brahma	Creator of the Trinity
Brahmacharya	Self-restraint; also celibacy
Brahman	God or the all-pervading Spirit from which Universe has emerged
Brahmanadi	Main channel of sushumna going towards Spirit
Buddhi	Intellect or judgment

C

Chaitanya	Consciousness that knows itself and knows others as absolute consciousness
Chhanda	Neurotransmitters and neurohormones that form a feedback system with the centers of awareness and consciousness within the brain and the spinal cord
Chakra	Wheel or plexus; seat of psychic energy in the human body Energy or prana flows through body through three channels Sushumna or spinal cord; Ida or parasympathetic moves up towards left nostril; Pingala or sympathetic moves up towards right nostril; These three nadis intersect at various chakras to regulate the body mechanisms.
Chakshu	Eye
Chit	Consciousness or individual Soul
Chitta	Awareness or a Sense of feeling through the mind, intellect and ego collectively
Chaturyuga	Four ages of the Hindu world-cycle: satya, treta, dvapara, and kali
Cheshta	Effort or endeavour
Chala	Quibble
Chidabhasa chaitanya	Reflection of Consciousness from Kutastha-chaitanya
Chidakasha	Brahman in Its aspect as limitless knowledge and intelligence
Chinmaya	Full of Consciousness
Chintana	Reflecting
Chit	Universal Intelligence
Chitta	Mind-stuff or subconscious mind

Chittavidya	Psychology
Chittavi mukti	Freedom from bondage of the mind

D

Daitya	Mighty beings with diabolic qualities; demons of Puranas
Darshana	A vision or discernment
Daiva	Lord who control all beings and gives them their due fate, destiny, justice, or controlling powers
Daivavani	Heavenly voice
Daivi	Divya or divine
Daivisampat	Divine wealth or qualities
Daksha	Expert or wise and intelligent
Dama	Control of outer senses or one of six-fold virtues of Niyama 0f Raja Yoga of Patanjali
Danda	Staff of a mendicant
Daana	Charity or giving
Darpa	Arrogance
Darshana	Insight
Dayaa	Mercy or compassion
Deha	Physical body
Dehaadhyaasa	False identification of the body
Dehashuddhi	Purity or purification of the body
Dehavidya	Physiology
Dehi	One conscious of being an embodied self
Devaloka	World of the celestials or higher subtler worlds
Devata	Deity who receives worship and gives them what they desire
Devayaana	Path of the gods after the soul leaves the body
Dhairya	Boldness or courage
Dhana	Wealth
Dhaaraa	Stream or continuous repetition
Dhaarana	Concentration with complete attention before dhyana and samadhi
Dharma	Moral merit or virtue of a thing or righteous way of living as enjoined by scriptures; characteristic or virtue
Dharma-megha-samadhi	Cloud of virtue; state of superconsciousness or samadhi; immortality through knowledge of Brahman when all vasanas are destroyed
Dharma-parishat	Assembly of the wise
Dharmi	Substratum of dharma
Dhatu	Metal or element; conservation of life-force

	through celibacy and development of Ojas and Tejas
Dhira	Steadfast
Dhriti	Patience -spiritual
Dhyana	Meditation
Dhvani	Tone or sound; the subtle vital shakti in Jiva as vibration
Doshaa	Fault
Dukha	Sorrow
Dvesha	Dislike
Dhyana	Meditation and contemplation
Dhyeya	Object of meditation or purpose of meditation
Diksha	Initiation or consecration
Dina	Humble or helpless
Dina-bandhu	Friend of the poor
Dinacharya	Daily conduct or activity
Dishtam	Unseen power in karma that links up the act with the fruit; destiny or fate
Divya	Divine or heavenly; sacred or luminous or supernatural
Divyachakshu	Divine eye
Divyadrishti	Divine vision
Divyagandha	Superphysical scent or smell
Dosha	Shortcoming or defect
Drdha	Unshaken or firm
Drk	Perceiver
Droha	Treachery
Drshta	Visible
Drshya	Perceived
Dvaanda-shaanta	Twelfth center or the pituitary center (Six centres within the brain and six below the brain)
Dvaita-advaita-vivarjita	Beyond monism and dualism
Dvaita-bhaava	Feeling of duality
Dvandvataa	State of duality
Dvayam	Two or a pair
Dvesha	Repulsion or hatred or dislike
Dvija	Twice born in baptism

E

EkaOne	
Ekadashi	Eleventh day of the lunar fortnight
Ekaagrata	One-pointedness
Ekam-eva-advitiyam	One alone without second or Brahman
Ekaanta	Solitude

Ekanta-bhava	Feeling of solitariness
Ekataa	Oneness or absoluteness
Ekatva	Unity or oneness
Evam	Thus or so; in this manner

G

Gagana	Sky
Gambhira	Deep and dignified or grave
Gambhirya	Gravity of demeanor
Ganapati	Ganesh of Cosmic Intelligence; deity of Hindus
Gandha	Smell
Garbha	Foots
Gayatri	Mother of Vedas; also a vedic hymn
Garva	Pride or arrogance
Gita	Sing
Gotra	Family lineage
Gu	First syllable of "guru"; darkness
Guda	Anus
Guha	Cave
Guhya	Secret or genital
Guna	Quality or dispositions born of Nature or Prakriti Sattva or good, pious, noble, calm, and tranquil Rajas or passionate, agitated, authoritative, and assertive Tamas or dull, inactive, sleepy, and ignorant
Gunatita	Beyond the three gunas
Guru	Remover of darkness or spiritual preceptor
Gurukrpaa	Guru's grace
Gurumantra	Guru given mantra at initiation

H

Hamsamantra	Automatic and involuntary utterance of hamsa-soham with every act of inspiration and expiration
Ham'saa	"I am He" used in pranayama
Hanuman	Powerful deity of Hindus; son of the wind-god; devotee of Rama; famous monkey who helped Rama fight with Ravana
Hari	Narayana or Krishna who destroys evil
Hatta yoga	Self-realization through physical discipline
Hetu	Cause or reason
Himsaa	Injury
Hiranyagarbha	Universal Soul invested in a subtle body;

	another name for Brahman as born from a golden egg; Cosmic Intelligence; Ganesh
Hrdayam	The heart of a being
Hrdaya-granthi	Knot of the heart of avidya, kaama, and karma
Hri	Modesty
I	
Icchaa	Desire
Ida	Psychic cooling nerve-current flowing through left nostril
Idam	This here
Indra	Lord of the senses, mind-soul; chief of the celestials
Indriya	Senses of perception and sense organ; external karma-indriyas or organs of action; or internal gyanaindriyas for cognition, knowledge or perception
Ishta	Object of desire
Ishtadevata	Chosen deity
Ishvara	God or Brahman
Itihaasas	Historical anecdotes centering around life and deeds of heroes as in the Ramayana and Mahabharata
J	
Jada	Insentient
Jagad-guru	World preceptor
Jagat	World; changing
Jagrat	Waking condition
Janma	Coming into being or birth
Japa	Prayer
Japamala	Rosary
Jaati	Specie
Jaya	Conquest
Jiva	Individual
Jivanmukta	Liberated in this life
Jivaatma	Individual soul
Jnaana	Knowledge or wisdom of Reality
Jyestha	Eldest or best
Jyoti	Illumination or effulgence
K	
Kaivalya	Transcendental state; moksha; final beatitude
Kaala	Time

Kaalachakra	Wheel of time
Kaali	Black
Kaliyuga	Age of Kali
Kalpa	A day of Brahma the Creator or code of rituals
Kalpana	Imagination or Creation
Kaama	Lust, passion or desire
Kaamyakarma	Action with desire for fruit of action
Kaanda	Root source
Kantha	Throat or neck
Kapha	Phlegm: one of three homours or doshas in Ayurveda
Karana	Cause or the unmanifested potential; cosmic energy in a potential condition
Kapaala	Skull
Kapaala-bhaati	Clearing the sinuses or Kriya yoga
Karma	Action. Action is of three kinds Sanchita accumulated actions of all previous births Praarabha or portion to be worked in this life Agaami or current karma being freshly performed Law of Karma or cause and effect binding the jiva to the wheel of birth and death Karma doctrine Law of Justice of cause and effect Is intertwined with the Doctrine of Reincarnation
Karmabandha	Bondage caused by karma
Karmabhumi	Land of action on earth-plane
Karmakanda	Section of vedas dwelling on rituals in the samhitas and Brahmanaas of the Vedas
Karmapara	Dependent on karma
Karmaphala	Fruit of action
Karmashaya	Aggregate of works done
Karmavaada	Doctrine of karma upholding that each deed [good or bad] is inevitably followed by pain or pleasure
Karmayoga	Yoga of selfless action
Karmendriya	Organs of action: tongue, hands, feet, genital, and anus
Kaarya	The physical body in contrast to causal body, the karana
Kaaryabrahma	The causal world or Hiranya-garbha
Kathaa	Narrative tale

Kaaya	Physical body
Kendra	Heart center
Kevala	Independent Absolute
Khyaati	Reputation; knowledge
Kirtana	Singing hymns of glory
Klesha	Affliction
Kosha	Sheaths; five concentric sheaths starting at the center: bliss, intellect, mind, life-force, gross-body
Krama	Rules of rituals
Kratu	Sacrifice or yagna
Kriya	Physical action; Cleansing rite in hatta yoga
Kriyaadvaita	Oneness in action
Kriyaanivrtti	Relief from action
Kriyayoga	Yoga of action of self-purification
Krodha	Anger
Krishna	Lord of all Yogas
Kshama	Forgiveness
Kshana	Moment
Kshara	World
Kshaya	Annihilation
Kshetra	Holy place; field; the physical body from a philosophical sense
Kshetrajna	Supreme Soul
Kshina	Powerless
Kuladharma	Particular duty pertaining to the family
Kumbha	Chalice
Kumbhaka	Intervals between inspiration and expiration; retention and suspension of breath
Kundalini	Coil of Primordial Energy lying dormant in the lowest Chakra; Making three and a half coils, it is said to lie dormant "like a coiled serpent" with the head towards the muladhara chakra. It is another term for Life-force roused with spiritual efforts. It rises up the sushumna and into the brahmanadi towards the sahasrahara
Kusha	Grass used in rites
Kutastha	Changeless Absolute found in all creatures from the Creator to the ant Who 'shines' and dwells as witness to the intellect of all creatures
Kutastha-chaitanya	Individual Consciousness free of all egoism; Universal Intelligence; Krishna or Christ Center

L

Laghimaa	Lightness; one of eight siddhis of Yoga practice
Lajjaa	Shame or shyness
Lakshya	Target
Laukika	Worldly
Laya	Dissolution
Layayoga	Absorption of individual soul into Supreme Soul
Lilaa	Cosmos looked upon as a divine play
Lina	Merged
Linga	Symbol
Lingadeha	Astral body
Lingasharira	Psychic body that becomes active during dream state; intellect, emotion and life-force constitute this body
Lingaatman	The subtle self
Lobha	Greed
Loka	World of names and forms

M

Mada	Pride
Madhura	Emotion between lover [devotee] and beloved [God]
Mahabhuta	Primordial element
Mahadbrahma	Hiranyagarbha; Cosmic Intelligence; Ganesh
Mahapralaya	The great deluge with destruction of the world at the end of a Cosmic Cycle or Yuga
Maharishi	Great sage
Mahat	Cosmic Intelligence in a Seed form; first product of prakriti according to Sankhyan Philosophy; Intellect
Mahavakya	Great Sentences Prajnanam Brahma: Consciousness is Brahman Aham Brahma-asmi: I am Brahman Tat Tvam Asi: That Thou Art Ayam Atma Brahma: This self is Brahman
Maheshvara	Shiva
Mahimaa	Glory
Maitri	Friendliness
Makara	Mystic 'm': the third letter that concludes Aum
Majja	Marrow
Maala	Impurity of the mind
Maalaa	Rosary
Mamakara	Thought 'this is mine'

Mamataa	Mineness
Maana	Respect
Manana	Constant reflection
Manas	Mind
Manda	Dull or thick
Manipura-chakra	Third yogic center in the navel region
Mantra	Sacred syllable or words which through repetition one attains perfection
Mantra-shakti	Potency of any mantra
Mantra-siddhi	Mastery over devata of a mantra for grace whenever invoked
Marga	Path
Mati	Thought directed towards revealing knowledge
Matsarya	Jealousy
Mamsa	Flesh
Mahabharata	Voluminous epic classified as Itihasa; composed by Valmiki in 24,000 stanzas 98 times the size of Odessey
Medas	Fat
Merudanda	Spinal column
Mimaamsa	Logical inquiry into Vedic Knowledge
Mithyaa	false
Moha	Infatuation or delusion
Moksha	Liberation
Mrtyu	Death or Lord Yama
Mrtyunjaya	Conqueror of death
Mudra	Sealing posture
Muhurtam	Auspicious moment; a period of 48 minutes
Mukhya	Primary or chief
Mukhyavritti	Power of words
Mukti	Liberation
Mula	Root
Muladhara chakra	Nerve plexus situated above the anus
Mulaprakriti	Ultimate subtle cause of matter
Muni	A sage
Murti	Idol

N

Naada	Inner mystical sound
Nadi	Psychic channels through which energy flows
Naivedya	Edible offering to deity at altar
Naama	Name
Narasimha	Man-lion manifestation of Vishnu
Narayana	Being that supports all beings or God

Neti	Hatta Yogic Kriya for cleansing nostrils
Neti-neti	'Not this-Not this'; Progressive analytical negation of names and forms in order to arrive at the eternal underlying Truth
Nidi-dhyaasana	Meditation; Third step in Vedantic sadhana after hearing and reflection
Nidra	Sleep or yoga-maya
Nirakaara	Formless
Niraa-lamba	Supportless
Niranjana	Spotless
Nirvana	Liberation from existence
Nirbhaya	Fearless
Nirbija	Seedless
Nirguna	Without attributes
Nirmala	Without impurity
Nirvikalpa	Without modification of the mind
Nischaya	Conviction
Nishkaama	Without desire
Nish-kriya	without action
Nitya	Eternal
Nityamukta	Eternally free
Nivrtti	Renunciation
Niyama	Second step of observances in Raja Yoga; internal and external purification, contentment, mortification, study, and worship
Nyaya	Logic
O	
Ojas	Physical essence or spiritual energy and vitality developed through the creative power of celibacy
Om	Pranava or sacred syllable symbolizing Brahman
Om tat sat	Benediction of divine blessing when invoked
P	
Pada	Foot or one quarter
Padartha	Substance or material
Padma	Lotus
Padmasana	Lotus pose or sitting cross-legged
Padya	One of 16 modes of formal worship: water for washing feet of deity
Pancha	Five
Pancha-akshara	Lord Shiva's mantra of five letters: [Om] Na-mah-shi-vaa-ya

Panchakosha	Five sheaths of ignorance enveloping the Self
Panchikarana	Quintuplation of 5 elements in the universe to form gross units of names and forms in the physical universe
Pandita	Scholar
Papa	Sin
Para	Supreme
Parama	Highest
Paramatma	Supreme Spirit
Parameshvara	Supreme Lord
Paraprakriti	Higher cosmic energy through which Brahman appears as individualized soul
Parpurna	Self-contained
Paroksha	Indirect
Parvati	Incarnation of Cosmic Mother; Shiva's consort
Pashu	Cattle
Pashupati	Shiva as Lord of individuals
Pashyanti	Second subtle state of sound manifesting as physical sound
Patanjali	Propounder of the Yoga Philosophy and author of The Yoga Sutras
Pavana	Wind-god
Phala	Fruit or effect
Pingala nadi	Sympathetic channel starting in the right nostril; ascends to the ajnaa of the brain and then descends towards the base of the spine
Pippala	Holy fig tree
Pitr	Departed ancestor
Pitrloka	Heaven occupied by divine hierarchy of ancestors
Pitryana	Path taken by souls who have done meritorious works; they ascend to the region of the moon to enjoy fruits of their action in dhumamarga or path of the smoke
Pitryagna	Oblations for gratifying departed ancestors
Prabhu	Lord
Pradakshina	Circumambulation around holy site or person
Pradhana	Prakriti according the sankhyan philosophy; the root base of all elements. Undifferentiated matter; material cause of world. Corresponds to Maya in Vedanta
Prajapati	Progenitor or Creator or Brahma
Pragnya	Awareness
Pragnya-atma	Intelligent self

Prakriti	Nature or Causal Matter
Pralaya	Dissolution with the merging of the cosmos into the unseen cosmic energy
Pramana	Proof or authority
Prameya	Object of proof or subject of inquiry
Prana	Breath or energy or soul
Pranamaya kosha	Prana sheath enveloping the Self
Pranava	Aum
Pranayama	Regulation and restraint of breath; fourth limb of Ashtanga Yoga of Raja Yoga
Praapti	One of eight major siddhis
Prarabdha	Karma that determines present life
Prasad	Food dedicated to deity and shared with faithful devotees as grace
Pratima	Image
Pratishta	Reputation or installation
Pratyahara	Withdrawal of mind from senses and organs of action; fifth limb of Patanjali's Ashtanga Yoga
Prayojana	Result
Prema	Divine love
Premabhava	Feeling of love
Prerana	Urging or prompting
Priya	Bliss derived from beloved object
Puja	Worship
Punya	Merit
Puraka	Inhalation
Purna	Full or complete
Purusha	Supreme Being lying in all hearts of all things; Universal psychic principle
Purushaartha	Human effort: dharma, artha, kama, and moksha Four aims of life: Ethics-Wealth-Desire-Liberation
Purushotama	Lord of Universe
Pushan	Sun-god
Pushti	Nourishment
Puranas	Texts divided into 3 categories dealing with Creation destruction and renovation of worlds

R

Raaga	Attachments
Ragadvesha	Attraction and repulsion; Likes and dislikes; love and hatred
Rajas	Passion; one of three aspects of or traits of cosmic energy; principle of dynamism in nature bringing about change; quality generates

	passion and restlessness
Raja yoga	Ashtanga Yoga propounded by Patanjali; system of meditation
Rakta	Blood
Rasa	Taste
Ramayana	Smaller of 2 epics of India which mirror highest ideals of Hindu tradition, culture and civilization; is classified as Itihasa
Ratna	Jewel
Rechaka	Exhalation of breath
Rig veda	contains hymns of praise Oldest book known to man with the ultimate Knowledge
Rishi	Sage
Ru	Second symbol of "guru" or Light
Ruchi	Taste
Rudraksha	Eye of Shiva; Seeds of berries used for rosaries
Rupa	Form

S

Sabda	Sound or word
Sat-chit-ananda	Absolute existence-knowledge-bliss
Sad-darshana	Six systems of thought or six philosophies of the Hindus: Nyaya, Vaishesika, Sankhya, Yoga, Mimamsa, and Vedanta
Sadhaka	Seeker
Saadhana	Quest or practice
Saadhu	Pious person
Sadvichara	Right inquiry
Sadvikara	Six bodily modifications: existence, birth, growth, change, decay and death
Saguna-brahma	Absolute conceived as mercy, omnipotence,., as distinguished from undifferentiated Absolute
Sah	He
Sahaja	True or native
Sahasrahara	Cerebral cavity of a thousand petals
Saakshi	Witness
Sakshibhava	Remaining as a witness
Shakti	Power or energy
Shaiva	Pertaining to Shiva
Sama veda	Most voluminous of 4 vedas. Pure liturgical collection of Chants and melodies
Samaadhi	State of Oneness of soul and Spirit
Samadrishti	Equal vision

Samasti	Integrated entity
Samhita	Collection of hymns and formulae from vedas
Sampat	Perfection; virtue
Samsara	Life through repeated births and deaths
Samsari	Transmigrating soul
Samkalpa	Mental resolve
Samskara	Impression; prenatal tendency
Samvritti	Relative truth
Samyama	Perfect restraint; a complete condition of balance, repose, concentration, meditation and samadhi
Sanatana Dharma	Faith of Eternal Values or popularly called Hinduism
Sankalpa	Desire
Sankhyan	One of six Hindu philosophies founded by Kapila;
Samshaya	Doubt
Santosha	Contentment
Sanyasa	Renunciation of social ties; last stage of Hindu life; Stage of spiritual meditation
Sanyasi	Monk
Sharanagati	Surrender
Sharira	Body
Sarasvati	Goddess of Learning who sits at the base of tongue
Shastra	Manual of rules
Sruti	God-revealed statements or Vedas
Smriti	Man-realized eternal principles with practical applications according to changing times
Sat	Truth or Supreme Spirit
Satsanga	Association with the wise
Sattva	Pure quality
Satya	Truth
Savikalpa	Without doubt
Savikalpa-samadhi	Samadhi with the triad of knower-knowledge-known
Shaucha	Cleanliness
Sidha	Sage
Siddhi	Supernatural powers
Shishya	Pupil
Shivoham	I am Shiva
Shloka	Verse of praise; usually containing 32 letters
Shodashi	Mother Nature conceived as 16 year old maiden
Sneha	Adhesiveness or friendship

Smriti	Memory
So'ham	"He I am" used in pranayama
Sphota	Manifestor
Sphurna	Throbbing or breaking up
Shradha	Faith
Shri Wealth	Lakshmi
Shrotra	Ear
Shravana	Hearing; first stage of self development
Shubha	Blessed
Shudha	Pure
Shudra	Varna or caste of servant
Sthita prajna	Firm of wisdom
Sthula sharira	Perishable body
Stuti	Praise
Sukshma sharira	Subtle body capable of heaving
Shunya	Empty
Sutra	Short aphorisms about a topic
Sushumna	Main central nervous system channel of energy
Svadhisthana	Chakra above the organs of procreation
Svah	Sky

T

Tamas	Ignorant or quality of darkness and indolence
Tanmatra	Atom
Tantra	Sadhana emphasizing on esoteric Upanishads
Tantrika	Worshipping of Divine Mother
Tapas	Austerity
Tapatraya	Three sufferings of mortal existence Adhyatmika from one's own body Adhibhautika from beings around him Adhidevika caused by devas
Tapaloka	Higher worlds
Tara	One form of Divine Mother
Tarka	Logic
Tattva	Element; essence
Tat tvam asi	That thou art
Tejas	Brilliance
Trigunamayi	Divine Mother who possesses three gunas
Trpti	Satisfaction
Trshna	Thirsting
Tulasi	Holy basil plant sacred to Vishnu and venerated

	by Hindus
Tushti	Contentment
Tyaga	Renunciation of ego and vasanas and the world

U

Udana	Vital air that fills thoracic cavity
Umadevi	Consort of Shiva who imparted knowledge to Indra
Upadhi	Superimposed thing giving a coloured view of substance beneath it
Upanishads	End philosophical portions of Vedas - together called Vedanata 1179 Upanishads exist 108 are considered authoritative Of these 10 are very important Upavedas Subordinates to vedas - 4 in number Ayurveda for science of longevity found in Atharva veda Dhanurveda for military science found in Yajur veda Gandharva-veda for science of music found in Sama veda Stapathya-sastra for science of mechanics found in Atharva veda

V

Vaada	Discussion
Vak	Speech
Vaanaprastha	Third stage of life as forest dweller
Vaikutha	Abode of Lord Vishnu
Vairagya	Dispassion
Vaishnava	Worshiper of Vishnu and his avatars
Vaishnavi	Power of Vishnu or Shakti or Energy
Varna	Class or caste
Varuna	Divine Intelligence presiding over water
Vasana	Desire or inclination
Vayu	Wind
Vasudeva	Krishna
Vata	One of three bodily humors
Vedas	Books of Knowledge or Hindu scriptures; four in number
Vedangas	Six in number: *siksha* or phonetics; *vyakarna* or grammar; *Nirukta* or vedic glossary; *kalpa*

	or religious rites; *Chhandas* or prosody; and *jyotisha* orastronomy
Vedanta	Philosophy of the Vedas located at the end of four vedas
Vedas	Books of knowledge or Hindu scriptures; four in number
	Essence of vedas classified under six schools based on same teachings
Veda-Upangas	Six in number; *nyaya* by Gautama deals with Logic; *vaisheka* by Kanada deals with theory of atoms and universe; *sankhya* by Kapil deals with Nature and Spirit; *yoga* by Patanjali deals with mastery of the soul; *mimamsa* by Jaimini deals with ritualism; and *vedanta* by Vyasa deals with philosophy and theology
Vidya	Knowledge of Brahman; there are two kinds of knowledge: Paravidya and Aparavidyas that assist in meditation and worship
Vighna	Obstacle
Vignesha	Ganesha
Vigyana	Pure Intelligence with knowledge of the Self
Vikalpa	Imagination or oscillating mind
Vikshepa	Wavering thoughts obstructing concentration
Viniyoga	Application
Virat	Macrocosm as Form of Lord in Manifested Universe
Vishva	Cosmos
Vishuddha chakra	Throat chakra
Viveka	Discrimination between Real and Unreal
Vrata	Resolution or vow
Vritti	Mental whirlpool
Vyana	One of five physiological functions of prana
Vyasa	Sage who wrote the Brahma Sutras
Vyadhi	Sickness

Y

Yagna	Rite
Yajur veda	Contains formulae for rituals and ceremonies
Yama	Lord of death and dispenser of justice
Yama	The first of the eight-fold paths *[ashtanga yoga]* in Yoga Sutras of Patanjali. - Raja Yoga Moral injunctions - the Don'ts of Behaviour
Yatra	Pilgrimage
Yuga	Cycle of Creation

Yoga	Union or to connect soul with Spirit
Yoga Sutra	Classical work written by Patanjali
Yogadanda	Wooden stick of 2ft with one end of U-shape; used for regulation of breath
Yogi	One who has erased his lower self and is identified with the Higher Self.
Yogamaya	Power of divine illusion
Yoganidra	Yogic sleep when individual retains slight awareness
Yogeshvara	Lord of Yoga or Krishna
Yoni	Womb
Yuga	Divisions of Time. There are four yugas: Kali, Dvapara; Treta; Satya. All four together are known as Chaturyuga. Kaliyuga is of 12,000 years; Dvapara- yuga is twice as long; Treta-yuga is thrice as long; and Satyayuga is four times as long. Chaturyuga or one cycle is of 1.2 million years.

Aum Tat Sat